THE PEDIATRIC CLINICS OF NORTH AMERICA

Pediatric Gastroenterology I

EMANUEL LEBENTHAL, MD, GUEST EDITOR

VOLUME 43 • NUMBER 1 • FEBRUARY 1996

W.B. SAUNDERS COMPANY
A Division of Harcourt Brace & Company
PHILADELPHIA   LONDON   TORONTO   MONTREAL   SYDNEY   TOKYO

W.B. SAUNDERS COMPANY
A Division of Harcourt Brace & Company

The Curtis Center • Independence Square West • Philadelphia, PA 19106-3399

The Pediatric Clinics of North America is also published in translated editions by the following:

Spanish   NEISA (McGraw-Hill/Interamericana de Mexico), Cedro 512, 06450, Mexico, D.F., Mexico

Portuguese Interlivros Edicoes Ltda., Rua Comandante Coelho 1085, CEP 21250, Rio de Janeiro, Brazil

Greek   Althayia SA, Athens, Greece

The Pediatric Clinics of North America is covered in *Index Medicus, Excerpta Medica, Current Contents, Current Contents/Clinical Medicine, Science Citation Index, ASCA, ISI/BIOMED,* and *BIOSIS*.

THE PEDIATRIC CLINICS OF NORTH AMERICA   ISSN 0031-3955
February 1996   Volume 43   Number 1

The opinions expressed in *The Pediatric Clinics of North America* are those of the contributors and/or editors of this issue and do not necessarily reflect the opinions or views of the Publisher. The ultimate responsibility lies with the prescribing physician to determine drug dosages and the best course of treatment for the patient. The reader is advised to check the current product information provided by the manufacturer of each drug to be administered, in order to ascertain any change in drug dosage, method of administration, or contraindications. Mention of any product in this issue should not be construed as endorsement by the contributors, editors or the Publisher. Clinicians are encouraged to contact the manufacturer(s) of these product(s) with any questions about their specific features or limitations.

The Pediatric Clinics of North America (ISSN 0031-3955) is published bi-monthly by W. B. Saunders Company, Corporate and Editorial Offices: The Curtis Center, Independence Square West, Philadelphia, PA 19106-3399. Accounting and Circulation Offices: 6277 Sea Harbor Drive, Orlando, FL 32887-4800. Second class postage paid at Orlando, FL 32862, and additional mailing offices. Subscription price per year is $72.00 (US residents), $83.00 (US individuals), $110.00 (US institutions), $117.00 (foreign individuals), and $132.00 (foreign institutions). To receive student/resident rate, orders must be accompanied by name of affiliated institution, date of term, and the signature of program/residency coordinator on institution letterhead. Orders will be billed at individual rate until proof of status is received. Foreign air speed delivery for all *Clinics* is $6.00 per issue. All prices are subject to change without notice. POSTMASTER: Send address changes to W. B. Saunders Company, Periodicals Fulfillment, Orlando, FL 32887-4800.

Customer Service: 1-800-654-2452.

The editor of this publication is Sandra Masse, and the production editor is Carrie Schaller, W. B. Saunders Company, The Curtis Center, Independence Square West, Philadelphia, PA 19106-3399.

Printed in the United States of America.

GUEST EDITOR

EMANUEL LEBENTHAL, MD, Professor and Chairman, Department of Pediatrics, Mount Scopus, Hadassah-Hebrew University Hospital, Jerusalem, Israel

CONTRIBUTORS

JOEL W. ADELSON, MD, PhD, Director, Division of Pediatric Gastroenterology and Nutrition, Hasbro Children's Hospital; and Professor of Pediatrics and Physiology, Brown University School of Medicine, Providence, Rhode Island

DAVID BRANSKI, MD, Professor and Chairman, Department of Pediatrics, Shaare Zedek Medical Center, Hebrew University Hadassah Medical School, Jerusalem, Israel

YORAM BUJANOVER, MD, Associate Professor, Pediatric Gastroenterology Unit, Dana Children's Hospital, Sourasky-Tel Aviv Medical Center; Tel Aviv, Israel

LAURIE N. FISHMAN, MD, Instructor, Department of Pediatrics, Harvard Medical School; and Assistant in Medicine, Children's Hospital, Boston, Massachusetts

A. CRAIG HILLEMEIER, MD, Director, Division of Pediatric Gastroenterology, and Professor, Department of Pediatrics, University of Michigan, Ann Arbor, Michigan

JEFFREY S. HYAMS, MD, Professor and Vice-Chairman, Department of Pediatrics, University of Connecticut School of Medicine; and Director, Division of Digestive Diseases, Connecticut Children's Medical Center, Hartford, Connecticut

MAUREEN M. JONAS, MD, Assistant Professor, Department of Pediatrics, Harvard Medical School; and Chief, Section of Hepatology, Children's Hospital, Boston, Massachusetts

BARBARA S. KIRSCHNER, MD, Professor, Departments of Pediatrics and Medicine, Pritzker School of Medicine, University of Chicago; and Section of Pediatric Gastroenterology, Hepatology, and Nutrition, Wyler Children's Hospital, Chicago, Illinois

JOEL E. LAVINE, MD, PhD, Associate Professor, Department of Pediatrics, University of California, San Diego; and Chief, Joint Program in Gastroenterology and Nutrition, University of California, San Diego, San Diego, California

EMANUEL LEBENTHAL, MD, Professor and Chairman, Department of Pediatrics, Mount Scopus, Hadassah-Hebrew University Hospital, Jerusalem, Israel

HANMIN LEE, MD, Research Fellow, Division of Research, Department of Surgery, Children's Hospital, Boston, Massachusetts

AARON LERNER, MD, Chairman, Department of Pediatrics, Pediatric Gastroenterology and Nutrition Unit, Carmel Medical Center, B. Rappaport Faculty of Medicine, Technion-Israel Institute of Technology, Haifa, Israel

VERA LOENING-BAUCKE, MD, Professor, Division of General Pediatrics, University of Iowa, Iowa City, Iowa

COLSTON F. McEVOY, MD, Assistant Professor, Pediatric Gastroenterology/ Hepatology Section, Department of Pediatrics, Yale University School of Medicine, New Haven, Connecticut

SHIMON REIF, MD, Lecturer, Pediatric Gastroenterology Unit, Dana Children's Hospital, Sourasky-Tel Aviv Medical Center; Tel Aviv, Israel

SARAH JANE SCHWARZENBERG, MD, Associate Professor, Department of Pediatrics, Division of Gastroenterology and Nutrition, University of Minnesota Hospital and Clinics, Minneapolis, Minnesota

LINDA B. SHALON, MD, Assistant Professor, Division of Pediatric Gastroenterology and Nutrition, Department of Pediatrics, Hasbro Children's Hospital; and Brown University School of Medicine, Providence, Rhode Island

HARVEY L. SHARP, MD, Professor, Department of Pediatrics, Division of Gastroenterology and Nutrition, University of Minnesota Hospital and Clinics, Minneapolis, Minnesota

FREDERICK J. SUCHY, MD, Professor, Pediatric Gastroenterology/Hepatology Section, Department of Pediatrics, Yale University School of Medicine, New Haven, Connecticut

JOSEPH P. VACANTI, MD, Director and Senior Associate, Division of Organ Transplantation, Department of Surgery, Children's Hospital; and Associate Professor, Department of Surgery, Harvard Medical School, Boston, Massachusetts

PETER F. WHITINGTON, MD, Professor and Chief, Section of Pediatric Gastroenterology, Hepatology, and Nutrition, Department of Pediatrics, University of Chicago, Pritzker School of Medicine, The Wyler Children's Hospital, Chicago, Illinois

JACOB YAHAV, MD, Lecturer, Pediatric Gastroenterology Unit, Sheba Hospital, Tel Hashomer, Israel

CONTENTS

from infection, and new immunomodulatory therapy with interferon-α is being used to eradicate disease in patients chronically infected with hepatitis virus B or C.

This article discusses congenital and acquired disorders of the bile ducts and gallbladder in infants and children. Problems, such as extrahepatic biliary atresia, that are unique to infants are covered as well as distinctive aspects of hepatobiliary disease in older children. Biliary tract disease in the fetus and neonate presents an important challenge in that not only is hepatic structure and function disturbed but also the process of normal development may be retarded or altered by the disease process.

Liver transplantation is an effective treatment for end-stage liver disease in the pediatric population. The 1-year survival rate in the United States is now approximately 80%, with some series showing a 90% 1-year survival rate. Most children who receive liver transplantation attain normal growth and development. Many pitfalls remain, however, in the treatment for pediatric liver disease with transplantation, including donor-organ scarcity and immunosuppression-related side effects. This article reviews indications for liver transplantation and clinical management of patients who receive liver transplantations.

The main congenital anomalies of the exocrine pancreas are reviewed, and several generalized and isolated hereditary pancreatic diseases are discussed. In contrast with adults, the most frequent causes of acute pancreatitis are viral infection, drug induction, and trauma. The dissimilarities between pediatric and adult acute and chronic pancreatitis are emphasized.

The gastrointestinal and nutritional complications of cystic fibrosis are diverse. As longevity improves in patients with cystic fibrosis, management of these complications is becoming increasingly important. This article provides overviews of the molecular aspects of the pathogenesis of cystic fibrosis, the current status of gene therapy, and a review of the gastrointestinal manifestations and nutritional care.

Gastroesophageal Reflux: Diagnostic and Therapeutic Approaches
A. Craig Hillemeier

The clinical challenge of determining the medical conditions that are associated with obvious symptoms of gastroesophageal reflux and what diagnostic tests are appropriate to define this relationship is substantial. To determine which infants may be suffering from pathologic conditions associated with subtle signs of gastroesophageal reflux is even more challenging. This determination is essential to avoid subjecting many healthy infants to costly and potentially invasive testing. This article focuses on the physiology, clinical presentations, diagnosis and evaluation, and therapy of gastroesophageal reflux.

Helicobacter pylori and Peptic Disease in the Pediatric Patient
Yoram Bujanover, Shimon Reif, and Jacob Yahav

The data accumulated on *Helicobacter pylori* infection in children suggests an important causative role of the organism in gastritis and peptic ulcer disease in this age group. The importance of eradication of *H pylori* in asymptomatic children in relation to its role in peptic disease and cancer in adults is debatable. This article describes the current data on bacteriologic features, pathologic spectrum, clinical significance, epidemiology, methods of diagnosis, and treatment of *H pylori* infection in children. Further studies will provide the information on the pathogenicity, mode of transfer, and optimal treatment of *H pylori* infection.

Ulcerative Colitis in Children
Barbara S. Kirschner

Chronic nonspecific ulcerative colitis remains a disease of unknown etiology, although much new information continues to be gleaned from basic research and clinical trials. In most instances, ulcerative colitis responds to medical therapy. Selecting appropriate drug therapy for a specific child depends on the extent and severity of the colitis. This article summarizes the clinical information, diagnostic studies, and approaches to management that should be considered when evaluating a child for ulcerative colitis.

Crohn's Disease in Children
Jeffrey S. Hyams

Crohn's disease is a chronic inflammatory condition that may affect any part of the gastrointestinal system and multiple extraintestinal organs. Although its exact pathogenesis remains unknown, increasing evidence suggests an abnormality in the control of "physiologic" inflammation caused by bacterial and other antigens. Diagnosis starts with a careful history and physical examination, and confirmation rests with radiologic and histologic studies. Newer treatments are more specifically targeting the cascade of cytokine-mediated events that perpetuate inflammation.

Constipation, encopresis, and fecal incontinence are common problems in children. Constipation can have a variety of causes, such as organic and anatomic causes or intake of medication. *Encopresis* is the involuntary loss of formed, semiformed, or liquid stool into the child's underwear in the presence of functional (idiopathic) constipation in a child 4 years of age or younger. *Fecal incontinence* is fecal soiling in the presence of an organic or anatomic lesion, such as Hirschsprung's disease, anal malformation, anal surgery or trauma, meningomyelocele, and some muscle diseases. This article reviews the symptoms of functional constipation in young children and the symptoms of functional constipation and encopresis in older children, presents the differential diagnosis of constipation with or without fecal incontinence, describes the evaluation and treatment of these children, and reports on treatment outcome.

FORTHCOMING ISSUES

April 1996
> PEDIATRIC GASTROENTEROLOGY II
> Emanuel Lebenthal, MD, *Guest Editor*

June 1996
> PEDIATRIC HEMATOLOGY
> George Buchanan, MD, *Guest Editor*

August 1996
> COMMON ORTHOPEDIC PROBLEMS
> Stephen P. England, MD, MPH, *Guest Editor*

RECENT ISSUES

December 1995
> PEDIATRIC NEPHROLOGY
> Uri Alon, MD, *Guest Editor*

October 1995
> PEDIATRIC RHEUMATOLOGY
> Michael L. Miller, MD, *Guest Editor*

August 1995
> PEDIATRIC NUTRITION
> Gerald E. Gaull, MD, *Guest Editor*

PREFACE

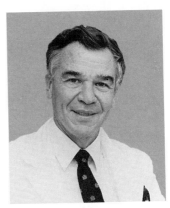

EMANUEL LEBENTHAL, MD
Guest Editor

The following two issues of *The Pediatric Clinics of North America*, dedicated to pediatric gastroenterology, were compiled in an attempt to advance knowledge and present new developments and challenges. During the past decade, pediatric gastroenterology has witnessed significant advances in our understanding of the etiophysiology of prevalent diseases and the genetic origin and gene mutations of some diseases. New diagnostic tools, better imaging, experience in endoscopy, colonoscopy, manometry, new serum and urine markers for disease activity have provided new dimensions in the quest for better definition of gastrointestinal diseases. In addition, new therapeutic modalities have been developed. The topics and authors were selected carefully on the basis of representing the most unique and important vantage points; however, readers are referred to books published on pediatric gastroenterology in the past decade[1-7] and the *Journal of Pediatric Gastroenterology and Nutrition* for further information.

In the first issue, the spectrum of liver diseases in infancy and childhood is presented. Whitington defines persistent hepatobiliary cholestasis starting early in life and considers its diagnostic and therapeutic challenges. The molecular mechanisms underlying hepatocellular cholestasis provide understanding of the etiology of various clinical syndromes, enabling their separation into those that are due to primary hepatocyte membrane injury, inhibition of active transport processes; those associated with subcellular anatomic changes, altered membrane fluidity with secondary membrane injury; and those due to secondary "cholestatic" bile acids, reduced bile salt pool, or disturbances in enterohepatic circulation. Diagnostic imaging is very helpful in the diagnosis of cholestasis, especially ultrasonography, biliary excretory scans, and cholangiography. Early diagnosis of biliary atresia is essential, because the outcome of patients treated by portoenterostomy before 2 months of age is much better than that of patients in whom intervention is delayed. Most patients ultimately require liver transplantation and account for 90% of transplantation candidates fewer than 2 years of age.

Our understanding of inherited metabolic diseases of the liver has accelerated thanks to current molecular diagnostics, as is discussed by Schwarzenberg and Sharp. For example, in patients with Wilson's disease, the liver's inability to transport and store dietary copper is due to an inability to secrete copper into the bile and circulation. The gene involved encodes the copper binding membrane spanning protein with P-type ATPase motifs that characterize metal transport proteins. The gene locus is on the long arm of chromosome 13 at 14q21, with the two most frequent defects being a point mutation or a frame shift. New developments in therapy of Wilson's disease include the use of pyridoxine, trientine, and triethylene tetramine hydrochloride, which are as effective as penicillamine. Another example of an advance in our knowledge is in genetic hemochromatosis, in which the defective gene has been localized to chromosome 6p close to HLA-A of the major histocompatability complex near the D6S105 locus. Very interesting data are presented on recent research in α_1-antitrypsin deficiency liver disease. It has been proposed that liver disease with the Z allele of α_1-antitrypsin deficiency is related to the effect of the inclusions in the endoplasmic reticulum of the hepatocyte. In addition, the potential for safe and effective gene therapy is discussed. Overall, an increasing number of genes responsible for metabolic liver diseases has been mapped and sequenced, leading to more rapid and precise diagnosis, family studies, prenatal diagnostic testing, and information that may lead to gene therapy.

The main viruses causing hepatitis have been identified as hepatitis A, B, C, D, and E. Fishman, Jonas, and Lavine define the clinical profile of these five viruses, and the taxonomy and characteristics of the agents, including the newly discovered hepatitis E virus. The past decade has witnessed the development of inactivated hepatitis A and recombinant hepatitis B vaccines and the Centers for Disease Control-ACIP recommendation for universal vaccination of newborns against hepatitis B. We have experienced new developments in the identification, cloning, diagnostic assays, and screening for hepatitis C, and the identification, cloning and diagnostic assays for hepatitis E. Interferon has been shown to be of benefit in the treatment of hepatitis B, C, and D.

Although neonatal cholestasis is presented at the beginning of this issue, a variation on the theme is presented by McEvoy and Suchy, whose article discusses the common cholangiopathies, such as extrahepatic biliary atresia, primary sclerosing cholangitis, choledochal cyst, Caroli's disease, and paucity of interlobular bile ducts. Conditions associated with cholelithiasis in the various pediatric age groups are discussed. The article also discusses gallstones found incidentally during the investigation of other problems. Treatment with ursodeoxycholic acid and cholecystectomy and other treatment modalities are presented.

Liver transplantation, the ultimate treatment in end-stage liver disease in children, is discussed in the article by Lee and Vacanti. Fifteen percent of all liver transplantations are performed in pediatric age groups, with a 65% 1-year survival rate. There are problems of rejection, opportunistic infections, immunosuppressive therapy, and donor-organ shortage, however. Children have unique issues of growth and development; indications for transplantation; and preoperative, intraoperative, and postoperative management.

New challenges of developing a bioartificial liver similar to a dialysis machine using porcine hepatocytes or a transformed line of hepatocytes for perfusion are presented. The article also discusses, on the other hand, the possibility of temporary liver replacement using xenografts from baboons for transplantation. It is emphasized that hepatocellular transplantation is a potential therapy for children with liver disease due to a single enzyme deficiency.

Diseases of the exocrine pancreas in childhood are discussed in the article by Lerner, Branski, and Lebenthal. The main problems in clinical practice are congenital malformations, pancreatic insufficiency, and acute pancreatitis. Most congenital anomalies of the pancreas are related to critical events that occur during morphologic development in the process of rotation and fusion. Pancreas divisum is found in 7.5% of patients undergoing endoscopic retrograde cholangiopancreatography and is perceived as a risk factor for the later development of pancreatitis. The causes of pancreatitis in children differ from those in adults and include primarily trauma, drugs, and viral infections. The use of pancreatic extracts in pancreatic insufficiency and new approaches to treatment are discussed.

The main cause of pancreatic insufficiency in children is cystic fibrosis, which is discussed in the article by Shalon and Adelson. Over the past years, great progress has been made toward understanding the molecular basis of cystic fibrosis. The mutated gene of cystic fibrosis encodes a chloride channel protein named *cystic fibrosis transmembrane conductance regulator,* located on the long arm of chromosome 7q31, which includes a cAMP-regulated chloride channel protein of 1480 amino acids. Three hundred fifty mutations have been described to date owing to amino acid substitutions, frame shift, and nonsense and mRNA-splicing mutations. The most common is F 508, representing a 3-nucleotide base-pair deletion that results in a missing phenylalanine at position 508. The common result of all of these defects is failure of chloride transport. Somatic gene therapy in patients with cystic fibrosis using retroviruses and adeno-associated viruses as vectors for integrating the gene to host cell genome by insertion of normal DNA has been tried. In addition, the authors describe a nonintegrative approach using liposomes and various molecular conjugates to insert extrachromosal DNA into the host cell nucleus. Such therapy has the potential for treating the lethal pulmonary manifestations of cystic fibrosis.

The first part of this issue emphasizes the advancement of frontiers of pediatric gastroenterology through more precise definition of the cellular mechanism of disease and gene therapy. The second part emphasizes the diagnostic and therapeutic challenge of common gestrointestinal problems in daily practice.

Practical developments related to gastroesophageal reflux, peptic ulcer disease, Crohn's disease, and ulcerative colitis in children include new diagnostic tools, such as endoscopy, colonoscopy, manometry, and imaging techniques, together with the new therapeutic modalities.

Hillemeier's article discusses approaches to diagnostic and therapeutic gastroesophageal reflux. Gastroesophageal reflux has no defined anatomic, metabolic, infectious, or neurologic etiology; however, spitting up and vomiting during the first year of life, associated with failure to thrive or respiratory symptoms, is a very important clinical problem. The pathophysiology is thought to be related to inappropriate relaxation of the lower esophageal sphincter.

The identification of a new development with practical clinical implication is *Helicobacter pylori* as the cause for peptic ulcer disease and gastritis. Recent developments in the diagnosis and treatment of *H pylori* are described in the article by Bujanover, Reif, and Yahav. *H pylori* is a spiral-shaped, gram-negative bacteria with flagella that has a urease enzyme that hydrolyzes urea into ammonium and bicarbonate. Ammonia and cytotoxins produced by *H pylori* can affect the production of mucin and damage epithelial cells, causing back diffusion of hydrogen ions that leads to submucosal injury, inflammation, and ulcer formation. In addition, other *H pylori* enzymes, such as mucinase and phospholipase, also might contribute to mucosal damage by degrading mucous.

In contrast with adults, in children the active antral inflammation in peptic ulcer disease consists of lymphocytes, with increased nodularity in the antral mucosa. Diagnostic tests for *H pylori* include mucosal and stool cultures, mucosal biopsy for urease and histology, urea breath test, and the ELISA test in saliva and serum for the bacteria. The multitude of tests provides the clinician with many tools for screening and diagnosis.

At present, no evidence indicates that *H pylori* infection is necessarily associated with a specific clinical picture. *H pylori* colonization in children can be asymptomatic. On the other hand, antimicrobial therapy can be of great benefit to symptomatic patients. The appropriate drugs and duration of treatment for symptomatic patients are discussed.

Another disease in which new developments are occuring is inflammatory bowel disease in children. With regard to children, there has been a rise in newly diagnosed Crohn's disease in the past four decades. Understanding concerning the alteration in the mucosal immune response and genetic predisposition has increased. Ulcerative colitis is presented in the article by Kirschner, and Crohn's disease in the article by Hyams. The importance of familial predisposition is illustrated by both authors. Family history is one of the most consistent risk factors for inflammatory bowel disease. Ulcerative colitis is considered a genetically heterogeneous disorder defined by genetic (HLA class II) and subclinical (antineutrophil cytoplasmic antibodies) markers. Mice rendered interleukin-2 or interleukin-10 deficient by gene targeting provide exciting new animal models for ulcerative colitis. In such animals, intestinal microflora seem to trigger or perpetuate disease.

Ulcerative colitis in children tends to be more severe than in adults. Despite this, the need for colectomy early in life has decreased significantly because of improved medical management. The goals of therapy are aimed at controlling the clinical complaints and providing adequate nutritional intake to secure normal linear growth and sexual maturation. The mainstay of treatment with sulfasalazine has been enhanced by the availability of newer 5-aminosalicylates. Corticosteroids are used in acute and severe attacks. Antibiotics are sometimes used in severe ulcerative colitis. However, the efficacy of aminoglycosides, metronidazole or second generation cephalosporins have not been proven. Immunosuppressive drugs, such as azathioprine, methotrexate, and cyclosporine, suppress disease activity in 70% of patients who are steroid dependent or have refractory disease, but the drugs should be used very carefully. The long period of time required to produce an effect, the risk of acute pancreatitis, and long-term malignant potential are important considerations mitigating against their use.

Loening-Baucke's article concludes the first issue with practical advice on constipation, encopresis, and fecal incontinence. The diagnostic role of anorectal manometry is presented. Management through education, disimpaction, prevention of reaccumulation of stools, pyschological treatment, and biofeedback treatment are evaluated. Information gained from the study of this seemingly mundane problem opens the door to new developments in understanding gut motility.

Overall, in this issue we have sought to define the state of the art of pediatric gastroenterology in 1996. In the past decade, advances in diagnostic imaging, microbiology, immunology, and, most importantly, molecular medicine have begun to shed light on diseases that have frustrated children and their physicians for many years. Most importantly, however, I hope we have managed to convey a sense of excitement as we look to the future of the field.

We stand on the verge of even more breakthroughs in the treatment of pediatric gastrointestinal diseases, particularly genetic diseases and inflammatory bowel disease. Further progress in these areas will depend on the efforts of the next generation of pediatricians and pediatric gastroenterologists, and it is to these physicians these issues are dedicated.

EMANUEL LEBENTHAL, MD
Guest Editor

Department of Pediatrics
Hadassah University Hospital
Mt. Scopus
Jerusalem
Israel

References

1. Lebenthal E (ed): Chronic Diarrhea in Children. New York, Raven Press, 1984
2. Lebenthal E (ed): Textbook of Gastroenterology and Nutrition in Infancy, ed 2. New York, Raven Press, 1989
3. Lebenthal E (ed): Human Gastrointestinal Development. New York, Raven Press, 1989
3a. Roy CC, Silverman A, Alagille D (eds): Pediatric Clinical Gastroenterology, ed 4. St. Louis, CV Mosby, 1995
4. Silverman A, Roy CC (eds): Pediatric Clinical Gastroenterology. St. Louis, CV Mosby, 1983
5. Suchy FJ (ed): Liver disease in children. St. Louis, Mosby Year Book, 1994
6. Walker WA, Durie PR, Hamilton JR, et al (eds): Pediatric Gastrointestinal Disease: Pathophysiology Diagnosis, Management. Philadelphia, BC Decker, 1991.
7. Wyllie R, Hyams JS (eds): Pediatric Gastrointestinal Disease: Pathophysiology, Diagnosis, Management. Philadelphia, WB Saunders, 1993

PEDIATRIC GASTROENTEROLOGY I   0031–3955/96 $0.00 + .20

CHRONIC CHOLESTASIS OF INFANCY

Peter F. Whitington, MD

This discussion focuses on a few disorders that can present within the first year of life and cause chronic cholestasis, which is defined as: (1) the principal manifestation of the hepatobiliary disease is cholestasis; (2) the hepatobiliary disease causing cholestasis and its consequences constitutes the principal health problem; and (3) cholestasis that is clinically evident for longer than 1 year or is expected to persist if not treated. By requiring cholestasis to be the main manifestation of the liver disease, most infectious hepatitis and inborn errors of metabolism, such as tyrosinemia, galactosemia, and hereditary fructose intolerance, are excluded from consideration. By requiring the cholestatic hepatobiliary process to be the principal problem, persistent, usually mild cholestasis that may be observed in association with a variety of systemic disorders, from cystic fibrosis to Alper's disease, are excluded from consideration. By requiring it to persist for more than 1 year if not treated, almost all patients with idiopathic neonatal hepatitis, drug-induced cholestasis, and inborn errors of metabolism, such as α1-antitrypsin deficiency, are excluded from consideration. Remaining is a small but important group of disorders that comprise those of the vast majority of infants with persistent and usually unremitting cholestasis.

DEFINITION AND PATHOPHYSIOLOGY OF CHOLESTASIS

Many reviews have been published concerning the mechanisms of cholestasis. These reviews and the author's own knowledge are used to

From the Section of Pediatric Gastroenterology, Hepatology and Nutrition, Department of Pediatrics, The University of Chicago, Pritzker School of Medicine, The Wyler Children's Hospital, Chicago, Illinois provide an overview of the subject. Readers are referred elsewhere for more details.[24, 26, 52, 53, 56, 61]

Cholestasis is defined as a pathologic state of reduced bile formation or flow. This definition applies more to the experimental situation, in which the rates of bile formation and flow can be measured, than to human cholestasis, in which neither can be assessed. The clinical definition of *cholestasis*, therefore, is any condition in which substances normally excreted into bile are retained. The serum concentrations of conjugated bilirubin and bile salts are the most commonly measured. Not all substances normally excreted into bile are retained to the same extent in various cholestatic disorders. In some conditions, serum bile salts may be markedly elevated while bilirubin is only modestly elevated, and vice versa. Retention of several substances should be demonstrable to establish a diagnosis of cholestasis. Only in rare disorders of bilirubin metabolism (e.g., Dubin-Johnson syndrome and Rotor's syndrome) does an isolated increase in the serum concentration of conjugated bilirubin occur, so increased serum conjugated bilirubin is taken to indicate cholestasis. The histopathologic definition of cholestasis is the appearance of bile within the elements of the liver, usually associated with secondary cell injury.

Although the mechanisms by which many diseases produce cholestasis are not clearly understood, most conditions can be classified as either obstructive cholestasis or hepatocellular cholestasis. The mechanism of obstructive cholestasis occurs when the reduction in bile flow and the retention of substance normally excreted into bile results from impedance of bile hydraulics. In other words, an anatomic or functional obstruction is present in the biliary system. This obstruction can be at the level of the large or extrahepatic bile ducts or the smaller intrahepatic bile ducts. Obstructive cholestasis, therefore, can be divided into two subclassifications: (1) extrahepatic biliary obstruction; and (2) intrahepatic obstructive cholestasis. In either case, the flow of bile within the bile ducts is the basis for disease, and the distinguishing histopathologic feature is the presence of bile plugs in interlobular bile ducts. Histologic evidence of secondary hepatocellular injury may be minimal to severe. Findings often involve central lobular hepatocytes and include hepatocyte cholestasis, ballooning, and necrosis. The principal causes of obstructive cholestasis in children are presented in Table 1. Of these, biliary atresia accounts for more than 90% of cases.

Hepatocellular cholestasis results from impairment of mechanisms of bile formation. It sometimes is called "hepatocanalicular cholestasis" in recognition of the canaliculus as the bile-forming apparatus of the hepatocyte. The typical histopathologic features of hepatocellular cholestasis include the presence of bile within hepatocytes and bile plugs in canalicular spaces. Histologic evidence of secondary hepatocellular injury is often severe. In most clinical forms of hepatocellular cholestasis, the molecular mechanism is unknown. The principal causes of hepatocellular cholestasis in children are listed in Table 1. Idiopathic neonatal giant cell hepatitis accounts for the majority of cases; however, the

Table 1. THE MAJOR CAUSES OF CHOLESTASIS IN INFANCY

Obstructive cholestasis
  Biliary atresia
  Congenital bile duct anomalies (choledochal cyst)
  Cholelithiasis
  Primary sclerosing cholangitis
  Infectious cholangitis
  Cholangitis associated with Langerhans'-cell histiocytosis
Cholestasis with ductal paucity
  Alagille's syndrome
  Nonsyndromic ductal paucity
  Ductopenic allograft rejection
Hepatocellular cholestasis
  Hepatitis
  α_1-Antitrypsin deficiency
  Inborn errors of bile acid synthesis
  Drug-induced cholestasis
  TPN-associated cholestasis
  Progressive familial intrahepatic cholestasis

last decade has brought an improved understanding of the causes of hepatocellular cholestasis in children and a reduction in the percentage of idiopathic cases.

Several mechanisms have been identified in experimental hepatocellular cholestasis and are thought to be important in human cholestasis also. These mechanisms are presented in Table 2. Primary hepatocyte membrane injury might result from chemical oxidative injury or ischemia-reperfusion injury, or the administration of substances, such as cyclosporine, that incorporate into membranes and alter their fluidity. Inhibition of active transport processes has been suggested as a mechanism of total parenteral nutrition—induced liver disease and cyclosporine-induced cholestasis. Subcellular anatomic alterations can interfere with important excretory mechanisms. For example, changes in the pericanalicular complex of microtubules may be a primary event in North American Indian cholestasis[77] and in some drug-induced cholestasis. Whatever the cause, once cholestasis begins, amplification by several mechanisms occurs, as is described later.

Table 2. MOLECULAR MECHANISMS OF HEPATOCELLULAR CHOLESTASIS

Primary hepatocyte membrane injury
Inhibition of active transport processes
Subcellular anatomic alterations
Amplification by several mechanisms
  Cholesterol retention with altered membrane fluidity
  Bile salt retention with secondary membrane injury
  Formation of secondary "cholestatic" bile acids
  Reduced bile salt-pool and enterohepatic recirculation

THE CONSEQUENCES OF CHOLESTASIS

The effects of cholestasis are profound and widespread.[8, 54] Although the principal effects involve the function of the liver and intestine, secondary effects can involve every organ system. Figure 1 provides a simplified overview of the consequences of cholestasis. The primary effects are bile retention and regurgitation into serum and reduction in bile delivery to the intestine. These effects cause secondary results that lead to worsening liver disease and systemic illness.

The retention of bile constituents results in several clinically important events. First is the retention of conjugated bilirubin and its regurgitation into serum. The excretion of conjugated bilirubin is the rate-limiting step of bilirubin clearance. The mechanism of excretion of bilirubin monoglucuronide and diglucuronide by the hepatocyte has not been exactly determined.[19] Although it possibly involves an ATP-dependent organic anion transporter, this is clearly not the only pathway. Recent data suggest that microtubules are involved in the excretion of conjugated bilirubin. Pathways may be redundant and overlapping. The rate of excretion of conjugated bilirubin by the liver directly correlates with the rate of bile salt transport and the rate of bile formation; therefore, any condition that results in reduced bile formation results in the retention of conjugated bilirubin. During cholestasis, conjugation of

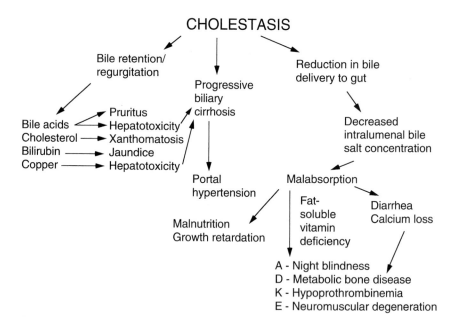

Figure 1. Some of the consequences of cholestasis. The major effects are bile retention, liver injury, and reduced delivery of bile into the intestine. These produce secondary effects, some of which amplify the cholestasis.

bilirubin continues, but excretion is reduced. The mechanism by which conjugated bilirubin regurgitates into serum is unclear but may differ according to the disease etiology. In hepatocellular cholestasis, in which bile formation is reduced, conjugated bilirubin likely effluxes directly from the hepatocyte via diffusion or vesicular exocytosis. On the other hand, in obstructive cholestasis, conjugated bilirubin may enter the canalicular space and efflux back through a weakened tight junction.

The presence of elevated serum concentration of conjugated bilirubin is a principal sign of cholestasis. It results in jaundice, which can be detected by scleral icterus at a concentration as low as 2 mg/dL, and dark urine. The concentration of conjugated bilirubin is affected by the rate of production of bilirubin, the degree of cholestasis, and alternate pathways of elimination, principally renal excretion. The magnitude of elevation is not diagnostically important because it does not reflect the type or degree of cholestasis. For example, although other investigations clearly indicate that the typical patient with neonatal giant cell hepatitis has more bile flow than a patient with biliary atresia, the serum conjugated bilirubin concentration is usually higher, which probably reflects an increase in bilirubin production in these patients. The absolute elevation of conjugated bilirubin is limited by alternate elimination pathways, principally the kidneys. A conjugated bilirubin concentration exceeding 30 mg/dL is unusual, although it can occur. Because conjugated bilirubin is bound relatively weakly to albumin, it can dissociate relatively easily and be filtered into the urine. Dark urine or stained diapers frequently are reported by the parents of children with cholestasis, and examination of the urine is a useful starting point in the evaluation of jaundiced infants.

Increased serum concentration of nonconjugated bilirubin is present in most patients with cholestasis. The rate of bilirubin conjugation is probably reduced by end-product inhibition or as the result of hepatocyte injury. The rate of bilirubin production may also be increased as the result of hemolysis that can accompany cholestasis. Newer methods of measuring bilirubin in serum have resulted in the discovery of a fraction of serum bilirubin that is covalently bound to albumin, known as *delta bilirubin* or *biliprotein*. This fraction may account for a large proportion of total bilirubin in patients with cholestatic jaundice, but it is absent in patients with nonconjugated hyperbilirubinemia. This complex is formed in plasma by a nonenzymatic process that involves acyl migration of bilirubin from its glucuronide ester with the formation of an amide link between one propionic acid side chain and a lysine residue of plasma albumin. The presence of large quantities of delta bilirubin indicates longstanding cholestasis. Any amount of delta bilirubin in cord blood or the blood of a newborn is an important sign indicating cholestasis that antedates birth.[79]

Hypercholeremia, or increased serum bile salt concentration, is a universal consequence of cholestasis. The transport of bile salts from plasma to bile is the principal driving force for bile formation.[25, 48] Failure to transport bile salts may be a principal mechanism of cholestasis or may be a consequence of the effects of cholestasis on hepatocyte function. In either case, retention of bile salts occurs by the liver cell, which results in down-regulation of new bile acid synthesis and an overall reduction in the total pool size. Bile salts are regurgitated from the hepatocyte, which results in an increase in the concentration of bile salts in the peripheral circulation. Furthermore, the uptake of bile salts entering the liver in portal vein blood is inefficient, which results in spillage of bile salts into the peripheral circulation. Reduced flux of bile salts into bile results in reduced delivery into the intestine and reduced enterohepatic recirculation. Because the movement of bile salts in the enterohepatic circulation represents the major driving force for bile formation, the degree of cholestasis is amplified by these events. Overall, the patient with cholestasis has an increase in serum concentration of bile salts, an increase in hepatocyte concentration of bile salts, a decrease of bile salts in the enterohepatic circulation, and a decrease in the total bile salt pool size.

One of the very common clinical consequences of cholestasis is pruritus. The mechanism of pruritus in liver disease is not entirely understood, and major debate exists concerning its relationship to the retention of bile salts.[33, 34] The serum or tissue concentrations of bile salts do not correlate well with the degree of pruritus, although all patients with pruritus related to liver disease have significant elevations of serum bile salts. Therapeutic approaches that reduce pruritus generally also reduce serum bile salt concentrations. New theories suggest that patients have differing sensitivities to elevated bile salt concentrations, which act on peripheral pain afferent nerves to produce the sensation of itching. This stimulation involves opiate-mediated pathways, and cholestasis-associated itching can be blocked by opiate antagonists.[11] Itching does not seem to be associated with histamine release, and antihistamine therapy is generally ineffective.

For the patient with cholestasis, pruritus may be a minimal problem or it may seriously impair the quality of life and indeed can be life-threatening. Scratching is the most measurable effect of pruritus. The degree of pruritus can be quantitated by clinical findings related to scratching, which has been useful in following response to therapy,[81] and more recently, computer-assisted "scratchometers" have been used in clinical research involving treatment of cholestasis-related pruritus.[75] Scratching leads to abrasions and skin mutilation in some patients. Secondary skin infections can occur. Constantly scratching the "unscratchable itch" has serious consequences. These children suffer loss of sleep, attention deficits, poor school performance, and a form of hyperkinesis that may be important regarding energy balance. Although the psychological ramifications have not been reported, older children express helplessness and can become suicidal. Unremitting and untreatable pruritus can be an indication for liver transplantation.[78, 80]

The effects of pruritus are age-dependent. Many parents and pediatricians ask why young infants with cholestasis do not itch. The author can confidently say that they do itch but are developmentally incapable of scratching. Scratching involves the use of arms, forearms, and fingers in a coordinated motion that occurs at a typical frequency.[75] It seems that the ability to scratch is not yet developed in the young infant. The cutaneous signs of scratching begin to appear in the 6- or 7-month-old baby, usually around the ears or the nasal bridge. From there they expand over the head, then the trunk, and finally to the limbs by the time the baby reaches 12 to 14 months of age. The mutilating scratching seen in older patients does not appear until well after the first birthday. That young infants do not scratch does not mean that they do not itch. Cholestatic babies are often irritable and do not socialize well. Young infants with those signs almost invariably proceed to scratching as they age, and irritability probably represents their response to pruritus.

Retention of bile salts results in injury of biologic membranes throughout the body. The liver is most affected. The retention of hydrophobic bile salts results in their incorporation into membranes, which alters membrane fluidity and function.[56] Bile salt injury of hepatocyte membranes is an important amplifier of cholestasis. The formation and retention of secondary "cholestatic" bile acids, such as lithocholic acid, result in further membrane injury. Bile salts may be a mediator of hepatic fibrosis also. Injury to red blood cells can result in spur-cell hemolytic anemia. Many patients with chronic cholestasis have an asthma-like syndrome, which may be quite severe and unresponsive to conventional asthma therapy.[83] Wheezing disappears with effective therapy of cholestasis, which suggests that it is a secondary event. The author's opinion is that retention of bile salts results in irritation of respiratory membranes and the asthma-like picture. Patients with chronic cholestasis also have frequent nosebleeds that are caused probably by the same mechanism. These patients may have life-threatening nosebleeds without abnormal coagulation parameters and with no clinically apparent anatomic problem in the nasal airway.

Hyperlipidemia is characteristic of some, but not all, cholestatic diseases.[59] Serum cholesterol is elevated in cholestasis because its metabolic degradation and excretion are impaired. Bile is the normal excretory pathway for cholesterol, and with reduced bile formation, cholesterol is retained. Cholesterol retention can cause an increase in membrane cholesterol content and a reduction in membrane fluidity and membrane function, thereby amplifying the cholestasis. Furthermore, bile salts are the metabolic products of cholesterol. In patients with cholestasis, synthesis of bile salts is reduced. Much of plasma cholesterol is in the form of lipoprotein-X, an abnormal lipoprotein seen only in the serum of patients with cholestasis. Although centrifugation density is similar to a low-density lipoprotein, the structure is very different. It has a high phospholipid and albumin content and a plate-like rouleau structure when viewed under the electron microscope. The marked elevation of serum cholesterol seen in children with cholestasis, which often exceeds 1000 mg/dL and sometimes can be as high as 4000 mg/dL, probably does not have as great an effect on the cardiovascular system as a similar elevation of low-density lipoprotein in familial

hypercholesterolemia. This may be because of the packaging of cholesterol into lipoprotein-X, which lacks the surface protein constituents
necessary to interact with vascular endothelium. Although it should be
considered in a therapeutic strategy, the potential for cardiovascular
disease is probably low.[54] Few studies of children with chronic cholestasis have demonstrated accelerated cardiovascular disease. The contribution of dietary cholesterol to the elevated serum cholesterol in patients
with cholestasis is probably minimal. Limiting the diet to reduce serum
cholesterol is not justified because that maneuver may have secondary
effects on nutrition. Furthermore, the use of oral bile salt–binding agents,
such as cholestyramine, has little effect on serum cholesterol in this
setting. The use of agents that block the synthesis of cholesterol has
been used sparingly in cholestasis and cannot be recommended at this
time. The proper approach to treating hypercholesterolemia in cholestatic liver disease is to treat the liver disease itself.

  Xanthomas may result from the deposition of cholesterol into the
dermis. The development of xanthomas is more characteristic of obstructive cholestasis than of hepatocellular cholestasis. They may develop
rapidly, over a few months in acute extrahepatic biliary obstruction.
Acutely developing xanthomas are usually the eruptive type, which are
pinpoint to 2-mm white pustular lesions that appear first on the trunk
and in the diaper area. Planar xanthomas that occur first around the
eyes but also in the creases of the palms and soles and on the neck
develop more slowly and are seen principally in chronic cholestasis
syndromes. Finally, tuberous xanthomas are associated with very long
duration of cholestasis and develop over the extensor surfaces, such as
the elbows, achilles tendons, and knees. They are unusual in pediatric
patients.[54]

  One of the major clinical effects of cholestasis, particularly chronic
cholestasis, is failure to thrive.[38, 63] The mechanisms of failure to thrive
include malabsorption, anorexia, poor nutrient utilization, hormonal
disturbances, and secondary tissue injury. Malabsorption in cholestatic
liver disease results from reduced delivery of bile salts to the intestine,
which results in inefficient digestion and absorption of fats. Digestion
is affected because bile salts are important for the function of bile-
salt–dependent lipase activity and the stabilization of the lipase-colipase
complex. Further, bile salts are important in stabilization of lipid emul-
sions, which is important for increasing the surface area on which
lipase works. Absorption is inefficient because of reduced formation of
intestinal micelles, which are important for removing the end products
of lipolysis and affecting their absorption. The result of these events is
the malabsorption of fat and fat-soluble vitamins.

  Malabsorption of fat results in the loss of a source of calories that
is important in infant nutrition.[38, 63] Further, the delivery of fat into
the colon can result in colonic secretion and diarrhea. Adults with fat
malabsorption often experience anorexia. This may also occur in the
infant, but more often, infants take in increased amounts of formula to
compensate for loss of calories. Finally, the loss of fat into the stool also

results in calcium wasting through the formation of calcium soaps of fatty acids. This may have an important role in bone disease in children and adults with chronic cholestasis. The treatment of fat malabsorption principally involves dietary substitution. In the older patient, a diet that is rich in carbohydrates and proteins can be substituted for a diet containing long-chain triglycerides. In the infant, that diet may not be possible, and the substitution of a formula containing medium-chain triglycerides may improve fat absorption and nutrition. This, however, has not clearly been proven, and therapeutic formulas containing medium-chain triglycerides may not be worth their expense. Bile salt therapy to replace missing bile salts is not practical. Ursodeoxycholic acid, which is used to treat some cholestatic conditions, does not form mixed micelles and has no effect on fat absorption.

The malabsorption of fat-soluble vitamins can result in vitamin deficiency states. Vitamins E, D, K, and A all are malabsorbed in cholestasis, and in that order. Vitamin E deficiency can result in peripheral neuropathy and possibly hemolysis. Vitamin D deficiency results in osteomalacia and rickets. Vitamin K deficiency causes coagulopathy and possibly reduced brain development. Vitamin A deficiency does not result in clinical disease in cholestasis. In chronic cholestasis, careful attention must be made to prevent fat-soluble vitamin deficiencies. This is accomplished by administering fat-soluble vitamins and monitoring the response to therapy.[54]

AN APPROACH TO DIAGNOSIS OF CHOLESTASIS IN INFANCY AND CHILDHOOD

The differential diagnosis of cholestasis in neonates and infants is much broader than in older children and adults,[3, 8, 27, 60, 71] because the immature liver is relatively sensitive to injury and the response of the immature liver is more limited. Cholestasis develops in response to a wide variety of insults. Although the reasons for this are not entirely clear, it is considered to be the result of immaturity of several critical mechanisms of bile formation. These are reviewed in detail elsewhere.[72] So-called "physiologic cholestasis" results from immaturity of these mechanisms.[73] This is better termed *physiologic hypercholeremia* and is characterized by the elevation of serum bile salt concentrations in normal infants to a level equal to that of many adults with pathologic cholestasis. This developmental condition probably helps to establish the infant's sensitivity to a variety of insults that would not produce cholestasis in the adult, such as gram-negative sepsis, heart failure, metabolic disease, and exposure to minimally toxic substances. Because of this, it is wise to look beyond the liver for the cause of cholestasis presenting in the newborn or young infant. If no other cause is found and liver disease is suspected, a more focused diagnostic investigation can be undertaken.

The differential diagnosis of hepatobiliary disease resulting in neonatal cholestasis is limited. Recent reference sources provide long lists of disorders that potentially produce cholestasis, some of which are more than two pages in length, but fewer than 15 disorders result in greater than 95% of neonatal cholestasis. The limited differential of neonatal cholestasis is presented in Table 1.

The first diagnostic concern should be the differentiation of hepatocellular from obstructive cholestasis, because it represents the differential between disorders of physiology and anatomy and medical versus surgical disease. All disorders that deserve surgical intervention in the first few months of life are obstructive disorders, and their timely identification can improve outcome. Differentiating acute cholestasis from chronic cholestasis, and secondary cholestasis from primary cholestasis also is useful. Acute secondary cholestasis is often the result of systemic bacterial infection. Although a patient cannot be diagnosed as having chronic cholestasis without the passage of time, some factors lead one to anticipate a chronic course. Unfortunately, few biochemical differences exist between hepatocellular cholestasis and obstructive cholestasis, and the diagnosis usually requires radiologic imaging and histology.

The tools that are useful in the diagnosis of cholestasis include liver enzymes, radiologic imaging, liver biopsy, and exploratory surgery.[71] The liver function tests that are useful include the cholestatic enzymes, γ-glutamyltranspeptidase (GGTP) and alkaline phosphatase (AP).[6] Alkaline phosphatase, an integral membrane protein of the canaliculi and bile duct epithelium, is elevated in virtually all cholestatic conditions. The serum elevation in obstructive cholestasis results from unregulated synthesis of AP by hepatocytes and movement of newly synthesized AP to the plasma membrane by vesicular transport. It is elevated in essentially all cholestatic conditions and in adults is a very useful test. It is less useful in infants and children, because it also emanates from bone. Values of as many as 500 U/L or more can be seen in normally growing children, and marked elevation into the thousands is observed in children with benign hyperalkaline phosphatemia. Measuring 5'nucleotidase, an AP found almost exclusively in the liver, can improve diagnostic efficiency, but it is not generally available. An AP level higher than 600 U/L in a neonate with other evidence of cholestasis suggests an obstructive lesion. GGTP is an integral membrane protein of the canaliculus and endoplasmic reticulum. It is elevated in patients with most cholestatic conditions and also by inducers of endosplasmic reticulum proliferation, such as phenobarbital or ethanol. Levels of GGTP correlate closely with those of AP and are elevated in virtually all obstructive cholestatic conditions; however, GGTP may be normal in some forms of hepatocellular cholestasis, which is discussed more fully later.

The author's experience with large numbers of infants with cholestasis have led to the adoption of a scheme for using AP and GGTP in diagnosis. If both are very high (> 600 U/L), the patient most likely has biliary atresia or other obstructive duct lesion, a primary ductal paucity syndrome, or α₁-antitrypsin deficiency. If AP is high and GGTP is low (< 100 U/L), the patient probably has progressive familial intrahepatic cholestasis or an inborn error of bile acid synthesis. If both are low or only modestly elevated (normal to 300 U/L), the patient probably has a primary hepatocellular disease, such as idiopathic neonatal hepatitis. Unfortunately, quite often values of both are mid-range (300–600 U/L) and, therefore, not terribly helpful.

Aminotransferases are not particularly helpful in the differential diagnosis of neonatal cholestasis. Markedly elevated levels, more than 800 U/L, indicate major hepatocellular injury and suggest primary hepatocellular disease as the cause of cholestasis. In some patients with acute biliary obstruction, however, aminotransferases are elevated similarly because of secondary hepatocyte injury. Aminotransferases used in tandem with cholestatic enzymes may be of more use. Relatively elevated aminotransferases indicate cellular disease.

The serum concentrations of conjugated bilirubin and bile salts are only markers for cholestasis and are not very helpful in differential diagnosis. In obstructive cholestasis, bilirubin and bile salts are elevated to roughly the same degree. In hepatocellular cholestasis, particularly in progressive familial intrahepatic cholestasis, and in cholestasis with ductal paucity, the serum bile salt concentrations are markedly elevated, whereas the bilirubin concentrations are sometimes only minimally elevated.

Radiologic imaging has assumed an important role in the diagnosis of cholestasis, but it is less valuable in the diagnosis of neonatal cholestasis than in older patients. Three entities—ultrasound, biliary excretory scan, and cholangiogram—are routinely used. In neonatal cholestasis, the ultrasound is used principally to exclude anatomic anomalies of the extrahepatic biliary system, the most common being choledochal cyst. It can be used to identify situs anomalies, vascular anomalies, and polysplenia and asplenia, which sometimes accompany biliary atresia. Otherwise, it is of little help in the diagnosis of biliary atresia despite the considerable literature to the contrary. The size and contractility of the gallbladder have been suggested to be helpful signs in diagnosing or eliminating the diagnosis of biliary atresia, but these findings have significant false-positive and false-negative errors. No study has been performed that blinded the radiologist to all other clinical findings, so the exact diagnostic precision is unknown. Ultrasound is very useful for the identification of biliary stones and sludge. Although it can probably accurately identify 90% of patients with gallstones, its accuracy in identifying significant biliary sludge or inspissated bile causing biliary obstruction is much less. Indeed, very small stones that can obstruct the common bile duct of a small infant may be easily missed by a competent ultrasonographer, and one should not hesitate to undertake exploratory surgery with operative cholangiogram to make this diagnosis.

Much has been written about the use of biliary excretory scan to diagnose biliary atresia.[44, 69] A variety of radiolabeled scintigraphic agents have been used, and the diagnostic precision of the test can be improved by administering phenobarbital for several days prior to imaging. The probable sensitivity for the diagnosis of biliary atresia is approximately 80%, and the specificity also is approximately 80%. Although this is fairly good for a single test, it is time-consuming and does have significant false-positive and false-negative results. Consequently, most experts do not use biliary excretory scan in this differential diagnosis.

Endoscopic retrograde cholangiogram (ERC) and percutaneous transhepatic cholangiogram are useful in the diagnosis of cholestasis in adults but have unproven value in the evaluation of neonatal cholestasis.[50, 65] Some literature is available concerning ERC for the diagnosis of biliary atresia. When used for that purpose, ERC poses many problems. Foremost is the fact that the diagnostic finding is the absence of demonstrable bile ducts. Because the test is difficult to perform and the risk for failing to demonstrate bile ducts is high due to technical reasons, the risk for false-positive diagnosis would seem to be very high. Demonstrating bile ducts would convincingly exclude biliary atresia, but very small bile ducts are common to several cholestatic conditions in which surgery is not indicated. Percutaneous transhepatic cholangiogram (PTC) is not useful because intrahepatic bile ducts often are not dilated in neonatal cholestatic disease, and if they are, they can easily be identified by ultrasound.

Percutaneous liver biopsy is the most useful test in the diagnosis of neonatal cholestasis; however, it has limitations.[13, 71] Despite the invasive nature of the procedure, it is associated with extremely low risk of significant morbidity or mortality. The biggest problem is that the interpretation of the histopathology requires experience and expertise, which many general pediatric pathologists lack. The interpretation of a single liver biopsy in a child with neonatal cholestasis is also limited by the dynamics of disease. Many cholestatic conditions express themselves differently over time. For example, patients with progressive familial intrahepatic cholestasis (see text to follow) frequently develop paucity of interlobular bile ducts, which could be misinterpreted as a primary ductal paucity syndrome. Liver biopsies from patients with biliary atresia, when obtained early in the course, sometimes seem to represent hepatitis. It is important to remember that a series of liver biopsies can provide useful information about the dynamics of the disease, which, in turn, can help develop a diagnosis.

While radiographic imaging is most useful in the diagnosis of surgical conditions, liver biopsy is very helpful in diagnosis of medical conditions. In addition to being able to visualize the hepatocanalicular cholestasis and cholate injury, the liver biopsy also can provide disease-specific findings, such as the periodic acid-Schiff–positive granules in α_1-antitrypsin deficiency. Disease-specific findings often are subtle, and expert interpretation is required to achieve the full potential of liver biopsy. Liver biopsy is helpful also in staging disease, in that secondary biliary injury and progressive fibrosis and cirrhosis can be identified.

Differentiating between idiopathic neonatal hepatitis and biliary atresia is a diagnostic challenge. In expert hands, no tool contributes as much to that differential diagnosis as does percutaneous liver biopsy. The landmark research of Brough and Bernstein[13] demonstrated the diagnostic usefulness of the percutaneous liver biopsy. In this study of 158 patients, the authors compared the original pathologic diagnosis with the ultimate diagnosis that included surgical findings and long-term follow-up evaluation. The original diagnosis was an error in 10 patients (6.3%), which makes it an excellent test. More importantly, however, was the type of error seen in these 10 patients. In 9 of the 10 patients, the pathologic diagnosis was obstructive disease, whereas the patient actually had neonatal hepatitis or α_1-antitrypsin deficiency. This error led to exploratory surgery that was performed to confirm the diagnosis. The surgery was of little harm to the patients. In only one patient with biliary atresia was the pathologic diagnosis that of hepatitis, which led to a delay in the diagnosis of this surgical obstructive disease. Thus, in only 1 of 158 patients (0.6%), a diagnostic error led to meaningful clinical consequences. Liver biopsy, therefore, has a very high sensitivity and specificity for the diagnosis of biliary atresia, with somewhat less specificity for the diagnosis of neonatal hepatitis.

Exploratory surgery is useful for diagnosing neonatal cholestasis. Although older literature suggested that exploratory surgery placed patients with neonatal hepatitis at risk, this is not true with modern anesthesia and surgical techniques. If there is a question about surgical disease, the patient undergoes exploratory surgery to provide a definitive demonstration of bile duct anatomy. In institutions with less experience and expertise, exploratory surgery should be performed more frequently, rather than less so. Operative cholangiogram is simple, straightforward, time-efficient, and definitive.

THE DIFFERENTIAL DIAGNOSIS OF CHRONIC CHOLESTASIS IN INFANCY

Chronic Obstructive Cholestasis

Biliary atresia, primary sclerosing cholangitis, and the biliary disease associated with Langerhans' cell histiocytosis are briefly considered.

Biliary Atresia

In patients with biliary atresia, the extrahepatic biliary tract is obstructed as the result of a process that obliterates the duct to the point at which no true lumen is present (atresia).[70] Although any part of the biliary tract may be involved, the most common finding is the obliteration of the entire extrahepatic ductal system, often with a microgallbladder.[16, 29, 74] It has a reported incidence of 1 in 15,000 to as many as 1 in 8000 live births and a female-to-male preponderance of 1.4 to 1.0. The etiology of biliary atresia is unknown. Many theories explain the etiology and pathogenesis of this disease, although none have adequately done so. Approximately 10% of patients have associated congenital anomalies, which suggests a developmental abnormality, and for years this was considered to be a congenital disorder. Considerable evidence has led to the current belief, however, that it is the acquired result of an inflammatory process that begins at approximately the time of birth and leads to destruction of the bile ducts. Some evidence suggests an infectious cause, but no agent has been identified. At this time, biliary atresia is classified as an idiopathic neonatal obliterative cholangiopathy.

Biliary atresia presents insidiously. Frequently, the only sign is hyperbilirubinemia that slowly increases during the first 4 to 6 weeks of life.[45, 47] Only rarely is jaundice noticed in the first few days of life, and almost never at birth. The baby usually is otherwise healthy, and the degree of jaundice causes little concern. Hepatomegaly is not prominent, and splenomegaly is either absent or minimal. Most patients have acholic stools, but new parents may not appreciate this abnormality and, therefore, do not bring it to the physician's attention. Meconium color is normal, indicating fetal bile duct patency. Persistent cholestasis and acholic stools in an otherwise healthy infant strongly suggest extrahepatic biliary atresia.

The laboratory evaluation of biliary atresia usually provides an inconclusive diagnosis.[17, 28, 45, 47, 66, 70, 84] The bilirubin usually plateaus in the range of 10 to 15 mg/dL, the majority being direct-reacting. Serum aminotransferases are moderately elevated (80–200 U/L). Alkaline phosphatase and GGTP are often very high; if both are more than 600 U/L, biliary atresia is a likely diagnosis. Although serum bile salt concentrations are elevated, neither the level nor the qualitative pattern offers any help with diagnosis.

Differentiation of biliary atresia from other causes of cholestasis is usually achieved by combining histopathology and diagnostic imaging. Initially, other surgical disorders, such as choledochal cyst, are excluded by ultrasound imaging. Percutaneous liver biopsy usually provides a sample that is adequate for diagnostic purposes. The findings of expanded portal areas, proliferation of interlobular bile ducts, and portal bile plugs are sensitive and specific for extrahepatic obstruction, which, in the neonate, is nearly always biliary atresia.[13] Percutaneous liver biopsy provides sufficient diagnostic discrimination to proceed to laparotomy if obstruction is evident, or to medical therapy and observation without further imaging. In centers without sufficient experience in evaluating liver biopsies, however, imaging using ^{99m}Tc agents can be used to diagnose biliary atresia.[69] Because some patients with intrahepatic cholestasis have essentially complete cessation of bile flow, falsely abnormal studies are significant. Pretreating with phenobarbital to stimulate bile flow may reduce error. Nasoduodenal intubation or passage of an absorbent string with observation of duodenal fluid for the presence of bilirubin has been presented as a practical, inexpensive, and safe diagnostic approach. It may, however, have significant potential for error.[30] When any combination of findings strongly suggests biliary atresia, laparotomy and operative cholangiogram are required for confirmation.

The early diagnosis of biliary atresia is essential, because the outcome of patients treated by portoenterostomy before 2 months of age is much better than that for patients with delayed intervention.[37, 42, 43] Several variations on the procedure described by Kasai and colleagues[37] are used, depending on the experience of the surgeon. This form of surgery is effective in providing bile drainage in a significant proportion of cases; however, long-term follow-up evaluation of patients successfully treated in this manner demonstrates that most have cirrhosis and many have significant abnormalities of liver function. Recurrent cholangitis is common and negatively affects outcome. Although few patients are truly cured by this procedure, it may improve the length and quality of life. Most patients ultimately require orthotopic liver transplantation (OLT), but a successful Kasai procedure can delay this for several years.[39, 43, 70]

Biliary atresia is, by far, the most common indication for OLT in children, constituting 50% to 75% of transplants performed. Approximately 400 to 600 new cases of biliary atresia are observed in the United States each year. Approximately half of these receive long-term benefit from a Kasai portoenterostomy that delays the need for transplant for patients more than 5 years of age. Patients with biliary atresia and failed Kasai procedures typically reach end stage between 9 and 18 months of age and may account for more than 90% of OLT candidates fewer than 2 years of age. The patient for whom the Kasai procedure failed or who has had no attempted surgical intervention has a clear indication for OLT and needs the procedure as an infant.[78, 80] Readers are referred to a recent review of this subject by Stein and Vacanti.[70]

Primary Sclerosing Cholangitis

This idiopathic chronic cholestatic disorder is characterized by inflammation of bile ducts, leading to their fibrosis or destruction.[9, 41] It can involve the larger bile ducts, both intrahepatic and extrahepatic, and the small bile ducts, down to the interlobular ducts, in any combination. It can involve the whole liver or it can be focal, involving only a single bile duct or diffusely involving the ductal system of a lobe or segment of the liver. The involved ducts become irregularly narrowed or obliterated, and proximal to tight narrowings, focal dilatations develop. This results in the characteristic beaded appearance on cholangiogram.

The prevalence of primary sclerosing cholangitis is 1 to 6 per 100,000 population; the average age at diagnosis is 39 years.[41] It is an uncommon condition among infants and children; however, its incidence may be underestimated because of underdiagnosis.[67] A well-established relationship exists between primary sclerosing cholangitis and inflammatory bowel disease (IBD), mainly ulcerative colitis. Patients with ulcerative colitis have a 2.5% to 7.5% risk of developing primary sclerosing cholangitis, and the majority of patients with primary sclerosing cholangitis can be found to have IBD if carefully studied. It can occur alone or in association with other disorders. The cause of primary sclerosing cholangitis is unknown, although genetic and immunologic factors seem to have a role. It is associated with other autoimmune diseases, a strong association exists with the autoimmune-associated HLA haplotypes B8 and DR3, and a familial incidence has been recorded. Autoantibodies can be found in the serum of a majority of patients. Other theories regarding the etiology of primary sclerosing cholangitis involve portal bacteremia, bacterial toxic products, and viral infections. Primary sclerosing cholangitis is classified as an idiopathic obliterative cholangiopathy, and in a neonate, it can be confused with biliary atresia.

The diagnosis of primary sclerosing cholangitis relies on cholangiography and histopathology.[41] It is suspected in any patient with IBD and abnormal liver biochemistries or other evidence of liver disease. It is suspected also in any patient with autoimmune liver disease, particularly if cholestatic features are present. The biochemical features of primary sclerosing cholangitis are not diagnostic. The disease often is accompanied by marked elevations of AP and GGTP. The average AP in 10 patients in the author's practice was 1418 ± 1056 (SD) U/L, and GGTP 2138 ± 1477 U/L.[83] This disease is one of only three disorders that the author has encountered in nontransplanted infants that are associated with very high GGTP (> 1500 U/L). The other two disorders are Alagille's syndrome and idiopathic granulomatous hepatitis. A super-high GGTP is not a very sensitive test for detecting any of these disorders, but if present, it limits the differential diagnosis. The presence of serum autoantibodies (perinuclear antineutrophil, antismooth muscle, and antinuclear antibodies are most frequently found) is suggestive of the diagnosis but is not sensitive or specific. Not all patients with primary sclerosing cholangitis are cholestatic. Fewer than 50% are jaundiced. This probably reflects the focal nature of the disease and the reserve excretory capacity of the liver.

Visualization of the biliary tree is essential for diagnosis. Visualization can be accomplished by ERC, PTC, and operative cholangiogram. The findings include irregular, focal, and segmental narrowing and dilatation of ducts, and sometimes complete obliteration of ducts. These findings are diagnostic of primary sclerosing cholangitis in the nontransplanted patient. Because a variant of primary sclerosing cholangitis, called *small duct cholangitis*, does not seem to affect the larger ducts, the diagnostic cholangiographic findings are absent, although "pruning" of the ductal system is often appreciated.

Liver biopsy pathology can aid in diagnosis. The findings are focused in the portal triads and include inflammation, edema, and fibrosis of the triads, pericholangitis, periductal fibrosis (including the diagnostic "onion-skinning" lesion), cholangitis, and duct loss. The histologic lesions are often not present and rarely are diagnostic.

No specific therapy exists for primary sclerosing cholangitis.[41] Anti-inflammatory and immunosuppressive drugs have been used with limited success. Although ursodeoxycholic acid administration seems to ameliorate symptoms and lower serum enzyme concentrations, the effect on the long-term course of disease is unknown. Although its course can be variable, it progresses slowly and relentlessly in most patients, leading to end-stage biliary cirrhosis, usually within 15 years of diagnosis. Despite its rarity, it is the fourth most common indication for OLT in adults. Readers are referred to two recent reviews of this subject by Lee and Kaplan[41] and Balistreri and Bove.[9]

Destructive Cholangitis Associated with Langerhans' Cell Histiocytosis

Langerhans' cell histiocytosis (until recently termed *histiocytosis-X*) comprises a complex spectrum of diseases, all of which are characterized by histiocytic lesions. The pathophysiology of the disorder is unclear, and whether the primary defect is in the Langerhans' cell or in a regulatory pathway is not known. Liver disease has been associated with Langerhans' cell histiocytosis. Some patients develop an acute hepatitis-like picture, and abnormal histiocytes can be demonstrated on liver biopsy. Others develop severe progressive cholestasis with duct lesions.[55] This has been classified as sclerosing cholangitis, and in a series of 78 pediatric patients with sclerosing cholangitis, 15% were associated with Langerhans' cell histiocytosis.[67] In the author's opinion, this lesion should not be classified as a sclerosing cholangitis, but rather as a destructive cholangitis. Once this process is initiated, it is inexorably progressive, leading to biliary cirrhosis. Control of the Langerhans' cell histiocytosis seems to have no effect on the progression of liver disease. It has been treated with liver transplantation.

The pathology of this lesion is dominated by destruction of bile ducts, usually the intrahepatic bile ducts. The gross morphology demonstrates necrosis of the walls of the major hepatic ducts with surrounding intense inflammation and fibrosis. Periductal bile lakes often are present, resulting from the extrusion of bile into the surrounding parenchyma. The cholangiogram picture in these patients is remarkable, demonstrating "puff-of-smoke" lesions in the parenchyma around major bile ducts. By the time these patients are evaluated for their liver disease, the liver biopsies often contain no abnormal histiocytes. The diagnosis, therefore, relies on the association of a destructive bile duct lesion with other clinical elements of Langerhans' cell histiocytosis.

No specific therapy exists for the destructive cholangitis in patients with Langerhans' cell histiocytosis. In fact, once this process has been initiated, there may be no therapy other than OLT. The course of disease, from onset to end-stage biliary cirrhosis, usually is fewer than 2 years.

Chronic Cholestasis in Association with Ductal Paucity

Alagille's syndrome and nonsyndromic ductal paucity cannot be classified easily as either obstructive or hepatocellular cholestasis. Whether the paucity of ducts is the cause of cholestasis, in which case it would be classified as an obstructive disease, or the result of a hepatocellular defect,[52] is debatable. Therefore, the author has given them a separate classification that acknowledges ductal paucity as the key histologic finding without inference to its role in the pathophysiology of cholestasis.

Alagille's Syndrome

This syndrome consists of chronic cholestasis in association with congenital heart disease, bone defects, ophthalmologic findings, and typical facies.[4, 5, 57, 58] It is also referred to as *arteriohepatic dysplasia, syndromic paucity of interlobular bile ducts, intrahepatic biliary hypoplasia,* and the *Watson-Alagille syndrome.* It is a genetic disorder inherited as an autosomal dominant trait, and the gene that is defective seems to be on chromosome 20.[23] The majority of patients, however, have no family history, and the rate of new genetic mutation or incomplete penetrance appears to be high.[64] It seems to occur throughout the world's populations. In the United States, it appears in the white, black, and Hispanic populations in a frequency proportional to their distribution in the population as a whole. It is one of the more common, if not the most common, causes outside of biliary atresia for chronic cholestasis in infants. Its estimated incidence is approximately 1 in 40,000 live births.[58]

Liver disease in Alagille's syndrome is characterized by variable degrees of cholestasis. Some patients present with severe unremitting cholestasis beginning at birth or shortly thereafter. These same patients often have the most severe degree of hypoplasia of major biliary ducts and the highest proclivity for progression to biliary cirrhosis. In other patients, jaundice is minimal, and they may present with severe pruritus and secondary skin changes later in life. Although the liver disease is most often nonprogressive, it may progress to biliary cirrhosis in some patients.

The diagnosis of Alagille's syndrome relies on demonstrating ductal paucity in a liver biopsy and the presence of other clinical features.[58] Congenital heart disease, usually peripheral pulmonic stenosis, is present in 50% to 90% of patients. Although the cardiac disease is not often clinically important, it may be the prominent finding in Alagille's syndrome and may complicate OLT. Skeletal abnormalities, usually butterfly vertebrae or hemivertebrae, are seen in 30% to 90% of patients. These are not usually clinically important. Joint deformities have been seen and can resemble rheumatoid arthritis. In one of the author's patients, a deforming, polyarticular arthritis was the prominent feature of disease. An important diagnostic finding is the presence of posterior embryotoxon, which is a thickening of Schwalbe's line.[12] This usually is not a clinically important defect, other than it helps in diagnosis. It is present in approximately 90% of patients with Alagille's syndrome and only 8% to 10% of the normal population. This defect rarely results in a deformed pupil and glaucoma. The face of the typical patient with Alagille's syndrome is unusual and characteristic.[4, 58] They look more like each other than they do their own family members. They have deep-set eyes, frontal bossing, a wide nasal bridge with a bulbous tip of the nose, a thin-lipped, turned-down mouth, and a small mandible with a pointed chin. Others have suggested that these are simply cholestatic facies, but in the author's experience, patients with Alagille's syndrome do have characteristic if not diagnostic facies.[68] Clinically significant renal disease is seen in a minority of patients.[31, 32] Growth failure is often profound and out of proportion to the liver and heart disease.[15] It seems to be a part of the syndrome and not the result of secondary malnutrition. These children often fail to grow despite efforts to hyperaliment them and to treat their liver disease, including after OLT.

The biochemical features of Alagille's syndrome are not diagnostic, but are characteristic. Marked elevations of AP and GGTP are observed in most cases. The average AP in 14 patients in the author's practice was 1148 ± 466 U/L, and GGTP 1893 ± 1534 U/L. This is one of the causes for very high GGTP (> 1500 U/L).[83] Approximately half of the author's patients have values exceeding 2000 U/L, and some reach as high as 4000 U/L. Serum cholesterol values also are often remarkably high. The average in 14 patients in the author's practice was 777 ± 439 mg/dL, and approximately 10% of patients have had serum cholesterol values exceeding 3000 mg/dL. HDL cholesterol values are low and lipoprotein-X is always present. Most patients are jaundiced, with serum bilirubin concentrations in the author's patients averaging 10.7 ± 5.4 mg/dL; however, some are minimally jaundiced or nonjaundiced. The serum bile salt concentrations are the highest observed in any cholestatic condition, averaging 346 ± 93 μmol/L in the author's patients (normal < 10).

Liver biopsy findings are characteristic and aid in diagnosis. The key finding is a paucity of ducts, which is quantitated by counting the percentage of portal triads containing an interlobular bile duct.[20, 35, 36, 46] One should be careful about identifying bile ducts, and a cytokeratin stain may be helpful.[76] Ductal paucity is defined as a ratio of ducts to portal triads of less than 0.5. Ductal paucity may not be demonstrated in the biopsies obtained early in the course of disease, and a destructive bile duct lesion, resembling small duct cholangitis, may be observed. The parenchymal architecture may be normal or may show such findings as cholate injury and giant cell transformation. Later in the course, some patients may have portal expansion, bridging fibrosis, and biliary cirrhosis.

No specific therapy exists for Alagille's syndrome, and careful attention is paid to preventing the complications of cholestasis, including deficiencies of fat-soluble vitamins. Ursodeoxycholic acid administration can dramatically improve the cholestasis in some patients, including reducing serum bile salt concentrations, improving pruritus, and lowering serum cholesterol.[10] Partial cutaneous biliary diversion can provide relief in patients with Alagille's syndrome, though not often complete elimination of clinical symptoms.[81] It can result in markedly reducing serum cholesterol values and disappearance of xanthomas. OLT is performed for the indication of Alagille's syndrome, both for cirrhosis and for the treatment of severe morbidity.[78, 80] Readers are referred to reviews of this subject by Riely.[57, 58]

Primary Nonsyndromic Ductal Paucity

Primary nonsyndromic ductal paucity is a rare condition, if it exists at all.[14] Ductal paucity commonly does occur out of the context of Alagille's syndrome, but it is nearly always, if not always, secondary to some other condition. Examples include progressive familial intrahepatic cholestasis (discussed later), small duct cholangitis (discussed earlier), graft-versus-host disease, and allograft rejection. It has even been observed in biliary atresia, in which ductal proliferation is a prominent early finding. It might even occur as a forme fruste of Alagille's syndrome, a possibility that cannot be tested before the development of genomic diagnosis. If ductal paucity is a prominent histologic feature in the liver biopsy of a patient with cholestasis, one should diligently look for another disease and only reluctantly call the process *primary nonsyndromic ductal paucity*. The author has made this diagnosis only once and believes the patient has Alagille's syndrome without other findings.

Chronic Hepatocellular Cholestasis

Infants rarely have chronic hepatocellular cholestasis, and the differential is very limited. The most confusion is with idiopathic neonatal giant cell hepatitis. Most patients with neonatal hepatitis experience complete resolution of clinical cholestasis by 6 to 9 months of age, and fewer than 10% in the author's series can be detected to have any degree of cholestasis by 1 year of age.[2, 21, 22, 40, 47] Likewise, most patients with α_1-antitrypsin deficiency resolve clinical cholestasis by 1 year of age.[49] The disorders that produce cholestasis beginning in infancy and chronic cholestasis as has been defined include: (1) progressive familial intrahepatic cholestasis; (2) inborn errors of bile acid synthesis; and (3) some disorders that seem to occur in limited, often isolated populations (e.g., Norwegian cholestasis,[1] North American Indian cholestasis,[77] and Greenland Indian cholestasis[51]). Benign recurrent cholestasis (Summerskill's disease) has been described in infants but does not meet the author's definition of *chronic cholestasis*.[58] Progressive familial intrahepatic cholestasis (PFIC) and inborn errors of bile salt synthesis are considered further later.

Progressive Familial Intrahepatic Cholestasis

Hereditary hepatocellular cholestasis was first described in an Amish kindred and called *Byler's disease* after the family's surname.[18] A similar or identical disorder has been described in many of the world's populations and the term *PFIC* has been used to describe the condition.[83]

The inheritance pattern is autosomal recessive. This not a rare disease; it occurs in approximately the same frequency in the author's practice as Alagille's syndrome.

The typical patient presents in the first 6 months of life with jaundice, itching, and growth failure. All of the author's patients presented with pruritus and direct hyperbilirubinemia. Although the jaundice may wax and wane, the pruritus is persistent and usually severe. Pruritus is often severe and out of proportion to the degree of bilirubin elevation. Approximately one fourth of patients have severe cutaneous mutilation, and most others have constant itching with significant excoriations. Symptoms referable to the airway are prominent. Approximately one fourth of patients have wheezing and cough, and three fourths have recurrent and severe epistaxis in the absence of coagulopathy or thrombocytopenia. Virtually all patients have significant hepatomegaly at the time of diagnosis, and splenomegaly can result from portal hypertension. Growth failure is severe in almost all untreated patients. Xanthomas are never observed. Cholelithiasis is observed in approximately one third of patients.

The serum biochemical studies in the patients with PFIC differ from children with cholestatic liver diseases owing to obstruction and ductal paucity. Although the majority of the abnormalities in PFIC patients reflect hepatocellular injury and cholestasis, values for GGTP and cholesterol are distinctly lower. GGTP levels in the author's patients with PFIC, when measured prior to the initiation of phenobarbital therapy, were 14.9 ± 11.8 IU/L and after phenobarbital therapy were 34.1 ± 21.1 IU/L.[83] Average serum GGTP levels in children with chronic cholestasis due to obstruction and ductal paucity are higher by at least a log order. A few PFIC patients have a GGTP level of more than 100 U/L while receiving inducers of microsome proliferation, such as phenobarbital and rifampicin. Also, the cholesterol level in PFIC patients is low relative to patients with cholestasis owing to obstruction and ductal paucity, averaging 156 ± 66 mg/dL. The diagnosis can be suspected in a cholestatic infant in whom pruritus is prominent and in whom laboratory evaluation reveals relatively low levels of GGTP and cholesterol. Other known disorders resulting in intrahepatic cholestasis should be specifically excluded.

Liver biopsy histopathology is helpful in the diagnosis of PFIC.[7] Hepatocellular and canalicular cholestasis are the most uniform findings. Hepatocellular injury, as evidenced by ballooning, giant cell formation, loss of normal liver plate architecture, and formation of pseudoacini, appears during the first few weeks of life and persists throughout the course. Giant cell transformation tends to regress with increasing age, but many patients with PFIC continue to have significant numbers of giant cells even late in childhood. Mallory hyalin and hepatocellular carcinoma are most often observed in advanced cases. Bile duct epithelial changes, including frank degeneration of duct epithelium, are prominent in PFIC and lead to ductal paucity. PFIC should be considered in the differential diagnosis of nonsyndromic paucity. Fibrosis appears first as pericentral sclerosis or portal fibrosis, or simultaneously in both areas. Bridging between tracts is followed by the development of stellate and lacy lobular fibrosis, a variable degree of inflammatory infiltrate, and complete loss of normal hepatic architecture. PFIC leads to a characteristic pattern of cirrhosis, consisting of micronodular, biliary cirrhosis with diffuse stellate, and lacy lobular fibrosis associated with severe cholestasis and pseudoacinar transformation.

No specific therapy exists for PFIC. Usual medical therapy, including the administration of ursodeoxycholic acid, has little effect. Partial biliary diversion, if performed prior to the development of bridging fibrosis, can eliminate pruritus and arrest the progression of disease in the majority of patients.[81, 83] In some patients, cellular cholestasis and fibrosis are markedly improved following the procedure.[7] Patients with moderate to severe cholestasis and minimal fibrosis are likely to benefit from partial biliary diversion. Patients with moderate fibrosis may benefit, but may fail to respond. Patients with extensive fibrosis, even without overt signs of liver failure, are unlikely to respond, and ultimately deteriorate and require OLT. Readers are referred to recent reviews of the subject by Whitington and coworkers[82, 83] and Alonso and coworkers.[7]

Errors of Bile Acid Synthesis

The pathway for bile acid synthesis is complex, and several inborn errors in this metabolic pathway have been described. Readers are referred to the detailed description of these defects by Setchell and O'Connell.[62]

Failure to synthesize bile acids that are capable of being conjugated and exported by the hepatocyte produces cholestasis because bile acid transport is the driving force for most bile formation. Defects early in the biosynthetic pathway produce profound neonatal cholestasis. Patients with these errors also may exhibit severe liver dysfunction and may present as having subacute hepatic failure. The key to diagnosis is to consider the possibility of an inborn error in any patient with cholestasis that is otherwise unexplained, particularly if it is severe and associated with severe hepatocyte dysfunction. Other hints are provided by routine liver biochemistries. The GGTP values in these patients are low as in PFIC, whereas AP and aminotransferases usually are elevated. Serum bile salt concentrations may be low or absent, depending on the method of analysis. Diagnosis is provided by qualitative assessment of bile acids in serum and urine, available in few specialized centers. This analysis should be requested for any infant with persistent or severe hepatocellular cholestasis, including patients thought to have PFIC.

These are rare disorders that produce rapidly progressive liver disease and hepatic failure. Early diagnosis permits therapy with exogenously administered bile acids, which have the effect of establishing the bile acid pool and bile formation, as well as down-regulating the synthesis of abnormal sterols that may be hepatotoxic. Orthotopic liver transplantation is an effective therapy also.

References

1. Aagenes O, Van der Hagan CB, Refsum S: Hereditary recurrent cholestasis with lymphoedema. Acta Paediatr Scand 63:465–471, 1974
2. Alagille D: Clinical aspects of neonatal hepatitis. Am J Dis Child 123:287–291, 1972
3. Alagille D: Cholestasis in the first three months of life. In Popper H, Schaffner F (eds): Progress in Liver Diseases, vol IV. New York, Grune and Stratton, 1979, pp 471–485
4. Alagille D, Estrada A, Hadchouel M, et al: Syndromic paucity of interlobular bile ducts (Alagille syndrome or arteriohepatic dysplasia): Review of 80 cases. J Pediatr 110:195–200, 1987
5. Alagille D, Odievre M, Gautier M, et al: Hepatic ductular hypoplasia associated with characteristic facies, vertebral malformations, retarded physical, mental and sexual development and cardiac murmur. J Pediatr 86:63–71, 1975
6. Allen K, Whitington PF: Evaluation of liver function. In Polin R, Fox W (eds): Fetal and Neonatal Physiology, ed 2. Philadelphia, WB Saunders, 1995, in press
7. Alonso EM, Snover D, Whitington PF, et al: Histologic pathology of the liver in progressive familial intrahepatic cholestasis. J Pediatr Gastroenterol Nutr 18:128–133, 1994
8. Balistreri WF: Neonatal cholestasis. J Pediatr 106:171–184, 1985
9. Balistreri WF, Bove KE: Sclerosing cholangitis. In Suchy FJ (ed): Liver Disease in Children. St. Louis, Mosby Year Book, 1994, pp 622–637
10. Balistreri WF, A-Kader HH, Ryckman FC, et al: Biochemical and clinical response to ursodeoxycholic acid administration in pediatric patients with chronic cholestasis. In Lentze MJ, Reichen J (eds): Falk Symposium No. 58, Pediatric Cholestasis: Novel approaches to therapy. Dordrecht, The Netherlands, Kluwer Academic, 1991, pp 323–333
11. Bergasa NV, Jones EA: Management of the pruritus of cholestasis: Potential role of opiate antagonists. Am J Gastroenterol 86:1404–1412, 1991
12. Brodsky MC, Cunniff C: Ocular anomalies in the Alagille syndrome (arteriohepatic dysplasia). Ophthalmology 100:1767–1774, 1993
13. Brough AJ, Bernstein J: Conjugated hyperbilirubinemia in early infancy: A reassessment of liver biopsy. Hum Pathol 5:507–516, 1974
14. Bruguera M, Llach J, Rodes J: Nonsyndromic paucity of intrahepatic bile ducts in infancy and idiopathic ductopenia in adulthood: The same syndrome? Hepatology 15:830–834, 1992
15. Bucavalas JC, Horn JA, Carlsson L, et al: Growth hormone insensitivity associated with elevated circulating growth hormone-binding protein in children with Alagille syndrome and short stature. J Clin Endocrinol Metab 76:1477–1482, 1993
16. Chandra IS, Altman RP: Ductal remnants in extrahepatic biliary atresia: A histopathologic study with clinical correlation. J Pediatr 93:196–200, 1978
17. Chiba T, Kasai M: An attempt to determine surgical indication for biliary atresia by laboratory examination. Tohoku J Exp Med 115:345–353, 1975
18. Clayton RJ, Iber FL, Ruebner BH: Byler disease: Fatal familial intrahepatic cholestasis in an Amish kindred. Am J Dis Child 117:112–124, 1965
19. Crawford JM, Gollan JL: Bilirubin metabolism and the pathophysiology of jaundice. In Schiff L, Schiff ER (eds): Diseases of the Liver, ed 7. Philadelphia, JB Lippincott, 1993, pp 42–84
20. Dahms BB, Petrelli M, Wyllie R, et al: Arteriohepatic dysplasia in infancy and childhood: A longitudinal study of six patients. Hepatology 2:350–358, 1982
21. Danks DM, Campbell PE, Smith AL: Prognosis of babies with neonatal hepatitis. Arch Dis Child 52:368–372, 1977
22. Deutsch J, Smith AL, Danks DM, et al: Long term prognosis for babies with neonatal liver disease. Arch Dis Child 60:447–451, 1985

23. Dhorne-Pollet S, Deleuze JF, Hadchouel M, et al: Segregation analysis of Alagille syndrome. J Med Genet 31:453–457, 1994
24. Elias E, Boyer JL: Mechanisms of intrahepatic cholestasis. In Popper H, Schaffner F (eds): Progress in Liver Diseases, vol IV. New York, Grune and Stratton, 1979, pp 457–470
25. Erlinger S: Recent concepts in bile formation and cholestasis. Medicina 81:387–391, 1990
26. Fallon MB, Anderson JM, Boyer JL: Intrahepatic cholestasis. In Schiff L, Schiff ER (eds): Diseases of the Liver, ed 7. Philadelphia, JB Lippincott, 1993, pp 343–361
27. Fitzgerald JF: Cholestatic disorders of infancy. Pediatr Clin North Am 35:357–373, 1988
28. Fung KP, Lau SP: Gamma-glutamyl transpeptidase activity and its serial measurement in differentiation between extrahepatic biliary atresia and neonatal hepatitis. J Pediatr Gastroenterol Nutr 4:208–213, 1985
29. Gautier M, Eliot N: Extrahepatic biliary atresia: Morphological study of 98 biliary remnants. Arch Pathol Lab Med 105:397–402, 1981
30. Greene HL, Helinek GL, Moran R, et al: A diagnostic approach to prolonged obstructive jaundice by 24-hour collection of duodenal fluid. J Pediatr 95:412–414, 1979
31. Habib R, Dommergues JP, Gubler MC, et al: Glomerular mesangiolipidosis in Alagille syndrome (arteriohepatic dysplasia). Pediatr Nephrol 1:455–464, 1987
32. Hyams JS, Berman MM, Davis BH: Tubulointerstitial nephropathy associated with arteriohepatic dysplasia. Gastroenterology 85:430–434, 1983
33. Jones EA, Bergasa NV: The pruritus of cholestasis: From bile acids to opiate agonists. Hepatology 11:884–887, 1990
34. Jones EA, Bergasa NV: The pruritus of cholestasis and the opioid system. JAMA 268:3359–3362, 1992
35. Kahn EI, Daum F, Markowitz J, et al: Arteriohepatic dysplasia, II: Hepatobiliary morphology. Hepatology 3:77–84, 1983
36. Kahn EI, Markowitz J, Aiges H, et al: Human ontogeny of the bile duct to portal space ratio. Hepatology 10:21–23, 1989
37. Kasai M, Kimura S, Asakura Y, et al: Surgical treatment of biliary atresia. J Pediatr Surg 3:665–675, 1968
38. Kaufman SS, Murray ND, Wood RP, et al: Nutritional support for the infant with extrahepatic biliary atresia. J Pediatr 110:679–686, 1987
39. Kobayashi A, Itabashi F, Ohbe Y: Long-term prognosis in biliary atresia after hepatic portoenterostomy: Analysis of 35 patients who survived beyond 5 years of age. J Pediatr 105:243–246, 1984
40. Lawson EE, Boggs JD: Long-term follow-up of neonatal hepatitis: Safety and value of surgical exploration. Pediatrics 53:650–655, 1974
41. Lee YM, Kaplan MM: Primary sclerosing cholangitis. N Engl J Med 332:924–933, 1995
42. Lilly JR, Karrer FM: Contemporary surgery of biliary atresia. Pediatr Clin North Am 32:1233–1246, 1985
43. Lilly JR, Karrer FM, Hall RJ, et al: The surgery of biliary atresia. Ann Surg 210:289–294, 1989
44. Majd M, Reba RC, Altman RP: Hepatobiliary scintigraphy with ^{99m}Tc-PIPIDA in the evaluation of neonatal jaundice. Pediatrics 67:140–145, 1981
45. Manolaki AG, Larcher VF, Mowat AP, et al: The prelaparotomy diagnosis of biliary atresia. Arch Dis Child 58:591–594, 1983
46. Markowitz J, Daum F, Kahn EI, et al: Arteriohepatic dysplasia, I: Pitfalls in diagnosis and management. Hepatology 3:74–76, 1983
47. Mowat AP, Pscharopoulos HT, Williams R: Extrahepatic biliary atresia versus neonatal hepatitis. A review of 137 prospectively investigated infants. Arch Dis Child 51:763–770, 1976
48. Nathanson MH, Boyer JL: Mechanisms and regulation of bile secretion. Hepatology 17:551–566, 1991
49. Nemeth A, Strandvik B: Natural history of children with alpha-1-antitrypsin deficiency and neonatal cholestasis. Acta Paediatr Scand 71:993–999, 1982
50. Nissenbaum MA, VanSonnenberg E, D'Agostino HB: Interventional radiology in the liver, biliary tract, and gallbladder. In Schiff L, Schiff ER (eds): Diseases of the Liver, ed 7. Philadelphia, JB Lippincott, 1993, pp 279–298

51. Ornvold K, Nielsen IM, Poulsen H: Fatal familial cholestatic syndrome in Greenland Eskimo children: A histomophological analysis of 16 cases. Virchows Archiv Pathol Anat 415:275–281, 1989
52. Phillips MJ: Mechanisms and morphology of cholestasis. In Suchy FJ (ed): Liver Disease in Children. St. Louis, Mosby-Year Book, 1994, pp 129–144
53. Radominska A, Treat S, Little J: Bile acid metabolism and the pathophysiology of cholestasis. Sem Liv Dis 13:219–234, 1993
54. Ramirez RO, Sokol RJ: Medical management of cholestasis. In Suchy FJ (ed): Liver Disease in Children. St. Louis, Mosby Year Book, 1994, pp 356–388
55. Rand EB, Whitington PF: Successful orthotopic liver transplantation in two patients with liver failure due to sclerosing cholangitis with Langerhans cell histiocytosis. J Pediatr Gastroenterol Nutr 15:202–207, 1992
56. Reichen J, Simon FR: Cholestasis. In Arias IM, Boyer JL, Fausto N, et al (eds): The Liver: Biology and Pathobiology, ed 3. New York, Raven, 1994, pp 1291–1326
57. Riely CA: Familial intrahepatic cholestatic syndromes. Sem Liver Dis 7:119–133, 1987
58. Riely CA: Familial intrahepatic cholestasis syndromes. In Suchy FJ (ed): Liver Disease in Children. St. Louis, Mosby Year Book, 1994, pp 443–459
59. Sabesin SM: Cholestatic lipoproteins: Their pathogenesis and significance. Gastroenterology 83:704–709, 1982
60. Sass-Kortsak A: Management of young infants presenting with direct-reacting hyperbilirubinemia. Pediatr Clin North Am 21:777–799, 1974
61. Sellinger M, Boyer JL: Physiology of bile secretion and cholestasis. In Popper H, Schaffner F (eds): Progress in Liver Diseases, vol IX. New York, WB Saunders, 1990, pp 237–259
62. Setchell KDR, O'Connell NC: Inborn errors of bile acid metabolism. In Suchy FJ (ed): Liver Disease in Children. St. Louis, Mosby Year Book, 1994, pp 835–851
63. Shepherd RW: Nutritional support of the child with chronic liver disease. In Suchy FJ (ed): Liver Disease in Children. St. Louis, Mosby Year Book, 1994, pp 389–400
64. Shulman SA, Hyams JS, Gunta R, et al: Arteriohepatic dysplasia (Alagille syndrome): Extreme variability among affected family members. Am J Med Genet 19:325–332, 1984
65. Siegel JH, Veerappan A: Gastrointestinal endoscopy in the diagnosis and management of hepatobiliary disease. In Schiff L, Schiff ER (eds): Diseases of the Liver, ed 7. Philadelphia, JB Lippincott, 1993, pp 299–333
66. Sinatra FR: The role of gamma-glutamyl transpeptidase in the preoperative diagnosis of biliary atresia. J Pediatr Gastroenterol Nutr 4:167–168, 1985
67. Sisto A, Feldman P, Garel L, et al: Primary sclerosing cholangitis in children: Study of five cases and review of the literature. Pediatrics 80:918–923, 1987
68. Sokol RJ, Heubi JE, Balistreri WF: Intrahepatic "cholestasis facies": Is it specific for Alagille syndrome? J Pediatr 103:205–208, 1983
69. Spivak W, Sarkar S, Winter D, et al: Diagnostic utility of hepatobiliary scintigraphy with ^{99m}Tc-DISIDA in neonatal cholestasis. J Pediatr 110:855–861, 1987
70. Stein JE, Vacanti JP: Biliary atresia and other disorders of the extrahepatic biliary tree. In Suchy FJ (ed): Liver Disease in Children. St. Louis, Mosby Year Book, 1994, pp 426–442
71. Suchy FJ: Approach to the infant with cholestasis. In Suchy FJ (ed): Liver Disease in Children. St. Louis, Mosby Year Book, 1994, pp 349–355
72. Suchy FJ: Bile formation: Mechanisms and development. In Suchy FJ (ed): Liver Disease in Children. St. Louis, Mosby Year Book, 1994, pp 57–80
73. Suchy FJ, Balistreri WF, Heubi JE, et al: Physiologic cholestasis: Elevation of the primary serum bile acid concentrations in normal infants. Gastroenterology 80:1037–1041, 1981
74. Suruga K, Nagashima K, Kono S, et al: A clinical and pathological study of congenital biliary atresia. J Pediatr Surg 7:655–659, 1972
75. Talbot TL, Schmitt JM, Bergasa NV, et al: Application of piezo film technology for the quantitative assessment of pruritus. Biomed Instr Technol 25:400–403, 1991
76. Treem WR, Krzymowski GA, Cartun RW, et al: Cytokeratin immunohistochemical examination of liver biopsies in infants with Alagille syndrome and biliary atresia. J Pediatr Gastroenterol Nutr 15:73–80, 1992

77. Weber AM, Tuchweber B, Yousef I, et al: Severe familial cholestasis in North American Indian children: A clinical model of microfilament dysfunction? Gastroenterology 81:653–662, 1981
78. Whitington PF: Advances in pediatric liver transplantation. *In* Barness LA (ed): Advances in Pediatrics, vol 37. Chicago, Year Book Medical Publishers, 1990, pp 357–390
79. Whitington PF, Alonso EM: Disorders of bilirubin metabolism. *In* Nathan DG, Oski FA (eds): Hematology of Infancy and Childhood, ed 5. Philadelphia, WB Saunders, 1995, in press
80. Whitington PF, Balistreri WF: Liver transplantation in pediatrics: Indications, contraindications, and pretransplant management. J Pediatr 118:169–177, 1991
81. Whitington PF, Whitington GL: Partial external diversion of bile for the treatment of intractable pruritus associated with intrahepatic cholestasis. Gastroenterology 95:130–136, 1988
82. Whitington PF, Freese DK, Alonso EM, et al: Progressive familial intrahepatic cholestasis (Byler's disease). *In* Lentze MJ, Reichen J (eds): Paediatric Cholestasis: Novel Approaches to Treatment. Dordrecht, The Netherlands, Kluwer Academic, 1992, pp 165–180
83. Whitington PF, Freese DK, Sharp HL, et al: Clinical and biochemical findings in progressive familial intrahepatic cholestasis. J Pediatr Gastroenterol Nutr 18:134–141, 1994
84. Wright K, Christie DL: Use of γ-glutamyl transpeptidase in the diagnosis of biliary atresia. Am J Dis Child 135:134–136, 1981

Address reprint requests to

Peter F. Whitington, MD
Department of Pediatrics
University of Chicago
The Wyler Children's Hospital
5841 South Maryland Avenue, #4065
Chicago, IL 60637-1470

PEDIATRIC GASTROENTEROLOGY I   0031–3955/96 $0.00 + .20

UPDATE ON METABOLIC LIVER DISEASE

Sarah Jane Schwarzenberg, MD, and Harvey L. Sharp, MD

The techniques of molecular biology have accelerated the knowledge concerning inherited disease to such a rapid pace that a textbook published today would be out of date. These elegant tools now provide accurate screening for metabolic liver disease but have failed to explain the variability with which these disorders present. One of the tasks of this article, however, is to reacquaint the reader with some of these rare disorders in an interesting way so that on presentation of such a patient, the diagnosis is entertained. For those readers interested in how to evaluate a child with metabolic liver disease, chapter 37 in the textbook *Liver Disease in Children*, edited by Suchy, is recommended. This article is limited to diseases that cause liver failure or cirrhosis that the authors are more familiar with as physicians in a liver transplantation center. In some instances, early diagnosis and treatment could have prevented the need for this life-saving procedure. Therefore, heavy metal storage diseases, protoporphyria, tyrosinemia, and α_1-antitrypsin deficiency are areas of concentration. For more details, see the above-mentioned textbook, plus the chapter on α_1-antitrypsin deficiency in *Diseases of the Liver*, ed. 7, edited by Schiff and his recently deceased father. Another textbook on liver pathology that includes color photos of slides is *Pathology of the Liver*, ed. 3, edited by MacSween and colleagues. Hopefully, this update will interest the reader in current molecular diagnostic techniques followed by brief exposure to the future application of human gene therapy.

This work was supported by contract NO1-DK-6-2274 from the National Institutes of Health.

From the Division of Gastroenterology and Nutrition, Department of Pediatrics, University of Minnesota Hospital and Clinics, Minneapolis, Minnesota

---

HEAVY METAL OVERLOAD

Copper Storage Disease

Indian childhood cirrhosis is a copper storage disease rarely observed in the United States. The etiology is primarily environmental, and whether a genetic defect is present is less clear with time.

Wilson's Disease

Wilson, a neurologist, described hepatolenticular degeneration, an autosomal recessive disorder, in 1912.[163] Although most patients initially present with liver disease during adolescence, clinical onset may be detected by 3 years of age without evidence of neurologic involvement. In contrast, adults usually present with neuropsychiatric symptoms, and the liver disease, although present, may be clinically silent. The copper-induced multiorgan systemic findings, particularly involving the central nervous system, are the result of the liver's inability to properly transport and store the normally absorbed dietary copper. Copper overload in the hepatocytes results from an inability to secrete copper into the circulation and into the bile. The gene recently has been identified to be a copper-binding membrane spanning protein with P-type ATPase motifs that characterize metal transport proteins.[19, 108, 149, 165] This recent investigative finding from multiple laboratories is a major advancement in understanding the transport defect. Detailed investigations are underway to more specifically explain the decreased hepatocyte copper biliary excretion and decreased serum levels of hepatocyte-produced ceruloplasmin.[28] Ultimately, better genetic identification of homozygous patients versus heterozygote carriers will be available. Although pencillamine remains the treatment of choice, other therapies are now available for patients who cannot tolerate this medication. Liver transplantation is curative for patients in whom detection of the disease is too late for a response to medical therapy.[121, 131]

Clinical Presentation

Hepatocellular Disease. Any patient between the ages of 5 and 20 years of age presenting with liver disease of unknown etiology should be evaluated for Wilson's disease, especially if evidence of Coombs' negative hemolytic anemia is present. Often, the initial hepatitis-like episode resolves with no therapy as does hemolytic anemia. A teenager with hepatosplenomegaly and other evidence of chronic liver disease is the most common clinical presentation. Although the liver pathology may have all of the characteristics of autoimmune hepatitis, the titers of the usual autoimmune markers are negative or unremarkable in Wilson's disease. Most patients have evidence of cirrhosis with or without inflammation on liver biopsy. A few patients may be detected because of a gallstone or elevated liver enzymes on screening tests. Acute fulminant liver failure is a less common presentation but more difficult to diagnose and treat. Again, the clues are hemolytic anemia and extremely low serum alkaline phosphatase levels and uric acid levels prior to renal failure. Patients found to be noncirrhotic may be precipitated by hepatitis.[125]

Neuropsychiatric Disease. The age range for neurologic presentation is from 6 years to the sixth decade, but it occurs predominantly in young adults; however, as many as 50% of teenagers may have some evidence of neurologic involvement.[141] Tremors, both resting and intentional, plus dysarthria that may progress to dysphagia, drooling, and an inability to self-feed are the most common presentations. Motor involvement is observed in more than 50% of these patients and may resemble Parkinson's disease, chorea, or various forms of ataxia. Sensory perception and intellect remain intact, leading the patient to become extremely frustrated and depressed. Psychiatric symptoms include personality changes and irritability, eventually leading to extreme uncontrolled anger and physical aggression. Psychiatric diagnoses have included organic dementia, obsessive-compulsive disorder, schizophrenia, manic-depressive psychosis, and antisocial behavior. Although cirrhosis of the liver usually is present, it may be difficult to detect because liver tests may be normal, especially in adults. Seizures are an uncommon late presentation, often occurring after the initiation of therapy.

Rare Initial Presentations. Renal tubular disease is a common complication of Wilson's disease, involving either proximal or distal tubular dysfunction or full-blown Fanconi's syndrome. The initial clinical presentation may be symptomatic urolithiasis in rare instances.[96]

Common Complications. Amenorrhea in women and gynecomastia in boys are common complications even when not on spironolactone for ascites or peripheral edema.[114] Nevertheless, pregnancy still can occur and is specifically addressed later. Cardiac abnormalities are common even in teenagers and rarely lead to death from ventricular fibrillation with or without cardiomyopathy. Electrocardiogram abnormalities are observed in one third of patients, with arrhythmias in 13%. Orthostatic hypotension is observed in 19% of patients, with 33% having an abnormal vascular response.[71]

Diagnosis. The pathognomonic finding for Wilson's disease is the brown Kayser-Fleischer ring reflecting copper deposits in the Descemet's membrane rimming the cornea. At early detection, a ring is not present. Initially, deposits are visualized at 11 to 1 o'clock and require a slit lamp examination by an experienced ophthalmologist for detection. This well-known sign is present in almost all neurologically impaired patients but may not be present in patients presenting with liver disease only.[160] The serum ceruloplasmin is below 20 mg/dL in 95% of homozygotes but may be low in heterozygotes and in patients with severe liver disease or malnourished patients. A level of more than 35 mg/dL rules out Wilson's disease. Serum copper levels are less helpful because they are high in fulminant disease instead of being low. The crucial measurement of essentially free poorly bound toxic copper attached to albumin and amino acids is not readily available.[103] One milligram of ceruloplasmin irreversibly binds 3 μg/dL of copper; ceruloplasmin binds 96% of normal circulating copper tightly.

A copper level of more than 250 μg/g wet weight of liver is diagnostic in the presence of compatible histology and in the absence of chronic cholestasis; however, when the sera is not diagnostic, appropriate liver tissue may not be readily available because of severely deranged coagulation factors or severe cirrhosis. These authors and others have found the baseline urine copper excretion more than 24 hours (> 100 μg or 1.5 μM/d) followed by the increase of copper excretion (1000 μg or 25 μM/d) during penicillamine therapy at a dose of 500 mg, twice a day 750 mg/m² is diagnostic of Wilson's disease.[30, 80]

Genetics. Wilson's disease is uncommon, 1 in 30,000 population universally, with a calculated gene frequency of 1 in 180.[145] The gene locus is on the long arm of chromosome 13 at 14q21. It is highly expressed in the brain and liver, the liver being important because the Menkes' gene, which encodes a protein with 76% amino acid homology, is barely expressed in the liver. The two most frequent defects are a point mutation resulting in C-to-A transversion or a frame-shift.[21] Therefore, these initial studies suggest numerous mutations of the gene, with most patients having two different mutations of the Wilson's disease gene by acquiring a mutation from each parent. At the present time, diagnostic molecular biologic studies can be performed only on complete families, and the disease incidence precludes universal screening. All family members are recommended to be screened with the currently available tests, including alanine aminotransferase or aminotransferase. This is cost-effective because early medical therapy prevents clinical disease. Early liver pathology includes microvesicular fat progressing to macrovesicular fat accumulation and an increased number of glycogenated nuclei in hepatocytes. Lifetime medical therapy prevents all disease complications.

Therapy. Failure of medical therapy is usually due to noncompliance either in adolescents detected by screening or young adults when they are no longer covered by their parents' health insurance. Injury begins in the hepatocyte, where free copper may cause direct chemical damage or promote lipid peroxidation of membranes.[142] Copper bound by metallothionein is stored both in the hepatocytes or prevented from systemic absorption in the intestinal cell.[26] Systemic free copper causes the injury previously described in other organs directly or via oxygenfree radicals.[1, 45] Cellular antioxidants recover during therapy.[103] Which types of oxidant injury are important remains to be resolved. Brain MR imaging can document neurologic involvement and improvement together with clinical findings.[122]

Chelators

One gram of penicillamine in divided doses (750 mg/m² in children) a half-hour before or 2 hours after meals remains the therapy of choice, except when life-threatening medication toxicity occurs. Future exceptions may include severe neurologic disease, 20% of patients initially deteriorate, and pregnancy because penicillamine is a known teratogen.[57] Early adverse reactions are common, often immune-mediated, and can be controlled by prednisone or reintroduction at an initially smaller penicillamine dose. Late complications include renal complications, Goodpasture's syndrome, lupus erythematosus, bone marrow suppression, pemphigus, and myasthenia gravis. Assumed to act as a chelator of free copper for urine excretion, recent evidence suggests induction of liver metallothionein. Pyridoxine (20–25 mg/d) continues to be recommended by experts. Trientine, triethylene tetramine hydrochloride, has been effective in the same doses as penicillamine (1.0–1.5 g) in patients unable to tolerate penicillamine. Toxicities include bone marrow suppression, nephrotoxicity, skin and mucosal lesions, and iron deficiency.[35, 130, 159] Ammonium tetrathiomolybdate complexes copper and proteins in the gastrointestinal tract as well as copper and albumin when absorbed.[14] Although proposed particularly for neurologic disease, clinical experience is not sufficient to define its role, and reversible pancytopenia has been a significant complication.[56] The dose is 30 mg/d, but animal skeletal toxicity studies suggest non-use in children and adolescents.[143]

Diet. From a practical standpoint, patients are recommended to avoid liver and shellfish. In difficult cases, further restrictions may be necessary. In such cases, the drinking water should be tested because patients with Wilson's disease can tolerate only 0.02 ppm, whereas Environmental Protection Agency regulations allow 1.0 ppm of copper contaminants from water pipes.[15]

Zinc. Zinc sulfate [150–220 mg, t.i.d. (nonprotocol)] or zinc acetate [50 mg, t.i.d. (protocol)] is increasingly being used as therapy for Wilson's disease, especially in patients not tolerating the previously mentioned medication. Its efficacy is based on induction of both gut and liver metallothionein. It is most effective when taken on an empty stomach. Whether it is best administered together with chelators is unclear to the authors. Advantages are its low toxicity, except for gastric distress and mild pancreatic enzyme elevations, and, presumably, cost. Disadvantages include its potential delayed benefit to neurologic disease.[15–17, 57, 60]

Pregnancy. Therapy is not to be interrupted during pregnancy because of the frequency of disease exacerbation plus fetal loss. The newborn liver may be affected when not on therapy. The incidence of teratogenesis is low (perhaps 2% with penicillamine) with cutis laxis (usually temporary) being the most common complication in newborns. Healing following cesarean section may be delayed. Data on other therapies are less extensive, although encouraging with regard to zinc. The zinc acetate dose is 25 mg, three times a day, during pregnancy and breast-feeding, pending follow-up evaluation of disease control.[18, 57, 102, 129, 141, 145, 160]

Liver Transplantation. The currently accepted indications for curative liver transplantation include those patients initially presenting with Wilsonian fulminant hepatitis and patients with severe hepatic insufficiency who are unresponsive to therapy within 3 months or developing after noncompliance with therapy.[131] Survival rate from one institution was 75%, with two deaths resulting from multiorgan failure and one death from B-cell lymphoma.[121] A survey of 15 transplant centers in the United States and 3 transplant centers in Europe retrospectively reviewed 55 transplants with a 1-year survival rate of 79%. Lymphoma was a complication in three patients, two of whom were treated at the authors' institution. This study also suggested a higher incidence in females of fulminant hepatitis.[131] Sufficient data are not available to recommend liver transplantation for primarily neurologic manifestation.[86]

Genetic Hemochromatosis

Blood loss by menstruation and pregnancy are the only good physiologic mechanisms available to compensate for the poor natural excretion of iron. Increased iron absorption characterizes genetic hemochromatosis, an autosomal recessive disorder seen earlier in males. Initially described by Trousseau in 1862,[154] epidemiologic data suggest that it is the most common inherited disorder in populations of northern European extraction. Screening for this disease is cost-effective.[4, 104] Bloodletting can prevent all systemic manifestations of disease. Olynyk[104] recently reviewed screening for and diagnosis of hemochromatosis. Diagnosis by the time the classic triad (i.e., cirrhosis, diabetes, and gray metallic skin) develops is too late. Hepatocellular carcinoma is the most frequent cause of death in adults and usually develops only after cirrhosis has been established.[33, 99] It is not detected by alpha-fetoprotein elevation. Although the incidence of this complication is 200 times that in the normal population, it is somewhat less clear that patients with genetic hemochromatosis are more predisposed to this fatal complication than other adult cirrhotics[33, 99] and that increasing age, alcohol abuse, and hepatitis B may be contributing factors.[44] Shockingly unacceptable are the mortality statistics following liver transplantation, and, thus, reevaluation is underway as to whether this iron-storage disorder is an indication for this procedure in the future.[65] For adult data, readers are referred to Bacon's review.[98]

Clinical

Estimates of disease prevalence range from 2.7 to 10.8 per 1000 individuals in numerous studies on white populations, suggesting a heterozygosity incidence of as many as 10% in this population.[38, 104, 110] In contrast, autopsy findings suggest an incidence of 0.2%. The youngest reported asymptomatic patient was diagnosed at 29 months of age,[7] whereas the youngest reported symptomatic patient was 4 years old.[62]

Seventy percent of patients present between 40 and 60 years of age. The most common cause of death in young patients is cardiac, although usually not suspected by the presenting signs and symptoms.[54] The chief specific complaint in young patients is decline in libido, secondary amenorrhea, and loss of sexual hair. Findings at this time include hepatomegaly in 83%, diabetes mellitus in 34%, and arthritis in 10% of patients.[54, 99] Rarely, adolescents may present with cardiac failure.[88] In such instances, the cause is often not suspected prior to an endomyocardial biopsy. Data subsequently obtained in the cited case report included a serum transferrin saturation of 99%, and ferritin was 4050 mg/mL. The liver contained 25.3 mg/g dry weight of iron, yet only demonstrated the development of mild fibrosis. Complete reversal of disease was accomplished with weekly phlebotomy of 450 mL of blood. The frequency of cardiomyopathy in young patients is 60%, and death may result from cardiac arrhythmia or rapidly progressive heart failure.[29, 45, 72]

Genetics and Screening

The elusive defective gene has been localized to chromosome 6p close to HLA-A of the major histocompatibility complex near the D6S105 locus.[61, 166] As a result, 75% of patients are HLA-A3, 47% are genotype B7, and 29% are genotype B14 because of tight linkage between these genotypes. Family members with the same genotype as the proband are predisposed to the disease, and haplotypes are carriers with no concerns for disease progression, despite mildly abnormal iron studies.[104]

Screening should be performed on siblings and children of known patients at 10 years of age unless both parents are known heterozygotes or homozygotes, respectively. Individuals with elevated transaminases, diabetes, or arthritis of unknown etiology should be considered for screening because 1% of the later diagnoses have iron overload. The initial test should be a *serum transferrin saturation* (TS), which is the percentage of iron divided by the total iron-binding capacity. An abnormal value is greater than 55%, with 90% of patients having a value greater than 60%. Less used is the *transferrin index*, which is the serum iron divided by the transferrin both calculated in μmol/L, which reportedly is 100% predictive of disease when the value is more than 1.0.[7] Serum ferritin values range from 400 to 6000 ng/mL in this disorder. The combination of TS and elevated ferritin has a sensitivity of 94% and a negative predictive value of 97%. A liver biopsy is recommended to confirm the diagnosis dividing the specimen for histology with iron staining plus a portion placed in a clean, dry container for determination of iron content. Normal values per gram of liver are up to 1200 μg or 21 μmol. Patients usually have at least ten times the normal documented iron stores. The hepatic iron index is the hepatic concentration in moles per gram divided by age in years with patients having a ratio of 0.9 or better. Fortunately, measurements can be performed on specimens recovered from paraffin blocks.[105]

Pathology and Pathogenesis

In the liver of young homozygous teenagers stained for iron by the Perls technique, early findings include pericanalicular hemosiderin and ferritin in lysosomes located in zone 1 (i.e., periportal hepatocytes), which is more marked in males than in females of comparable age.[137] This type of iron-staining pattern persists with progression to involvement to central hepatocytes. Fibrosis begins in the portal triad, progressing ultimately to micronodular cirrhosis. Eventually, Kupffer's cells, other macrophages, and bile duct cells accumulate iron.

Cirrhosis, hypogonadism, and arthritis are irreversible pathologic conditions. Deferoxamine rarely is necessary for this condition because phlebotomy is more effective. Toxicity relates to iron levels in the liver plus good evidence for reactive oxidant species contributing to cell injury.[98] Mean survival in adults with therapy is 92% at 5 years and 49% at 20 years.[99]

In this condition, iron absorption via the small intestinal cell is extremely high despite evidence of iron overload. The poorly understood feedback mechanism from the liver governing the rate of iron absorption is defective. Inadvertently, a donor liver from a patient with hemochromatosis was transplanted into a well-documented patient with primary biliary cirrhosis.[69] Iron overload persisted 4 years later, secondary to an increased iron absorption. The recipient's major histocompatibility complex (MHC) haplotype was A3A26B7B15. In two previous patients receiving livers from donors with hemochromatosis, the iron overload did not persist, but the MHC recipients' haplotypes are unknown. Irreversible cardiomyopathy has been reported following successful liver transplantation despite completely normal iron studies in one patient 1 year postoperatively.[94, 162] Cardiac complications may be a contributing factor to the high mortality rate following transplantation.[44] Fifty-six patients have undergone liver transplantation with a 1-year survival rate of only 53% and the expected survival rate decline at 5 years of 43%.[65]

Neonatal Hemochromatosis

Neonatal hemochromatosis results in intrauterine liver failure and has no relationship with genetic hemochromatosis or any of the other secondary causes of iron storage. Most recently, this disorder was summarized by Knisely,[68] a pathologist who has written extensively on this condition. The first cases were probably described by Dible in 1954.[34] The first criteria for definition, which included recurrence in siblings and liver disease evident within hours after birth, came 3 years later.[25] Thirty years later, Knisely used the following criteria[69]: (1) a rapidly progressive clinical course with death in utero or in the early neonatal period; (2) increased tissue iron deposited in many organs with reticuloendothelial system relatively unaffected; and (3) no evidence for hemolytic disease syndromes associated with hemosiderosis or exogenous iron overload from transfusions. All children in a family may be affected. Reported in abstract form are two families with more than one father involved. Iron studies have been unremarkable in the few survivors or parents. Large placentas may be present. Oligohydramnios is common, although polyhydramnios has been reported. The presenting signs are those of liver failure with lethargy, poor feeding, jaundice, nonpalpable livers to mild hepatomegaly, hypoglycemia, hypoproteinemia, and abnormal coagulation studies. Most patients are either premature or small for gestational age. Transaminase levels are low because most affected newborns have massive necrosis.

Residual hepatocytes are iron overloaded and may exhibit giant cell transformation or pseudoacinar formation. Regenerative nodules may be present. Mild inflammation or steatosis may be present. Pertinent extrahepatic organs with iron storage include the pancreas, heart, parathyroid glands, and mucosal glands of the oronasal pharynx. While on antibiotics, an infectious cause is sought focusing on viruses, particularly intrauterine parvovirus β19.[89] Other liver diseases that have demonstrated iron storage include tyrosinemia, Zellweger syndrome, α_1-antitrypsin deficiency, and leprechaunism. D4-3 Oxosteroid 5B reductase deficiency has been suggested as a cause of late-onset neonatal hemochromatosis,[132] but the urinary bile acid excretion of 7a hydroxy-3-oxo-4-cholenoic acid and 7a,12a dihydroxy-3-oxo-4-cholenoic acid have been documented in other known disorders of severe hepatocyte damage, although it does not persist when the patient recovers.[22, 23] The diagnosis of neonatal hemochromatosis is one of exclusion, with most cases diagnosed by the postmortem pathologist from death in utero or before 4 months of age. Liver biopsy usually is not performed because of the severe coagulopathy routinely present. Other diagnostic tests under evaluation include biopsy of salivary glands[67, 118] or MR imaging of the liver, pancreas, and heart for iron storage without iron increase in the spleen.[58, 118]

Therapy

Supportive medical treatment or, occasionally, liver transplantation rarely has been successful.[24, 84, 118] One therapy has been devised by Freese[47] on the basis that antioxidant therapy might be beneficial. Rapid response was initially reported in three patients.[138] Although which components are necessary is unknown, such therapy may be helpful for multiple causes of acute liver failure. The regime includes N-acetyl cysteine (200 mg/kg/d in 17–21 doses), Liqui E (25 IU/kg/d), selenium (2–3 µg/kg/d), prostaglandin E Ia (0.6 mg/kg/h for 3–4 weeks), and deferoxamine (30 mg/kg/day IV) until the ferritin decreases to 500 ng/mL.

Erythropoietic Protoporphyria

Erythropoietic protoporphyria, an inherited metabolic disorder, presents in childhood, with photosensitive skin because of an enzyme defect in the erythroblast that results in a fatal black liver disease in a very small percentage of patients. The enzymatic defect results from ferrochelatase deficiency, the final step in heme synthesis.[13] The first case was reported in 1926, with further dermatologic definition in 1961, and the liver disease was initially reported 30 years ago.[27, 51, 85] There is no racial or sex predilection, and prevalence is 1 in 75,000 to 200,000. Inheritance is usually autosomal dominant but may be autosomal recessive. An excellent review has been published by Todd.[150] Gene therapy is a reasonable hope for these patients in the future.

Clinical

Photosensitivity begins before 6 years of age, presenting as an extreme burning sensation that may keep the child up for nights, accompanied by erythema and swelling. Repetitive sun exposure eventuates into waxy thick skin resembling premature aging. Unpredictably, liver disease occurs in 1% to 5% of patients.[3, 101] Although the liver disease can present in teenagers, most cases are detected after 30 years of age. Clinical detection begins with right upper quadrant pain radiating to the back. Usually no evidence of biliary obstruction is found.[120] Death occurs within 3 to 5 months (range 1 month to 2 years) following the development of jaundice. Gallstones can be ruled out by liver ultrasound. A microcytic hypochromatic anemia occurs in 20% to 50% of patients. Although most patients are iron-deficient, ineffective hemoglobin synthesis is the most likely cause, with ring sideroblasts characterized by iron present in erythroblast mitochondria found by bone marrow examination in some patients.[117] Elevated red-cell–free protoporphyrin with normal urine porphyrins in a child with acute photosensitivity is diagnostic.

Genetics

The gene for ferrochelatase is on the long arm of chromosome 18. With a size of approximately 4.5 kilobases and located in the mitochondria, it is composed of 11 exons and 10 introns, with multiple mutations causing defective enzyme activity. Mutations have been documented in exons 1 and 10 and intron 9.[73, 97, 126, 133, 151] Ferrochelatase catalyzes the insertion of iron into protoporphyrin as the final step in heme synthesis.[13] Functional enzyme levels in patients usually are less than 50%; however, inheritance may also be autosomal recessive[126] instead of autosomal dominant with variable expression despite very few documented cases in both parents and children. Recent data still suggest autosomal dominant inheritance in most families, and liver disease can be observed with both inheritance patterns.[49]

Pathogenesis and Pathology

Excess protoporphyrin accumulates secondary to the enzyme deficiency. The bone marrow contributes 80% of the protoporphyrins, and the liver, up to 20%.[112, 135] Protoporphyrin is poorly water soluble and is only secreted by the hepatocyte into bile. When the liver and biliary system are overwhelmed, protoporphyrin becomes insoluble and begins to aggregate and form crystals in hepatocytes, canaliculi, and small bile ducts, resulting in black liver disease.[9] The liver demonstrates dark brown pigment in interlobular bile ducts, canaliculi, connective tissue, and Kupffer's cells, which are birefringent with a centrally located Maltese cross.[27, 66]

Skin Therapy

Violet light in the 400 to 410 nm wavelength photo excites the accumulated cutaneous protoporphyrin ultimately to a stable triplet state, producing reactive oxygen species and activating complement. Mast cells are degranulated and membranes are damaged. Local treatment consists of reflective sun screens with iron oxide.[150] The only effective systemic treatment is beta-carotene, a free radical scavenger, dosed according to age to obtain a serum level of 800 mg/dL. Special transparent filters to block these wavelengths can be placed over windows and especially over operating room lights to prevent serious damage, especially during laparotomy.[12]

Liver Disease Therapy

No single therapy has been found to be routinely effective for liver disease. Various therapies have been tried to decrease the production of protoporphyrin. Iron therapy unfortunately has not always decreased protoporphyrin levels, but instead increased the protoporphyrin load in some patients since it was initially proposed in 1986.[11, 87, 91] Blood transfusions to suppress the bone marrow red cell and thus protoporphyrin production have also produced mixed results.[152, 158] Hematin has been the most successful medical therapy although it works primarily on hepatic production of porphyrin.[10] Although coagulopathy routinely occurs acutely after hematin, thrombophlebitis rather than bleeding has been a more common complication and requires hematin administration into a large vein.[50, 93] Heme arginate, if available, is safer and usually is as effective.[95]

Cholestyramine has been used to bind protoporphyrin in the gut and interfere with the enterohepatic circulation.[8] Further reports concerning its efficacy have not appeared. Chenodeoxycholic acid has been used on the basis of increasing protoporphyrin secretion in bile but may work by other mechanisms.[116, 156] Ursodeoxycholic acid has not been used on the basis of lack of change in protoporphyrin excretion in the isolated rat liver.[6]

Liver transplantation has saved lives, but for how long and at what cost is less clear because it does not correct the main source of protoporphyrin.[12, 59, 64, 113] Postoperative complications, including cutaneous and visceral burns, hemolysis, and porphyric neurologic crises, hopefully will be avoidable in the future by using operating room light filters. Biliary tree complications prolong cholestasis and result in protoporphyrin reaccumulation. Unfortunately, liver disease has already recurred in some patients, especially teenagers.

Future Therapy

Bone marrow transplantation should be curative with the earlier-mentioned complications avoided. Unfortunately, most patients with liver disease die following attempts at bone marrow transplantation.[120] Thus, this particular procedure must be performed after a successful liver transplantation because significant bone marrow chimerism has not been documented in this disorder.[144] Bone marrow transplantation has been successful in reducing the porphyrins and eliminating photosensitivity in a patient with congenital erythropoietic porphyria who did not have liver disease.[63] The success of bone marrow transplantation and the availability of a mouse model[155] provide the necessary ingredients to anticipate successful gene therapy in the future.

Tyrosinemia

Tyrosinemia (hereditary tyrosinemia type I) is a hepatorenal disease characterized by progressive liver disease often not reflected in routine liver function tests.[47, 74] The first good clinical description was in 1956.[5] Unique features of tyrosinemia include renal tubular dysfunction resulting in hypophosphatemic rickets that usually is responsive to dietary and medical therapy.[148] However, the marked coagulopathy,[42, 74] neurologic complications simulating porphyria,[92] and predisposition to hepatocellular carcinoma[161] are not responsive to currently available medical therapy. Therefore, most institutions recommend early liver transplantation.[47] Inheritance is autosomal recessive. The enzyme deficiency, fumarylacetoacetate hydrolase, has been known since 1977 when reported by Lindblad and colleagues.[79] To date, further enzyme characterization has not explained the variation in progression of this disorder. A new medical therapy has been proposed by Lindstedt and colleagues[81] in part related to their intimate knowledge of the enzyme pathway and who participated in clarifying the confusion concerning the original enzymatic defect.[79]

Clinical

The earlier that symptoms present in infancy, the poorer the ultimate prognosis.[157] However, the heterogeneity of presentation, including age in the first year of life, does not predict the subsequent course and outcome despite initiation of dietary restrictions and N-acetylcysteine.[47] This is particularly true for patients diagnosed in Canada,[106] where clinical experience has been best observed and elegant screening has been accomplished.[53, 106] Although patients who present within 2 months of age have a poor prognosis,[157] unfortunately the same may be true for patients detected at birth because a sibling was diagnosed previously. Therefore, evaluation of any medical therapy is difficult.

Common symptoms include vomiting, diarrhea, failure to thrive, abdominal distension, anemia, bleeding, and rickets. Common findings include ascites, hepatosplenomegaly, peripheral edema, hypoglycemia, and urinary symptoms compatible with renal tubular changes as bad as Fanconi's syndrome. Hypoproteinemia and severe coagulopathy are quite common. Liver crises typically present in the first 2 years of life[106] and are characterized by worsening of the earlier mentioned liver findings, with jaundice heralding the terminal event. Often precipitated by an infection, coagulation tests worsen and are not responsive to vitamin K, despite low levels of vitamin K responsive factors in contrast to factor V levels. Bleeding can respond to fresh frozen plasma.[106]

Diagnosis

A diagnostic clue is finding markedly elevated alpha-fetoprotein (AFP) levels in the presence of nearly normal liver tests. Screening for tyrosinemia is best accomplished by testing the urine for an elevated level of succinylacetone. The diagnosis can be confirmed by red cell, lymphocyte, cultured fibroblasts, or liver analysis for fumarylacetoacetate hydrolase (FAH). Prenatal diagnosis by amniotic fluid after 15 weeks can detect succinylacetone in the amniotic fluid or FAH in the cells. Although chorionic villous biopsy can be performed by 10 weeks of age for FAH determination, differentiating heterozygotes or pseudo-deficiency mutant homozygotes may be difficult.[124] DNA testing is necessary for a firm diagnosis[111] or to identify the mutations.[123]

Pathophysiology

FAH is the last enzyme in the tyrosine degradation pathway resulting in nonspecific elevation of tyrosine, phenylalanine, and methionine. Just prior to this defective enzyme, maleylacetoacetate, fumarylacetate and their derivatives succinylacetoacetate and succinylacetone accumulate. The first two may contribute to the initiation of liver cell injury. Maleylacetoacetate is more likely to be involved with renal tubular injury. Succinylacetone is a potent inhibitor of the enzyme delta-amino levulinic acid dehydratase in the heme synthesis pathway, resulting in delta-amino levulinic acid nerve toxicity.[92, 147]

Other Complications

Neurologic crises[92, 147] are often precipitated by an infection. These children become irritable, less active, and develop severe pain, often localized to the legs. Paresthesias, hypertension, tachycardia, and paralysis may develop. The paralysis may progress to complete flaccid quadriplegia, including bilateral diaphragm paralysis, and require mechanical ventilation. The gastrointestinal tract may also be involved. Liver function may not change. Cerebral spinal fluid analysis is unremarkable. Intravenous hematin (see section on protoporphyria) to suppress the first step in heme synthesis may have minimal or no effect in severe cases.[100, 119] Both reported patients[100, 119] took more than a year to completely recover neurologic function following liver transplantation. Usually cases are less severe with the acute phase lasting up to a week; however, death is a common result.[92]

Renal Disease

Renal tubular disease and rickets are common complications. Nephromegaly is observed in more than 80% of patients, and 33% have nephrocalcinosis. Glomerular function may be reduced. Glomerular sclerosis and interstitial fibrosis may develop. No unusual acceleration of the renal disease has been documented following transplantation of the liver.[106]

Hepatocellular Carcinoma

The rate of development of hepatocellular carcinoma has been reported to be as high as 37%,[161] is associated with cirrhosis, and may be observed as early as 2.5 years of age[90] or as late as adulthood. Alpha-fetoprotein levels have been useless because they are usually elevated but still are followed for a dramatic rise. This complication has been seen with normal AFP levels.[107] Radiographic imaging studies including angiography are of little help and may be misleading.[31]

Uncommon Complications

Clinical hypertrophic cardiomyopathy has been documented in three infants.[39, 78]

Genetics

Fumarylacetoacetate hydrolase is mapped to chromosome 15q 23–25.[109] Mutations continue to emerge.[53, 123, 124] The incidence in most populations is 1 in 100,000 population. In the Saguenay-Lac St. Jean area of Quebec, however, the carrier frequency is estimated to be as low as 1 in 16 to 1 in 22.[32] A splice mutation in intron 12 can identify all of the patients from this region. Thus, an allele-specific oligonucleotide hybridization test on a filter paper blood spot from newborn infants could be used as a screening test in Quebec.

Therapy

Dietary restrictions of phenylalanine and tyrosine have been proven to be effective for the renal tubular disease. Otherwise, it is intuitively helpful in regard to improving liver tests, but no evidence suggests that it prevents cirrhosis or the development of hepatocellular carcinoma. The addition of methionine restriction when levels are high also may improve laboratory parameters. On the basis of decreased sulfhydryl compounds in liver and kidneys, Lindblad[77] suggested the use of N-acetylcysteine to replete tissue glutathione content (see section on neonatal hemochromatosis). No data yet support its usefulness acutely or chronically.[52] Liver transplantation is currently the treatment of choice with excellent results. It may be combined with kidney transplant when renal function is severely impaired.

In 1992, Lindstedt and colleagues[81] proposed that an inhibitor of an early enzyme in the tyrosine degradation pathway, 4-hydroxyphenyl pyruvate dioxygenase, prevents the accumulation of proposed toxic products in tyrosinemia. Five patients, one with the acute neonatal form, were treated orally at 0.1 to 0.6 mg/kg two or three times a day of 2 -(2 nitro 4- trifluoromethylbenzoil)-1; 3-cyclohexanedione. Succinyl acetone decreased to barely detectable levels. Five-aminolevulinate decreased to slightly above normal. The complete inhibition of porphobilinogen synthetase was almost totally abolished, suggesting that neurologic crises might be prevented in the future in these patients. Alpha-fetoprotein has steadily decreased in all but one patient, in whom hepatocellular carcinoma already may have been developing. Prothrombin time is normal in all patients, and the platelet count improved in three. Computed tomography heterogeneity presumably reflecting, in part, regenerative nodules improved in three patients. Improvement was observed in two liver tests. No toxicity occurred. No long-term therapeutic results are currently available. Hopefully, this treatment will decrease the need for liver transplantation; however, the development of hepatocellular carcinoma remains a concern.

α_1-Antitrypsin Deficiency

α_1-Antitrypsin deficiency (A1AT) predominantly presents as liver disease in children and early-onset emphysema in adults. A serum A1AT level should be obtained from all infants presenting with cholestasis of infancy and all children and adults with undefined liver disease. Family protease inhibitor (PI) phenotyping is obtained when low levels are encountered. The most common genotype associated with disease is homozygous *PiZ*. Only a small percentage of patients develop cirrhosis. No treatment is available other than liver transplantation.

Z-A1AT has a single amino acid substitution in the A1AT polypeptide chain, glutamic acid replaced by lysine at position 342. Z-A1AT is not secreted normally and is retained within the endoplasmic reticulum of the hepatocyte.[136] A1AT is a serine protease inhibitor that functions predominately as an inhibitor of leukocyte elastase.

Recent research in A1AT deficiency-associated liver disease has focused on two areas: (1) the mechanism by which the A1AT produced by the Z allele (Z-A1AT) is retained in the endoplasmic reticulum of the hepatocyte and (2) the pathogenesis of liver disease associated with Z-A1AT deficiency. These two areas of research are related, because it has been proposed that liver disease in Z-A1AT deficiency is related to the effect of the inclusions of Z-A1AT in the endoplasmic reticulum of the liver. In this event, studies in these areas are essential precursors to the development of safe and effective gene therapy for Z-A1AT-deficiency–associated liver disease.

The mechanism of Z-A1AT retention within the endoplasmic reticulum has been clarified by the work of Lomas and coworkers.[83] Understanding their work requires some understanding of the structure of normal or M-A1AT. A1AT acts as a pseudosubstrate for its target protease. Elastase is captured by A1AT when it cleaves the reactive center peptide bond at methionine 358-serine 359 (the P1-P1' amino acids). This peptide bond is accessible to elastase because the N-terminal portion of the reactive center is inserted into another portion of the A1AT protein, which forms the β-pleated sheet designated A. This allows exposure of the P1-P1' residue and provides a "stressed loop" conformation necessary to the inhibitor's function.[82] Lomas and colleagues[83] showed that the mutation resulting in Z-A1AT disturbs the relationship between the reactive center loop and the β-pleated sheet. In this situation, the reactive center loop of one Z-A1AT molecule can insert into the β-pleated sheet of a second molecule, resulting in polymerization of Z-A1AT. This polymerized Z-A1AT is retained in the endoplasmic reticulum. PiZZ individuals (homozygotes for Z-A1AT) generally have circulating levels of A1AT of approximately 10% of those of normal individuals, which may represent the approximately 15% of Z-A1AT that remains monomeric. As inflammation and increased temperature can increase polymerization of Z-A1AT, the authors speculate that controlling fever or inflammation in patients homozygous for Z-A1AT might prevent sudden increases in retained Z-A1AT. If retained Z-A1AT is, in fact, responsible for liver disease associated with this genetic defect, this therapy might reduce injury to the liver.[83, 139]

Other investigators have been interested in the mechanism by which retained A1AT is targeted by the hepatocyte for degradation. Calnexin, a molecular chaperone protein, is found in the endoplasmic reticulum in mammals. One function proposed for this phosphoprotein is that of "quality assurance" in protein synthesis, recognizing abnormal proteins and retaining them in the endoplasmic reticulum. Le and coworkers[75] found calnexin associated with A1AT null_{Hong Kong}, a very rare allele of A1AT that encodes a truncated protein that is retained in the endoplasmic reticulum. It lacks the amino acid sequences of the reactive center, and thus is unlikely to polymerize in the same way as Z-A1AT. Whether Z-A1AT is similarly associated with calnexin is not yet known, but studies of this type will expand the understanding both of the mechanism of Z-A1AT retention in the endoplasmic reticulum and of the mechanism by which the retained Z-A1AT is subsequently routed for degradation. Such studies may permit strategies to be developed for reducing the amount of retained Z-A1AT in the hepatocyte to prevent any injury caused by this material. They also may allow the development of strategies for mobilizing the Z-A1AT, which functions normally in the serum, out of the hepatocyte.

Explaining the pathogenesis of Z-A1AT associated-liver disease has been difficult. As previously stated, only a few infants and adults homozygous for Z-A1AT have liver disease despite the fact that they all have the same genetic mutation in A1AT. This has led some investigators to suggest that either another genetic defect exists in those infants who develop liver disease or that individuals who develop liver disease are exposed to an environmental stress. Studies to elucidate these putative differences have come from cell culture systems, transgenic mouse models, and epidemiology.

Studies in skin fibroblasts from patients with Z-A1AT deficiency have been used as a model system by Wu and coworkers[164] to investigate factors contributing to the development of liver disease. Human fibroblasts from PiZZ individuals with and without liver disease were studied. Fibroblasts do not express the A1AT gene; therefore, cells from each group were transduced with the Z-A1AT gene in a vector designed for constitutive expression. Fibroblasts from ZZ individuals with liver disease had a delay in degradation of the gene product of the transduced gene, compared with fibroblasts from ZZ individuals without liver disease. The authors suggest that this study uncovers a genetic difference in PiZZ individuals with and without liver disease. They speculate that individuals susceptible to liver disease may have a defect in the endoplasmic reticulum degradation pathway. This would allow an increased amount of Z-A1AT to accumulate in the hepatocyte and, assuming that this material damages the hepatocyte by an as yet undetermined mechanism, would result in increased hepatocyte damage in these individuals.[164]

Other investigators have made progress in transgenic mouse models of human A1AT deficiency. Previous investigators have suggested that transgenic mouse models bearing the human Z-A1AT gene develop a clinical and histopathologic picture similar to that of human neonates with liver disease associated with Z-A1AT deficiency.[36] Unfortunately, the histopathologic characteristics of the liver disease seen in these transgenic mice are mild, usually develop only in older animals, and do not resemble the histopathology of A1AT deficiency.[20, 48] The failure to thrive observed in these animals is far in excess of that seen in affected human infants.[36] In addition, studies by Sifers and colleagues[139] in mice transgenic for the normal or M-A1AT showed that human M-A1AT trapped in the endoplasmic reticulum hindered secretion of mouse A1AT from the hepatocytes.[140] If this is also true for mice transgenic for Z-A1AT, they may not have normal levels of circulating A1AT, which means that the current models might not distinguish effectively between hepatic injury attributable to intrahepatic inclusions and that attributable to decreased circulating or local antielastase activity.

A recent study of a Z-A1AT transgenic mouse line developed by Ali and coworkers[2] concluded that no mouse model currently available developed liver disease similar to that of a human neonate. They suggested that the available models might be useful for studying the development of liver disease in deficient adults, especially because they offer the opportunity to study the interaction of the Z-A1AT with the effects of other genetic defects or environmental factors that might predispose to the development of liver disease.

Some investigators have suggested that other hepatotoxins might be an environmental influence that could be a factor in the development of liver disease in only a small subgroup of Z-A1AT adults. One group has examined the association between viral hepatitis, alcoholism, and autoimmune markers and liver disease associated with Z-A1AT. Propst and coworkers[115] measured antibody to hepatitis C and B, hepatitis B surface antigen, and hepatitis B core antigen, as well as antinuclear and antimitochondrial antibodies in 164 patients homozygous or heterozygous for the Z allele. They also assessed alcohol abuse by history. They found that patients with cirrhosis and the Z-allele (i.e., PiMZ, SZ, FZ, or ZZ) had a very high incidence of antibodies to hepatitis C (41%) compared with their PiMM population with cirrhosis (20%). Patients with the Z allele and no liver disease had no evidence of antibodies to HCV. Patients with liver disease and the Z allele also had more frequent evidence of hepatitis B virus and excess alcohol use than did patients without liver disease. This observation may suggest that adult patients with liver disease associated with the Z allele have their liver disease precipitated by a secondary environmental factor.[115] It would suggest that patients with Z-A1AT deficiency should be protected from other hepatotoxins, including hepatitis and alcohol ingestion. This study is relevant only to adults and may explain the increase in cryptogenic cirrhosis in heterozygotes.

In conclusion, the pathogenesis of Z-A1AT-deficiency–associated liver disease remains unclear. The currently available models, including cell culture studies and transgenic mouse models, may elucidate the interaction between the effects of the endoplasmic reticulum inclusions and the effects of other genetic or environmental factors. Most importantly, several lines of evidence suggest the need for an aggressive stance toward prevention of liver disease in adults by avoiding the effects of fever and inflammation in the PiZZ individual and avoiding other hepatotoxins in both homozygotes and heterozygotes for Z-A1AT. A model Z-A1AT-associated neonatal liver disease does not seem to have been developed.

Molecular Biology: Advances in Diagnosis of Metabolic Liver Disease

As an increasing number of the genes for metabolic liver diseases are mapped and sequenced, molecular biology techniques assume a dominant role in diagnosis. These techniques permit more rapid and precise diagnosis and a basis for family studies and prenatal diagnostic testing. Ultimately, they provide information that may lead to gene therapy. Polymerase chain reaction (PCR) technology also is essential to the development of preimplantation genetic disease diagnosis. Individual blastomeres are removed from a human embryo at the 6–8 cell stage, and PCR is used to amplify the DNA of interest. Subsequent analysis of the amplified DNA can be used to determine whether the embryo is affected by the disease of interest. Embryos found to be free of disease can be implanted in the uterus. This technique has resulted in successful pregnancies in one sex-limited disease.[40, 55]

Variations on PCR technology provide rapid screening for multiple genetic defects in a single gene and determination of previously unknown defects in a gene of interest. Analysis of the PCR-amplified DNA may include nucleic acid sequencing, oligonucleotide probe hybridization, restriction enzyme analysis, or gel analysis (single-strand confirmation polymorphism studies).

Polymerase Chain Reaction

For diagnostic purposes, PCR amplification begins with a known segment of DNA, which has been previously isolated and sequenced (Fig. 1). Oligonucleotide primers that are expected to flank the defective area of the gene are synthesized. When more than one genetic defect can result in similar disease (e.g., as is the case in cystic fibrosis), the primers may be separated by a large span of DNA to incorporate any previously described gene defect. When the defect is well localized or unique (e.g., the single base pair change resulting in Z-α_1-antitrypsin), a single exon or even less may separate the primers.

The duplex DNA, extracted from cells of the individual presumed to be affected by the disease, is denatured to separate the strands and each primer anneals to one of the complementary strands of DNA. DNA polymerase is used to extend the primers using the patient's DNA, to which the primers are annealed, as the template. This sequence of denaturation, primer annealing, and primer extension defines one PCR cycle. This cycle is then repeated until amplication produces enough DNA for further analysis. If the primers are selected carefully, the newly synthesized strand of DNA initiated by one primer extends through the region complementary to the other primer. In this event, the newly synthesized DNA also can serve as primers in subsequent PCR cycles, which permits a rapid accumulation of copies of the desired segment of DNA. The availability of thermostable DNA polymerases, derived from bacteria living under conditions of high heat, means that DNA polymerase is not inactivated during the denaturation phase of the PCR cycle. This has resulted in improvements in both speed and specificity of DNA synthesis.[40]

Analysis of PCR Products

Several methods are available to analyze DNA amplified by PCR. Direct DNA sequencing provides complete analysis of the product.

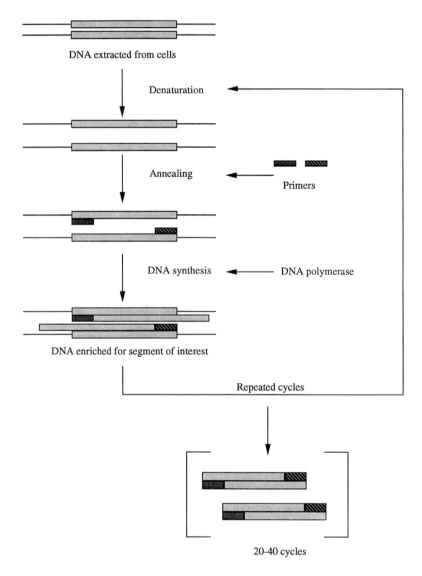

Figure 1. DNA is extracted from the cells of the patient, denatured, and annealed to the oligonucleotide primers. Addition of DNA polymerase permits the primers to direct DNA synthesis, using the patient's DNA as the template and the primers as the starting points. This cycle of denaturation, primer annealing, and primer extension is repeated, resulting in exponential accumulation of the DNA of interest.[40]

Although this may be useful to characterize newly discovered mutations, it is not usually necessary and may be quite tedious for rapid diagnosis of a well-described defect. Polymerase chain reaction products can be subjected to restriction enzyme digest, which, if the DNA amplified contains an informative sequence, can give a rapid result. Using carefully chosen and controlled hybridization conditions, oligonucleotide probes that are specific for wild-type and mutant genes can be used to probe the amplified DNA. Although these techniques could be used on DNA directly extracted from tissues, the PCR technology allows analysis of orders of magnitude less DNA than standard Southern blot technology.[40]

Single-strand confirmation polymorphism studies take advantage of the mobility of a strand of DNA (or RNA) in a native polyacrylamide gel and the change in mobility that occurs in a mutated sequence. Using PCR, large amounts of the DNA of interest can be amplified. The amplified nucleic acids are run on a native polyacrylamide gel. Because the mobility changes are usually quite small, conditions for electrophoresis are quite exacting. In addition, this technique can only be used with very short stretches of DNA (200–300 bp). The bands produced by the nucleic acids of the patient are compared with those amplified from a known wild-type and mutant allele. In this way, rapid diagnosis is possible in a disease with a characterized mutation, as is diagnosis of the carrier state. Single-strand conformation polymorphism can be used to detect regions of a gene that vary in mobility from the wild-type, thus pinpointing regions for further study by more time-consuming methods, including sequencing.[127]

Fluorescence in situ Hybridization

Fluorescence in situ hybridization is a technique that allows visualization of specific DNA sequences or DNA deletions in metaphase or interphase cells. In this technique, a probe with a fluorescent reporter tag is hybridized to a chromosome spread or to a whole-cell preparation. The results are visualized by fluorescence microscopy.[153]

This technique has many research applications. Because it is a very rapid technique, its primary application in the diagnosis of metabolic liver disease would be in prenatal diagnosis or in other conditions when rapid diagnosis would be of value.[157] This technique has the capacity to detect submicroscopic deletions of DNA and thus might be used to detect those forms of Alagille's syndrome associated with deletions in chromosome 20.[134]

Liver-Directed Gene Therapy

Pediatricians who manage patients with metabolic liver disease have seen great advances in diagnosis and treatment during the past 15 years with the advent of molecular biologic diagnosis and the availability of liver transplantation. We are likely on the threshhold of an even more important advance in therapy for these patients, the advent of gene therapy. Although some physicians find themselves at institutions pioneering this area of medicine, many nonacademic pediatricians likely will be involved in these protocols in some way. Some may be asked to refer patients for the protocols or will be asked by patients and parents to explain these protocols. It is necessary to compare the risks and benefits of this new therapy with those of conventional therapy for metabolic liver disease (including liver transplantation). Physicians involved in the care of children with life-threatening metabolic diseases will, in some cases, be asked to administer the therapy. Therefore, pediatricians must understand this type of therapy and be available to patients and to institutional review boards and biomedical ethics committees to resolve the issues arising from the use of these methods for treatment.

A full discussion of this issue is beyond the scope of this text. Several reviews are available.[76, 146] This update highlights only selected issues: the selections of liver diseases that are most amenable to gene therapy, the choice of short-term or long-term gene therapy, and the timing of clinical trials of gene therapy in metabolic liver disease.

Gene therapy involves the addition of a normal, wild-type gene to the nucleus of liver cells containing a mutant form of the gene. Depending on the vector used for delivery of the gene to the hepatocyte, the gene may integrate itself into the individual's genome and be duplicated with cell division, or it may not be incorporated into the genome, in which case it is lost with the next cell division cycle. Again, depending on the vector used and delivery method, the gene may be expressed in cells outside the liver or may be expressed in the liver only. In both cases, the mutant gene continues to be transcribed and translated along with the new, wild-type gene. This may be of concern if the genetic disease is a storage disease, because the mutant gene product is still produced. Several methods allow specific deletion of a mutant gene or specific inhibition of translation. Studies are being conducted that would allow these techniques to be used in conjunction with conventional gene therapy.[128] If patients are being recruited for experimental gene therapy protocols, each of these factors should be outlined for the referring physician.

An ideal metabolic liver disease for gene therapy would result from a single gene defect, with expression of the gene limited to the liver. This disease would result from an enzyme deficiency state. Treatment by gene therapy would precede the development of irreversible structural damage to any organ (e.g., cirrhosis resulting from α_1-antitrypsin deficiency). A more conventional therapy with lower risk would not be available for the disease. Putative candidate diseases in the area of metabolic liver disease include the urea cycle defects (in particular, ornithine transcarbamylase deficiency) and hereditary tyrosinemia. Certainly, several other diseases are targets for hepatic gene therapy (e.g., phenylketonuria or familial hypercholesterolemia).

The ideal hepatic gene therapy would make it necessary to develop a method for delivering the new gene to a large number of hepatocytes, have it stably expressed at high levels, and have it regulated in a manner physiologically similar to that of the normal gene. In fact, the first protocols likely will make available gene therapy to provide a modest level of unregulated hepatic enzyme production that will be short-term and not necessarily organ-specific. Liver-directed gene therapy has been suggested to be suitable as emergency therapy for certain metabolic diseases. Even a modest amount of enzyme activity in a disease such as ornithine transcarbamylase deficiency may improve the patient's life expectancy by reducing the incidence of hyperammonemic crises associated with common childhood illness. Thus, especially in the early phase of the development of gene therapy, short-term delivery of ornithine transcarbamylase during hyperammonemic crisis in a deficient individual might be used to maintain stability until a suitable transplant organ is found or until more definitive long-term gene therapy is developed. A potential complication of such therapy could be the development of antibodies to the product of the transplanted gene. Protocols of this type may be available in fewer than 5 years.

SUMMARY

Metabolic liver disease can be screened in a cost-effective manner to allow earlier, more effective therapy. Liver transplantation for these disorders should be continually re-evaluated. Gene therapy is being investigated as a therapy for the future with animal models as a prototype.

The following organizations are available for your patients: American Liver Foundation, 1425 Pompton Avenue, Cedar Grove, NJ 07009; and American Porphyria Foundation, PO Box 22712, Houston, TX 77227.

ACKNOWLEDGMENT

Acknowledgment goes to Cindy Sharp for her help in preparing the manuscript.

References

1. Aaseth J, Ribarov S, Bohev P: The interaction of copper (Cu + +) with the erythrocyte membrane and 2,3-dimercaptopropanesulphonate in vitro: A source of activated oxygen species. Pharmacol Toxicol 61:235, 1987
2. Ali R, Perfumo S, della Rocca C, et al: Evaluation of a transfenic mouse model for alpha-1-antitrypsin (AAT) related liver disease. Ann Hum Genet 58:305, 1994
3. Baart de la Faille H, Bijlmer-Iest JG, van Hattum J, et al: Erythropoietic protoporphyria: Clinical aspects with the emphasis on the skin. Curr Probl Dermatol 20:123, 1991
4. Balan V, Baldus W, Fairbanks V, et al: Screening for hemochromatosis: A cost-effectiveness study on 12,258 patients. Gastroenterology 107:453, 1994
5. Barber MD: A case of congenital cirrhosis of the liver with renal tubular defects akin to those in the Fanconi syndrome. Arch Dis Child 3:335, 1956

6. Berenson MM, Marin JJG, Gunther C: Effect of bile acid hydroxylation on biliary protoporphyrin excretion in rat liver. Am J Physiol 255:G382, 1988
7. Bielb J, Olynyk J, Ching S, et al: Transferrin index: An alternative method for calculating the iron saturation of transferrin. Clin Chem 38:2078, 1992
8. Bloomer JR: Pathogenesis and therapy of liver disease in protoporphyria. Yale J Biol Med 52:39, 1979
9. Bloomer JR, Enriquez R: Evidence that hepatic crystalline deposits in a patient with protoporphyria are composed of protoporphyrin. Gastroenterology 82:564, 1982
10. Bloomer JR, Pierach C: Effect of hematin administration to patients with protoporphyria and liver disease. Hepatology 2:817, 1982
11. Bloomer JR, Brittenham GM, Hawkins CW, et al: Iron therapy for hepatic dysfunction in erythropoietic protoporphyria. Ann Intern Med 105:27, 1986
12. Bloomer JR, Weimer MK, Bossenmaier IC, et al: Liver transplantation in a patient with protoporphyria. Gastroenterology 97:188, 1989
13. Bonkowsky HL, Bloomer JR, Ebert PS, et al: Heme synthetase activity in human protoporphyria. Demonstration of the defect in liver and cultured skin fibroblasts. J Clin Invest 56:1139, 1975
14. Brewer GJ, Dick RD, Yuzbasiyan-Gurkin V: Initial therapy of patients with Wilson's disease with tetrathiomolybdate. Arch Neurol 48:42, 1991
15. Brewer GJ, Yuzbasiyan-Gurkan V: Wilson's disease. Medicine 71:139–164, 1992
16. Brewer GJ, Hill GM, Dick RD, et al: Treatment of Wilson's disease with zinc III. Prevention of reaccumulation of hepatic copper. J Lab Clin Med 109:526, 1987
17. Brewer GJ, Yuzbasiyan-Gurkan V, Lee DY: Use of zinc-copper metabolic intractions in treatment of Wilson's disease. J Am Coll Nutr 9:487, 1990
18. Brewer GJ, Yuzbasiyan-Gurkan V, Young AB: Treatment of Wilson's disease. Seminars in Neurol 7:209, 1987
19. Bull PC, Thomas GR, Rommens JM, et al: The Wilson disease gene is a putative copper transporting P-thpe ATPase similar to the Menkes gene. Nat Genet 5:327, 1993
20. Carlson JA, Rogers BB, Sifers RN, et al: Accumulation of PiZ a1-antitrypsin causes liver damage in transgenic mice. J Clin Invest 83:1183, 1989
21. Chelly J, Monaco HP: Cloning the Wilson's disease gene. Nat Genet 5:317, 1993
22. Clayton PT: Inborn errors of metabolism. J Inherit Metab Dis 14:478, 1991
23. Clayton PT, Patel E, Lawson AM: 3-oxo-delta-4 bile acids in liver disease. Lancet 1:1283, 1988
24. Colletti PB, Clemmons JJW: Familial neonatal hemochromatosis with survival. J Pediatr Gastroenterol Nutr 7:39, 1988
25. Cottier VH: Ueber ein der Hamochromatose vergleilchbares. Krankheuts bild bei Neugeboren. En Schweiz Med Wochenscher 37:39, 1957
26. Cousins RJ: Absorption, transport and hepatic metabolism of copper and zinc: Special reference to metallothionein and ceruloplasmin. Physiol Rev 65:238, 1985
27. Cripps DJ, Scheuer PJ: Hepatobiliary changes in erythropoietic protoporphyria. Arch Pathol 80:500, 1965
28. Czaja MJ, Weiner FR, Scharzenberg SJ, et al: Molecular studies of ceruloplasmin deficiency in Wilson's disease. J Clin Invest 80:1200, 1987
29. Dabestani A, Child JS, Perloff JK, et al: Cardiac abnormalities in primary hemochromatosis. In Hemochromatosis. Proceedings of the First International Conference. Ann NY Acad Sci 526:234, 1988
30. DaCosta CM, Baldwin D, Portmann B, et al: Value of urinary copper excretion after penicillamine challenge in the diagnosis of Wilson's disease. Hepatology 15:609, 1992
31. Day DL, Letourneau JG, Allan BT, et al: Hepatic regenerating nodules in hereditary tyrosinemia. AJR 149:391, 1987
32. DeBraekeleer M, Larochelle J: Genetic epidemiology of hereditary tyrosinemia in Quebec and in Saguenay-Lac-St. Jean. Am J Hum Genet 48:525, 1991
33. Deugnier YM, Guyader D, Crantock L, et al: Primary liver cancer in genetic hemochromatosis: A clinical, pathological, and pathogenetic study of 54 cases. Gastroenterology 104:228, 1993
34. Dible JH, Hunt WE, Pugh WW, et al: Foetal and neonatal hepatitis and its sequelae. J Path Bacteriol 67:195, 1954

35. Dubois RS, Rodgerson DO, Hambridge KM: Treatment of Wilson's disease with triethylene tetramine hydrochloride (trientine). J Pediatr Gastroenterol Nutr 10:77, 1990
36. Dycaico MJ, Grant SGN, Felts K, et al: Neonatal hepatitis induced by α1-antrypsin: A transgenic mouse model. Science 242:1409, 1988
37. Dycaico MJ, Felts K, Nichols SW, et al: Neonatal growth delay in alpha-1-antitrypsin disease: Influence of genetic background. Mol Biol Med 6:137, 1989
38. Edwards CQ, Dadone MM, Skolnick MH, et al: Hereditary hemochromatosis. Clin Haematology 11:411, 1982
39. Edwards MA, Green A, Colli A, et al: Tyrosinemia type I and hypertrophic obstructive cardiomyopathy. Lancet 1:1437, 1987
40. Erlich HA, Arnheim N: Genetic analysis using the polymerase chain reaction. Ann Rev Genet 26:479, 1992
41. Escobar GJ, Heyman MB, Smith WB, et al: Primary hemochromatosis in childhood. Pediatrics 80:549, 1987
42. Evans D, Sanharwalla IB: Coagulation defect of typrosinemia. Arch Dis Child 59:1088, 1984
43. Fargion S, Fracanzani AL, Piperno A, et al: Prognostic factors for hepatocellular carcinoma in genetic hemochromatosis. Hepatology 20:1426, 1994
44. Farrell FJ, Nguyen M, Woodley S, et al: Outcome of liver transplantation in patients with hemochromatosis. Hepatology 20:404, 1994
45. Fernandes A, Mira ML, Azevedo MS, et al: Mechanisms of hemolysis induced by copper. Free Radic Res Comm 4:291, 1988
46. Finch SC, Finch CA: Idiopathic hemochromatosis: An iron storage disease. Medicine 34:381, 1955
47. Freese DK, Tuchman M, Schwarzenberg SJ, et al: Early liver transplantation is indicated for Tyrosinemia Type I. J Pediatr Gastroenterol Nutr 13:10, 1991
48. Geller SA, Nichols WS, Dycaico MJ, et al: Histopathology of α1-antitrypsin liver disease in a transgenic mouse model. Hepatology 12:40, 1990
49. Goen G, Bolson K, Binsel Meyer S, et al: Recessive inheritance of erythropoietic protoporphyria with liver failure. Lancet 344:337, 1994
50. Goetsch CA, Bissell DM: Instability of hematin used in the treatment of acute hepatic porphyria. N Engl J Med 315:235, 1986
51. Gray AMH: Hematoporphyria congenita with hydro vacciniforme and hirsuities. QJ Med 19:381, 1926
52. Gray RGF, Patrick AD, Preston FE, et al: Acute hereditary tyrosinemia type I: Clinical, biochemical and haematological studies in twins. J Inherit Metab Dis 4:37, 1981
53. Grompe M, St.-Louis M, Demers SI, et al: A single mutation of the fumarylacetoacetate hydrolase gene in French Canadians with hereditary Tyrosinemia Type I. N Engl J Med 331:353, 1994
54. Gruen JR, Goei VL, Capossela A, et al: Hemochromatosis in children. *In* Suchy F, et al (eds): Liver Disease in Children. St. Louis, Mosby, 1994, p 773
55. Handyside AH, Kontogianni EH, Hardy K, et al: Pregnancies from biopsied human preimplantation embryos sexed by Y-specific DNA amplication. Nature 344:768, 1990
56. Harper PL, Walshe JM: Reversible pancytopenia secondary to treatment with tetrathiomolybdate. Brit J Haematol 64:851, 1986
57. Hartand C, Kuzz K: Pregnancy in a patient with Wilson's disease treatment with D-pencillamine and zinc sulfate. Eur Neurol 34:1337, 1994
58. Hayes AM, Jaramillo D, Levy HL, et al: Neonatal hemochromatosis: Diagnosis with MR imaging. Am J Roentology 159:623, 1992
59. Herbert A, Corbin D, Williams A, et al: Erythropoietic protoporphyria; unusual skin and neurologic problems after transplantation. Gastroentrol 100:1753, 1991
60. Hill GM, Brewer GJ, Prasad AS, et al: Treatment of Wilson's disease with Zinc I, oral zinc therapy regimens. Hepatology 7:522, 1987
61. Jazwinska EC, Lee SC, Webb SI, et al: Localization of the haemochromatosis gene close to D 65105. Am J Hum Genet 53:347, 1993
62. Kaltwasser JP, Shalk KP, Werner E: Juvenile hemochromatosis. *In* Hemochromatosis:

Proceedings of the First International Congress, New York. Ann NY Acad Sci 526:274, 1988

63. Kauffman L, Evans DIK, Stevens RF, et al: Bone-marrow transplantation for congenital erythropoietic porphyria. Lancet 337:1510, 1991

64. Key N, Rank JM, Freese D, et al: Hemolytic anemia in protoporphyria: Possible precipitating role of liver failure and photic stress. Am J Hematol 39:202, 1992

65. Kilpe VE, Krakauer H, Wren RE: An analysis of liver transplant experience from 37 transplant centers as reported to Medicare. Transplantation 55:554, 1993

66. Klatskin G, Bloomer JR: Birefringence of the hepatic pigment deposits in erythropoietic protoporphyria. Gastroenterology 67:294, 1974

67. Knisely AS: Neonatal hemochromatosis. Adv Pediatr 39:383, 1992

68. Knisely AS: Neonatal hemochromatosis. In Suchy FJ, et al (eds): Liver Disease in Children. St. Louis, Mosby, 1994, p 784

69. Knisely AS, Mugid MS, Dische MR, et al: Neonatal hemochromatosis. In Gilbert EF, et al (eds): Genetic Aspects of Developmental Pathology (National Foundation of the March of Dimes). New York, Alan R. Liss, 1987, p 75

70. Koskinas J, Portman B, Lombard M, et al: Persistent iron overload 4 years after inadvertent transplantation of a hemochromatic liver in a patient with primary biliary cirrhosis. J Hepatol 16:351, 1992

71. Kuan P: Cardiac Wilson's disease. Chest 91:579, 1987

72. Lamon JM, Marynick SP, Roseblatt R, et al: Idiopathic hemochromatosis in a young female: A case study and review of the syndrome in young people. Gastroenterology 76:178, 1979

73. Lamoril J, Boulechfar S, de Verneuil H, et al: Human erythropoietic protoporphyria: 2 Point mutations in the ferrochelatase gene. Biochem Biophys Res Comm 181:594, 1991

74. Larochelle J, Mortezai A, Belanger M, et al: Experience with 37 infants with tyrosinemia. Can Med Assoc J 97:1051, 1967

75. Le A, Steiner JL, Ferrell GA, et al: Association between calnexin and a secretion-incompetent variant of human α1-antitrypsin. J Biol Chem 269:7514, 1994

76. Ledley FD: Hepatic gene therapy: Present and future. Hepatology 18:1263, 1993

77. Lindblad B: Treatment with glutathione and other sulfhydryl compounds in hereditary tyrosinemia. In Larson, et al (eds): Functions of Glutathione: Biochemical, Physical, Toxological and Clinical Aspects. New York, Raven Press, 1983, p 337

78. Lindblad B, Fallstrom SP, Hoyer S, et al: Cardiomyopathy in fumarylacetoacetase deficiency (hereditary tyrosinemia): A new feature of the disease. J Inherit Metab Dis 10(suppl 2):319, 1987

79. Lindblad B, Lindstedt S, Steen G: On the enzymatic defects in hereditary tyrosinemia. N Engl J Med 322:423, 1977

80. Lindahl J, Sharp HL: Screening asymptomatic family members for Wilson's disease. Minn Med 65:473–475, 1982

81. Lindstedt S, Holme E, Lock EA, et al: Treatment of hereditary tyrosinemia type I by inhibition of 4-hydroxyphenylpyruvate dioxygenase. Lancet 340:813, 1992

82. Lomas DA: Loop-sheet polymerization: The structural basis of Z α1-antitrypsin accumulation in the liver. Clin Sci 86:489, 1994

83. Lomas DA, Evans DL, Finch JT, et al: The mechanism of Z α1-antitrypsin accumulation in the liver. Nature 357:605, 1992

84. Lund DP, et al: Liver transplantation in newborn liver failure: Report of successful liver transplantation. Transplant Proc 25(1PE 2)1068, 1993

85. Mangus IA, Jarrett A, Prankerd TAJ: Erythropoietic protoporphyria: A new porphyria syndrome with solar urticaria due to protoporphyrinemia. Lancet ii:448, 1961

86. Mason AL, Marsh W, Alpers DH: Intractable neurological Wilson's treated with orthotopic liver transplantation. Dig Dis Sci 38:174, 1993

87. McClements BM, Bingham A, Callender ME, et al: Erythropoietic protoporphyria and iron therapy. Brit J Dermatol 22:423, 1990

88. Menahem S, Salmon AP, Dennett X: Hemochromatosis presenting as severe cardiac failure in an adolescent. Int J Cardiol 29:86, 1990

89. Metzman R, Anand A, DeGuilo PA, et al: Hepatic disease associated with intrauterine

parvovirus B19 infection in a newborn premature infant. J Pediatr Gastroenterol Nutr 9:112, 1989

90. Mieles LA, Esquivel CO, Van Thiel DH, et al: Liver transplantation for tyrosinemia: A review of 10 cases from the University of Pittsburgh. Dig Dis Sci 35:153, 1990
91. Milligan A, Grapahaun-Brown RAC, Sarkany I, et al: Erythropoietic protoporphyria exacerbated by oral iron therapy. Brit J Dermatol 119:64, 1988
92. Mitchell G, Larochelle J, Lambert M, et al: Neurologic crisis in hereditary tyrosinemia. N Engl J Med 322:432, 1990
93. Morris DL, Dudley MD, Pearson RD: Coagulopathy associated with hematin treatment for acute intermittent prophyria. Ann Int Med 95:700, 1981
94. Mosemain F, Gardaz JP, Gillet M: Fatal cardiomyopathy after liver transplantation for genetic hemochromatosis. Transplant Proc 26:3635, 1994
95. Mustajoki P, Normann Y: Early administration of Heme Arginate for acute porphyric attacks. Arch Int Med 153:2004, 1993
96. Nakada SY, Brown MR, Rabinowitz R: Wilson's disease presenting as symptomatic urolithiasis: A case report and review of the literature. J Urol 152:978, 1994
97. Nakanashi Y, Miyazuki H, Kadota Y, et al: Molecular defect in human erythropoietic protoporphyria with fatal liver failure. Hum Genet 91:303, 1993
98. Nichols GM, Bacon BR: Hereditary hemochromatosis: Pathogenesis and clinical features of a common disease. Am J Gastroenterol 84:851, 1989
99. Niederau C, Fischer R, Sonnenberg A, et al: Survival and causes of death in cirrhotic and in noncirrhotic patients with primary hemochromatosis. N Engl J Med 313:1256, 1985
100. Noble-Jamieson G, Jamieson N, Clayton P, et al: Neurologic crisis in hereditary tyrosinemia and complete reversal after liver transplantation. Arch Dis Child 70:544, 1994
101. Nordmann Y: Erythropoietic protoporphyria and hepatic complications. J Hepatol 16:4, 1992
102. Oga M, Matsui N, Anai T, et al: Copper deposition of the fetus and placenta in a patient with untreated Wilson's disease. Am J Obstet Gynecol 169:196, 1993
103. Ogiharu H, Ogiharu T, Miki M, et al: Plasma copper and antioxidant status in Wilson's disease. Pediatr Res 37:219, 1995
104. Olynyk JK: Genetic haemochromatosis—preventable rust. Aust NZ J Med 24:711, 1994
105. Olynyk JK, O'Neil R, Britton RS, et al: Determination of hepatic iron concentration in fresh and paraffin-embedded tissue, diagnostic implications. Gastroenterology 106:674, 1994
106. Paradis K, Mitchell G, Russo P: Tyrosinemia. In Suchy FJ, et al (eds): Liver Disease in Children. St. Louis, Mosby, 1994, p 803
107. Paradis K, Weber A, Seidman EG, et al: Liver transplantation for hereditary tyrosinemia. The Quebec experience. Am J Hum Genet 47:338, 1990
108. Petrikhin K, Fischer SG, Pirastu M, et al: Mapping, cloning, and genetic characterization of the region containing the Wilson disease gene. Nat Genet 5:338, 1993
109. Phaneuf D, LaBelle Y, Berube D, et al: Cloning and expression of the cDNA encoding human fumarylacetoacetate the enzyme deficient in hereditary tyrosinemia: Assignment of the gene to chromosome 15. Am J Hum Genet 48:525, 1991
110. Phatak PD, Cappuccio JD: Management of hereditary hemochromatosis. Clin Haematol 11:411, 1982
111. Ploos van Amstiel JK, Janesen RPM, Verjael M, et al: Prenatal diagnosis of Type I hereditary tyrosinemia. Lancet 344:336, 1994
112. Poh-Fitzpatrick MB: Protoporphyrin metabolic balance in human protoporphyria. Gastroenterology 88:1239, 1985
113. Polson RM, Lim CK, Rolles K, et al: The effect of liver transplantation in a 13-year-old boy with erythropoietic protoporphyria. Transplantation 46:386, 1988
114. Potter C, Willis D, Sharp H, et al: Primary and secondary amenorrhea associated with spirolactone therapy in chronic liver disease. J Pediatr 121:141–143, 1993
115. Propst T, Propst A, Dietze O, et al: High prevalence of viral infection in adults with homozygous and heterozygous alpha1-antitrypsin deficiency and chronic liver disease. Ann Int Med 117:641, 1992

116. Rademakers LHPM, Cleton MI, Kooijamn C, et al: Early involvement in hepatic parenchymal cells in erythropoietic protoporphyria? An ultrastructure study of patients with and without overt liver disease and effect of chenodeoxycholic acid treatment. Hepatology 11:449, 1990
117. Rademakers LHPM, Koningsberg JC, Sorber CWJ: Accumulation of iron in erythroblasts of patients with erythropoietic protoporphyria. Eur J Clin Invest 23:130, 1993
118. Rand IB, McClenathan DT, Whitington PF: Neonatal hemochromatosis: Report of a successful orthotopic liver transplantation. J Pediatr Gastroenterol Nutr 15:325, 1992
119. Rank JM, Pasqual-Leone A, Payne W, et al: Hematin therapy for the neurologic crisis of tyrosinemia. J Pediatr 118:136, 1991
120. Rank JM, Straka JG, Bloomer JR: Liver in disorders of porphyrin metabolism. J Gastroenterol Hepatol 5:573, 1990
121. Rela R, Heaton ND, Vougas V, et al: Orthotopic liver transplantation for hepatic complications of Wilson's disease. Br J Surg 80:909, 1993
122. Rol JK, et al: Initial and followup brain MRI findings and correlation with the clinical course in Wilson's disease. Neurology 44:1064, 1994
123. Rootwelt H, Kristensen T, Berger R, et al: Tyrosinemia type I—complex splicing defects and a missense mutation in the fumarylacetoacetase gene. Hum Genet 94:235, 1994
124. Rootwelt H, Brodtkorb E, Kvittingen EA: Identification of a frequent pseudodeficiency mutation in the fumarylacetoacetase gene, with implications for the diagnosis of Tyrosinemia type I. Am J Hum Genet 55:1122, 1994
125. Sallie R, Chiyende J, Tan KC, et al: Fulminant hepatic failure resulting from co-existent Wilson's disease and hepatitis E. Gut 35:849, 1994
126. Sarkany RPE, Alexander GJMA, Cox TT: Recessive inheritance of erythropoietic protoporphyria with liver failure. Lancet 343:1394, 1994
127. Sarker G, Yoon MS, Sommer SS: Screening for mutations by RNA single-strand conformation polymorphism (rSSCP): Comparison with DNA-SSCP. Nucleic Acids Res 20:871, 1992
128. Savransky E, Hytiroglou P, Harpaz N, et al: Correcting the PiZ defect in the α1-antitrypsin gene of human cells by targeted homologous recombination. Lab Invest 70:676, 1994
129. Schagen van Leewen JH, Christaens GCML, Hoegenraad TV: Recurrent abortion and the diagnosis of Wilson's disease. Am J Obstet Gynecol 169:196, 1993
130. Scheinberg IH, Jaffe ME, Sternlieb I: The use of trientine in preventing the effects of interrupting penicillamine therapy in Wilson's disease. N Engl J Med 317:209, 1987
131. Schilsky ML, Scheinberg IH, Sternlieb I: Liver transplantation for Wilson's disease: Indications and outcome. Hepatology 19:583, 1994
132. Schneider BL, Setchell KDR, Whitington PF, et al: Delta 4-3-oxosteroid 5B-reductase deficiency causing neonatal liver failure and hemochromatosis. J Pediatr 124:234, 1994
133. Schneider-Yin X, Schafer B, Mohr P, et al: Molecular defects in erythropoietic protoporphyria with terminal liver failure. Hum Genet 93:711, 1994
134. Schnittger S, Hofers C, Heidemann P, et al: Molecular and cytogenetic analysis of an interstitial 20p deletion associated with syndromic intrahepatic ductular hypoplasia (Alagille syndrome). Hum Genet 83:239, 1989
135. Scholmek P, Marver HS, Schmid R: Erythropoietic protoporphyria: Evidence for multiple sites of excess protoporphyrin formation. J Clin Invest 50:203, 1971
136. Schwarzenberg SJ, Sharp HL: α1-antitrypsin deficiency. In Schiff L, Schiff ER (eds): Diseases of the Liver, ed 7. Philadelphia, JB Lippincott, 1993, p 692
137. Searle J, Kerr JFR, Halliday JW, et al: Iron storage disease. In MacSween RNM, Anthony PP, Scheuer PJ (eds): Pathology of the Liver, ed 3. Hong Kong, Churchill-Livingstone, 1994, p 219
138. Shamieh I, Kibort PK, Suchy FJ, et al: Antioxidant therapy for neonatal iron storage disease (NISD). Pedatr Res 33:109a, 1993
139. Sifers RN: Z and the insoluble answer. Nature 357:541, 1992
140. Sifers RN, Rogers BB, Hawkins HK, et al: Elevated synthesis of human α1-antitrypsin hinders the secretion of murin α1-antrypsin from hepatocytes in transgenetic mice. J Biol Chem 264:15696, 1989

141. Sokol RJ: Wilson's disease and Indian childhood cirrhosis. *In* Suchy FJ (ed): Liver Disease in Children. St. Louis, Mosby, 1994, p 747
142. Sokol RJ: At long last: An animal model of Wilson's disease. Hepatology 20:533, 1994
143. Spence JA, Suttle NF, Wonham G, et al: A sequential study of the abnormalities which develop in rats given a small dietary supplement of ammonium tetrathiomolybdate. J Comp Pathol 90:139, 1980
144. Starzl TE, Demetris AJ, Trucco M, et al: Chimerism after liver transplantation for type IV glycogen storage disease and type I Gaucher's disease. N Engl J Med 328:745, 1993
145. Sternlieb I, Scheinberg IH: Wilson's disease. *In* Schiff L, Schiff ER (eds): Diseases of the Liver. Philadelphia, JB Lippincott, 1993, p 659
146. Strauss M: Liver-detected gene therapy: Prospects and problems. Gene Ther 1:156, 1994
147. Strife CF, Zuroweste EL, Emmett EA, et al: Tyrosinemia with acute intermittent porphyric aminolevulinic acid dehydratase deficiency related to elevated urinary aminolevulinic acid levels. J Pediatr 90:400, 1977
148. Suzuki Y, Konda M, Imai F, et al: Effect of dietary treatment on the renal tubular function in a patient with hereditary tyrosinemia. Int J Pediatr Nephrol 8:171, 1987
149. Tanzi RE, Petrukhin K, Chernov I, et al: The Wilson disease gene is a copper transporting ATPase with homology to the Menkes disease gene. Nature Genet 5:344, 1993
150. Todd DJ: Erythropoietic protoporphyria. Br J Dermatol 131:751, 1994
151. Todd DJ, Hughes AE, Ennis KT: Identification of a single base pair deletion (40 del G) in exon 1 of the ferrochelatase gene in patients with erythropoietic protoporphyria. Hum Mol Genet 2:1495, 1993
152. Todd DJ, Callender ME, Mayne EE, et al: Erythropoietic protoporphyria, transfusion therapy and liver disease. Brit J Dermatol 127:534, 1992
153. Trask BJ: Fluorescence in situ hybridization: Applications in cytogenetics and gene mapping. Trends Genet 7:149, 1991
154. Trousseau A: Clin Med de Hotel de Paris (2nd ed). 1865, p 663
155. Tutois S, Montagutelli X, DaSilva V, et al: Erythropoietic protoporphyria in the house mouse: A recessive inherited ferrochelatase deficiency with anemia, photosensitivity and liver disease. J Clin Invest 88:1730, 1991
156. Van Hattum J, Baart de la Faille H, van den Berg JWO, et al: Chenodeoxycholic acid therapy in erythrohepatic protoporphyria. J Hepatol 3:407, 1986
157. van Spronsen FJ, Thomasse Y, Smit GPA, et al: Hereditary tyrosinemia type I: A new clinical classification with difference in prognosis on dietary treatment. Hepatology 20:1187, 1994
158. van Wijk HJ, Van Hattum J, Baart de la Faille H: Blood exchange and transfusion therapy for acute cholestasis in protoporphyria. Dig Dis Sci 33:1621, 1988
159. Walshe JM: Treatment of Wilson's disease with trientine (triethylene tetramine) dihydrochloride. Lancet 1:643, 1982
160. Walshe JM: Wilson's disease (hepatolenticular degeneration). *In* Haubrich WS, Schaffner F, Berk JE (eds): Bockus Gastroenterology, ed 15. Philadelphia, WB Saunders, 1994, p 234
161. Weinberg AG, Mize CE, Worthen HG: The occurrence of hepatoma in the chronic form of hereditary tyrosinemia. J Pediatr 88:434, 1976
162. Westra WH, Hruban RH, Baughman KL, et al: Progressive hemochromatotic cardiomyopathy despite reversal of iron deposition after liver transplantation. Am J Clin Path 99:39, 1993
163. Wilson SAK: Progressive lenticular degeneration: A familial disease associated with cirrhosis of the liver. Brain 34:295, 1912
164. Wu Y, Whitman I, Molmenti E, et al: A lag in intracellular degradation of mutant α1-antitrypsin correlates with the liver disease phenotype in homozygous PiZZ α1-antitrypsin deficiency. Proc Natl Acad Sci USA 91:9014, 1994
165. Yamaguchi Y, Heinz ME, Gitlin JD: Isolation and characterization of a human liver cDNA as a candidate gene for Wilson's disease. Biochem Biophys Res Com 197:271, 1993

166. Zheng H, Bhavsar D, Volz A, et al: Exclusion of ferritins and iron-responsive element binding proteins as candidates for the hemochromatosis gene. Hum Genet 94:159, 1994

Address reprint requests to

Sarah Jane Schwarzenberg, MD
Department of Pediatrics
Division of Gastroenterology and Nutrition
University of Minnesota
420 Delaware Street SE
Minneapolis, MN 55445

UPDATE ON VIRAL HEPATITIS IN CHILDREN

Laurie N. Fishman, MD, Maureen M. Jonas, MD,
and Joel E. Lavine, MD, PhD

The past decade has been a time of rapid acquisition of knowledge regarding the agents known as hepatitis viruses. Vaccines have been produced that can safely and effectively prevent the occurrence of hepatitis A (HAV) and B (HBV). Molecular biology has provided powerful tools, revealing new etiologic agents, hepatitis C (HCV) and E (HEV) viruses. Epidemiologic features and natural history of these infections have been defined. Treatments of chronic HBV and HCV infections have been initiated and refined. These exciting advances are summarized as follows:

Development of an inactivated HAV vaccine
Development of a recombinant HBV vaccine
Universal vaccination of newborns against HBV
Identification and cloning of HCV
Development of diagnostic assays for HCV
Screening of blood products for HCV
Interferon treatment of HBV, HCV, and HDV
Identification and cloning of HEV
Development of diagnostic assays for HEV

This work was supported in part by grants from the Glaxo Institute for Digestive Health (JEL) and the American Liver Foundation. Dr. Lavine is the Dr. W. Stanley Mooneyham Research Scholar of the American Liver Foundation.

From the Center for Childhood Liver Disease, and the Combined Program in Pediatric Gastroenterology and Nutrition (LNF), Children's Hospital; and Harvard Medical School, Boston, Massachusetts

Table 1. TAXONOMY AND CHARACTERISTICS OF VIRAL HEPATITIS AGENTS

Virus	Classification	Genome	Gene Products
HAV	Picornavirus	Linear SS (+) RNA 7.5 kb	Capsid proteins, VPg, protease, polymerase
HBV	Hepadnavirus	Circular partially DS DNA 3.2 kb	Surface Ag, eAg, core Ag, X and polymerase proteins
HCV	Flavivirus-like	Linear SS (+) RNA 9.4 kb	Core and envelope proteins, helicase, replicase
HDV	Unclassified (defective)	Circular rod-like SS (+) RNA 1.7 kb	HDAg
HEV	Calicivirus	Linear SS (+) RNA 7.6 kb	Undergoing characterization

Hepatitis A, B, C, D, and E have a common feature: hepatotropism. They have widely varying physical and molecular characteristics (Table 1), however, and clinical features of infection with these agents may be very different (Table 2). This article presents recent developments that enhance understanding and promote control of infection, and it highlights pediatric issues in viral hepatitis.

HEPATITIS A

The incidence of 40,000 cases per year of HAV reported to the Centers for Disease Control (CDC) is believed to be an underestimate; 136,000 cases are considered a more accurate estimate for 1991.[3] Pediatric infections account for more than one third of recognized incidents but likely are under-reported because 90% of children fewer than 5 years of age are anicteric, compared with 20% to 30% of adults. The total cost of

Table 2. CLINICAL PROFILE OF VIRAL HEPATITIS

Virus	Transmission	Active Immunization	Passive Immunization	Chronicity	Incubation Period (d)
HAV	Fecal-oral Parenteral rare	Yes	Yes	No	15–49
HBV	Perinatal Sexual Parenteral	Yes	Yes	Common	60–180
HCV	Parenteral Perinatal rare Sexual infrequent	No	No	Common	14–160
HDV	Parenteral Sexual Perinatal rare	Indirect, against HBV	Indirect, against HBV	Common	21–42
HEV	Fecal-oral	No	No	No	21–63

HAV infection in the United States is estimated to be more than $200 million per year.

Transmission of hepatitis A is predominantly fecal-oral; crowded or unsanitary areas are commonly implicated. In 1992, the CDC detailed the source of reported HAV cases as follows: personal contact in 25% to 30% of HAV cases; day care centers with children in diapers in 10% to 15% of cases; contaminated food and water in 3% to 8% of cases; and travel to endemic areas in 9% of cases.[55] In 50% of cases, the sources were unknown.[10] The incubation period for HAV is 28 days. A patient is infectious in the prodromal stage, 1 to 2 weeks prior to the clinical illness, precluding enteric precautions even in overt cases. Parenteral transmission, although rare, is possible because transient viremia occurs in the prodromal period. Cases of post-transfusion hepatitis A are documented in hemophiliacs[33] and in neonatal nurseries. In one instance, a single unit of packed red blood cells given to 11 neonates in an intensive care unit led to 55 cases of HAV among the neonates, staff, and relatives.[41] Vertical transmission has been documented on one occasion.[62]

Clinical manifestations of HAV may go unrecognized. Some children remain completely asymptomatic, whereas others exhibit nonspecific symptoms, such as nausea, vomiting, or diarrhea, and the self-limited infection is often misdiagnosed as gastroenteritis. Typically, jaundice and intestinal symptoms resolve 2 to 3 weeks after onset; however, atypical courses include cholestatic hepatitis, with jaundice and severe pruritus, lasting more than 12 weeks, and relapsing hepatitis, in which a second or third recrudescence of signs and symptoms occurs after initial abatement. This latter form is seen in 5% to 10% of adult cases. Neither chronic hepatitis nor a carrier state result from HAV infection. Although children generally experience a mild clinical course, they infect adults who may experience overt disease and higher mortality rates; patients more than 40 years of age have a mortality rate of 1.1%, whereas those fewer than 14 years have a rate of 0.1%.[9]

Hepatitis A virus exists as a single serotype. Exposure to virus induces a humoral immune response that confers lifelong protection. Due to the reasonably high prevalence of HAV antibody (38%) among adults in the United States, pooled immunoglobulin contains titers of anti-HAV that are protective. Thus, HAV infection can be prevented by the administration of immune serum globulin (ISG). Prophylaxis with 0.02 mL/kg of body weight given intramuscularly (IM) is recommended when travel to an endemic region is planned. This provides protection for 3 months. For patients with postexposure prophylaxis to household or intimate contacts, this dose must be administered within 2 weeks of exposure.[22] If given early in the incubation period, ISG has 80% to 90% efficacy in preventing infection.

The first vaccine against HAV was licensed in the United States in February 1995 (Havrix-SmithKline Beecham).[35] The vaccine is prepared in cell culture and is subsequently inactivated with formalin. The manufacturer recommends its use for travelers going to areas of high prevalence and groups at high risk for exposure, such as military personnel,

Native Alaskans, Native Americans, homosexuals, intravenous (IV) drug users, and residents of communities with HAV epidemics. Other appropriate vaccine candidates include residents of institutions for the developmentally disabled, day-care providers, laboratory personnel working with HAV, and handlers of primates. The vaccine can be administered with ISG for postexposure prophylaxis if given in separate syringes at different sites.

The vaccine dose for adults is 1440 U IM, followed by a booster of the same dose 6 to 12 months later. The dose for children aged 2 to 18 years is 360 U IM for each of two initial injections 1 month apart, followed by a booster 6 to 12 months after the first injection. An adult dose costs approximately $43 and a pediatric dose, $15.

Side effects include soreness at the injection site (in 50% of adults and 15% of children) and headache (in 14% of adults and < 5% of children). Induration and redness at the injection site, fatigue, malaise, and anorexia were each reported in 1% to 10% of those receiving the vaccine.

Response to the vaccine is evaluated by quantifying the titer of antibody to HAV (anti-HAV). Levels greater than 20 mIU/mL are protective. In 99% of adults receiving the 1440-U dose, titers of 335 to 667 mIU/mL were observed at 1 month. Similarly, 99% of children receiving 2 doses seroconverted, with titers of 3000 to 4000 mIU/mL after one month. Specific antibodies become evident as early as 2 weeks after immunization. Duration of protection is unknown because current studies document follow-up evaluation for fewer than 4 years; however, one group of investigators analyzed the rate of decay of anti-HAV more than 48 months and extrapolated that protective titers could last for 20 years. In naturally occurring HAV infection, the amnestic response provides protection despite undetectable titers of antibody.

Another inactivated HAV vaccine (Merck), awaiting licensure in the United States, also seems effective in preventing childhood infection. A study of 1037 healthy seronegative children aged 2 to 16 years living in a New York City area known for a high incidence of HAV were randomized to receive either a single vaccine dose or placebo.[63] Seven infections developed between 5 and 18 days after the vaccinations, and none developed after day 21. Three cases of HAV infection in placebo recipients occurred during the 5- to 18-day period, but 34 cases developed after day 21. Early cases likely represented exposure prior to vaccine administration. Of the 305 children who received vaccine and did not develop HAV, all but one had detectable antibody (mean titer, 42 mIU/mL) 1 month after vaccination. Follow-up evaluation 10 months later demonstrated no further cases in vaccinated children.

Vaccines for HAV and HBV have demonstrated excellent immunogenicity when combined into a single injection. Hepatitis A virus vaccine has not been studied in combination with other childhood vaccines. The efficacy of postexposure vaccination has not yet been assessed.

Recommendations regarding target populations for receipt of HAV vaccine have not yet been made. Initially, immunization may be recommended only for high-risk groups, such as day-care workers and travelers. Universal childhood HAV immunization might be considered. This would target a relatively asymptomatic but accessible group to prevent more serious disease in adults, as has been done for rubella. Recommendations need to take cost into account and may reflect the extent to which HAV is viewed as a public health priority in the United States.

HEPATITIS B

More than 1 million people in the United States are chronic carriers of HBV, and 200,000 to 300,000 new cases of HBV infection occur each year.[34] Children account for a small portion of new cases; 8% occur in children fewer than 10 years of age, and an additional 10% in those aged 11 to 19 years.[10] The vast majority of pediatric HBV infections are asymptomatic; however, a disproportionate number of pediatric cases become chronic.

Several HBV proteins and the antibodies produced in response to them have important clinical ramifications. Surface antigen (HBsAg) is the major protein of the viral envelope that circulates in serum as a complex particle and indicates current infection. Antibody-to-surface protein (anti-HBs) indicates either resolved infection or past immunization (Table 3). Although the core protein is not routinely measured in serum, antibody-to-core antigen (anti-HBc) indicates either current or past natural infection. Hepatitis B e antigen (HBeAg) is considered a marker of active viral replication; the development of antibody to e Ag (anti-HBe) usually indicates cessation of this process.

Risk factors for acquisition of HBV include parenteral exposure to blood and blood products, parenteral drug use, heterosexual and homosexual activity, living or working in an institution for the developmentally disabled, and occupational exposure to blood. Horizontal spread (i.e., infection acquired from living with a chronic HBV carrier) and perinatal transmission are important additional routes of infection in children. No risk factors are identified in 40% of cases.

The risk of developing chronic HBV infection is inversely propor-

Table 3. SEROLOGIC FINDINGS IN HBV AND HDV SUPERINFECTION

Marker	Immunized	Resolved	Acute	Chronic	HDV Superinfection
HBsAg	−	−	+	+	+
Anti-HBs	+	+	−	Usually −	−
Anti-HBc	−	+	+*	+	+
Anti-e	−	+	−	Usually −	Usually −
eAg	−	−	+	Usually +	Usually +
Anti-HDV	−	−	−	−	+

*IgM subtype.

tional to age at acquisition. Persistent infection develops in 90% of neonates, compared with 20% to 50% of young children and 5% of adults.[36] The presence of e antigen (eAg) in maternal serum is a predisposing factor for neonatal HBV infection, presumably because eAg correlates with active viral replication and higher viral titers. In mothers producing eAg, transmission of HBV to her offspring occurs in 70% to 90% of cases, whereas perinatal transmission occurs in 10% to 40% of cases in eAg-negative women.[22]

Although HBV transmission occurs at, and not before, parturition in more than 95% of infected newborns, the dramatically high rate of chronic infection in neonates is thought to be due to the immune tolerance produced by exposure in utero to viral antigens. Tolerance induced to eAg or related core antigen is particularly significant because epitopes in these viral proteins seem to provide key targets for cytotoxic T-cell mediated immune responses required for viral clearance. Transplacental transfer of HBeAg, but not HBsAg or HBcAg, has been demonstrated. HBeAg can be detected in cord blood of 54% to 88% of newborns born to HBV-infected, eAg-positive mothers. To assess the effect of fetal exposure to eAg on neonatal tolerance, Milich and colleagues used mice expressing eAg transgenes.[37, 38] These studies demonstrate that T cells, but not B cells, are made tolerant by eAg, and that this transient tolerance extends to the T-cell response to core antigen. These investigators speculate that transfer of eAg in utero leads to functional deletion of major histocompatibility complex class II-restricted HBeAg-specific T cells in the fetal thymus, equivalent to the way that immune responses to self-antigens are deleted. Thus, prenatal exposure of the fetus to eAg contributes to chronicity in the perinatally infected newborn by inactivating T-cell responses vital for viral clearance.

The HBV genome undergoes constant evolution during replication, and certain mutants are selected in this process. These mutants likely have a role in chronic disease, contributing to persistence and pathogenesis. Mutations in the surface (S), core, and X genes of HBV have been described; however, the "precore" mutant is best characterized. A precore, or e-, mutant, in contrast with wild-type virus, cannot produce eAg during active viral replication. Absence of eAg may confer a selection advantage by allowing escape from immune surveillance. In addition, in vitro studies show that these mutants replicate more efficiently. Immune selection pressure can cause rapid emergence of mutation; in 23 patients with only wild-type at the onset, 9 were found to have e- mutants after 2 years.[20] The e- mutant has been associated with fulminant hepatitis in several series[30] and was associated with disease exacerbation in a series of 106 patients with chronic HBV infection[8]; however, these mutants arise also in patients with stable chronic HBV disease.

Chronic HBV infection has been linked to the development of hepatocellular carcinoma (HCC). The relative risk for acquiring HCC is increased more than 100-fold in chronic HBV carriers. Usually this complication is late in onset, occurring more than 20 years after the onset of HBV infection. The majority of cases occur in patients with cirrhosis, and based on the prolonged interval between infection and malignant transformation, the virus is conjectured to generally contribute to oncogenesis indirectly. Presumably, persistent infection leads to rapid cell turnover, accumulation of errors in replication, and instability in the host genome; however, HBV-associated HCC cases have been described in young children without cirrhosis. In these instances, HBV may have a more direct role in tumorigenesis; occasional viral insertion into the host genome, a unique feature of HBV among hepatitis viruses, may inactivate a tumor suppressor gene or activate a cellular proto-oncogene. Rarely, in adult HBV-associated HCC, viral integrations have demonstrated near-critical growth control genes. Direct effects of HBV on growth control have also been demonstrated through the HBV X protein, a potent pleiotropic stimulator of essential cellular genes. Although unique site integration of HBV in pediatric liver tumors has been found, further investigation is required to evaluate whether HBV contributes to early-onset HCC in children by such direct oncogenic mechanisms.[17]

The incidence of HCC in children is unknown; cases have been reported in various populations and in children as young as 8 months of age. No current guidelines exist for monitoring children with chronic HBV infection, although in chronically infected adults, periodic ultrasound and serum alpha-fetoprotein protein levels are followed. The cost-benefit ratio in screening children is likely very high.

Evaluation of patients with chronic HBV infection must take into account the divergent natural history that exists in differing populations. In Asian populations with a high rate of perinatal acquisition, infected individuals often have minimal clinical disease. These patients have a higher rate of positive eAg serology and higher HBV DNA levels. In Western populations in which individuals tend to acquire HBV later in life, more severe clinical symptoms and a lower carrier rate are observed. In a series of 51 Chinese children followed for 4 years, the spontaneous clearance rate of eAg was 7%.[32] This can be compared with an Italian series of 76 children who had an eAg clearance rate of 50% to 70% after more than 5 years.[6] The difference between Western and Asian populations, demonstrated in many studies, probably reflects the longer duration of infection in the Asian population and the effect of eAg on immune tolerance. Genetic factors may also have a role.

Limited treatment options exist for HBV infection at the present time. Recombinant interferon (IFN) alfa-2b is effective and is the only approved in the United States antiviral agent for chronic HBV in adults. It is usually administered subcutaneously as 5 million U daily or 10 million U three times per week for 16 weeks.

Response to therapy has been defined in terms of viral replication suppression (i.e., loss of HBeAg and serum HBV DNA) and improvement of liver disease (normalization of alamine amniotransferase [ALT] and improvement in histologic findings). Several studies indicate an overall response rate of 40% to 50% with sustained results in the vast majority.[24,44] Elevated ALT (greater than twice normal) and low serum HBV DNA titers seem to be the most important predictors of response. Other factors that favor a response include eAg positivity, active hepatic inflammation, female sex, and recent acquisition of infection.

Side effects of IFN include transient flu-like symptoms of fever, headache, fatigue, and malaise in the majority of patients. Thrombocytopenia and leukopenia occur frequently and may necessitate dose reduction or cessation. Alopecia, prolonged fatigue, and depression are less common effects of IFN therapy. Development of autoantibodies is not uncommon but usually is of no clinical significance.[44]

To date, no approved treatments exist for children. The limited number of clinical trials of IFN in children show response rates similar to those in adults. In 29 Belgian children treated with 9 mU/m^2 of IFN alfa-2b for 16 weeks, 48% had persistent loss of HBV DNA, 38% lost HBeAg, and 7% lost HBsAg at 8 months after treatment.[54] In 77 Italian children treated with high-dose (7.5 mU/m^2) or low dose (3 mU/m^2) IFN alfa-2a, the seroconversion rate for HBeAg was 30% in the high-dose group and 21% in the low-dose group compared with 13.5% in the untreated control group at 18 months.[5] In another controlled study, 3 mU/m^2 IFN alfa-2a was administered for 12 months after a month-long course of prednisone to 22 Italian children. At 20 months, 41% of treated patients had cleared HBV DNA and seroconverted from HBeAg to anti-HBe, compared with 9% of the 21 untreated controls.[59] Similarly, in a series of 36 Spanish children treated with IFN alfa-2b for 6 months, 50% of treated patients demonstrated loss of HBV DNA, and 92% seroconverted to anti-HBe[52]; however, a series of 90 Chinese children treated with 5 mU/m^2 IFN alpha-2b with and without prednisone pretreatment demonstrated a lower response rate. In the IFN treatment group, 3% lost HBV DNA and seroconverted to anti-HBe, whereas in the IFN with steroid group, 16% lost HBV DNA and 13% seroconverted to anti-HBe.[26]

The availability of a safe and effective HBV vaccine provides protection from this potentially fatal disease; however, targeting of high-risk individuals to receive the vaccine has been problematic. They are often unrecognized or lack consistent access to medical care. Although health care workers are more likely to obtain the HBV vaccine, occupational exposure accounts for only 5% of HBV infections. Thus, in 1991, the Advisory Committee on Immunization Practices of the CDC recommended screening all pregnant women for HBsAg, with appropriate treatment of their newborns, and incorporation of HBV into the current childhood immunization schedule for all infants. In addition, selected adolescents and adults in high-risk situations should be vaccinated.

The initial vaccine, prepared by isolating HBsAg from pooled donor plasma, is no longer available. Current vaccines are prepared from recombinant HBsAg particles purified from baker's yeast that express a plasmid containing the DNA sequences for HBsAg. These new vaccines are safe; no serious adverse effects have been reported. The incidence of minor reactions, such as soreness at the injection site and low-grade fever, match that of placebo. The two recombinant vaccines, Recombivax (Merck) and Engerix-B (SmithKline, Philadelphia), are formulated differently and thus require different dosages; however, the vaccines can be interchanged within a vaccination series. Both require three IM injections. Newborns of HBsAg-positive mothers receive the first immunization within 12 hours of birth, together with hepatitis B immune globulin (HBIG). The second dose is administered at 1 month, and the third dose at 6 months of age. Newborns of HBsAg-negative mothers may receive immunizations at birth, 1 to 2 months, and 6 to 18 months or alternatively at 1 to 2 months, 4 months, and 6 to 18 months. A delay in vaccination does not require restarting the series. Postimmunization serologic screening is recommended for infants of HBsAg-positive mothers at 1 year of age, because 4.8% become carriers despite appropriate vaccination and HBIG administration.[56] Prevaccination screening is cost-effective only for children and adults in high prevalence contexts, such as Native Alaskans, Pacific Islanders, children of immigrants from countries with high endemicity, and family members of chronic HBV carriers.

Following the three-dose immunization, protective levels of anti-HBs (greater than 10 mIU/mL) are demonstrated in 90% to 95% of adults[15, 23] and 95% of children.[45] Lower levels are noted when the vaccine is administered in the buttock or intradermally. Protection has been confirmed for at least 5 years in children[31] and 9 years in adults.[19, 61] In vitro studies prove that an amnestic response still occurs in B cells from those responders whose antibody levels have diminished to the undetectable range at 7 to 8 years after vaccination. Booster shots are not recommended.

The results of the new immunization recommendations require long-term evaluation. Controversy regarding the need and cost of universal newborn HBV vaccination has contributed to a slower-than-desired increase in immunized children. In the future, combined vaccines may help to offset concern about multiple injections.

HEPATITIS C

The major agent of parenterally transmitted non-A, non-B hepatitis eluded discovery for many years because the low titers of virus in infectious serum prohibited detection by traditional techniques, such as immune electron microscopy and antigen immunoprecipitation. A novel approach uncovered a component of the pathogenic agent, first, by isolating viral nucleic acid from infectious chimpanzee sera, then, after reverse transcription, cloning it into bacteria. The protein expressed by a single bacterial clone was recognized exclusively by antisera obtained from infected individuals. A complementary DNA then was used to create assays for antibody to viral antigens.[42]

Diagnosis of HCV has become increasingly sensitive and specific. The enzyme-linked immunosorbent assay (ELISA), developed in 1989, detected antibody to a single HCV antigen (C100).[25] The relative insensitivity and high false-positive rate of this test led to refinements in a second-generation ELISA, which detects antibody to multiple core and nonstructural HCV antigens.[39] The recombinant immunoblot assay (RIBA) was introduced as a confirmatory test to address the lack of specificity and sensitivity of the early ELISA tests.[13] The second-generation test (RIBA-2) detects antibody to four HCV antigens.[60] Although RIBA-3 and ELISA-3 are now available, in most instances, the ELISA-2 is performed with RIBA-2 as the confirmatory test. ELISA-1 sensitivity is approximately 90%, whereas ELISA-2 is estimated as 97% to 100% sensitive; however, anti-HCV titers may be undetectable in early infection (prior to 16 weeks) and in immunocompromised individuals, leading to false-negative results. A positive result does not distinguish between resolved and current infection. It also may represent passive transfer of maternal or exogenously administered antibody rather than actual HCV infection.

A reverse-transcriptase polymerase chain reaction (RT-PCR), recently released commercially, detects low amounts of HCV RNA genome in serum and tissue samples within days of infection.[7] This method detects active HCV infection and is particularly useful in those patients with recent or perinatal acquisition, hypogammaglobulinemia, or immunosuppression, in whom antibody results are unreliable. A branched DNA signal amplification assay[28] and modified PCR techniques may soon permit molecular testing and viral quantitation in routine clinical settings. Quantitative measurements of HCV RNA may be useful in determining prognosis or evaluating response to therapy.

Prior to the incorporation of routine testing for anti-HCV in donated blood, 25% of HCV infections were acquired through transfusions. Since then, infection by this mode has been significantly decreased. Currently, at least 40% of new adult HCV cases result from IV drug use, 6% from heterosexual contact, 3% from household contact, 2% from occupational exposure, and less than 1% from transfusions. Almost 40% of patients infected with HCV deny all known risk factors.[4]

The epidemiology of HCV in the pediatric population is unknown. Prevalence in healthy children ranges from 0% in Japan[57] to 14% in Camaroon.[40] Hepatitis C virus prevalence has not yet been studied in a healthy United States pediatric population. The majority of HCV infections are identified in children with repeated exposure to blood products. Conditions associated with HCV infection in children include the following:

Thalassemia
Sickle cell disease
Hemophilia
History of malignancy
Hemodialysis
Solid organ transplants
IV drug use
Multiple sexual partners

Mother with chronic HCV
Household contact with an HCV carrier

The prevalence of HCV in children with thalassemia is as high as 60%[27, 47]; with hemophilia it is as high as 98%,[58] and in those undergoing hemodialysis, it is 15% to 20%. Contaminated intravenous immune globulin (now withdrawn from the market) has been implicated as the source in some cases of HCV.[29]

Although household and sexual transmissions have been demonstrated, the mechanism remains enigmatic. HCV RNA has not been found in saliva, semen, urine, stool, or vaginal secretions by most investigators.[16, 21] Duration of sexual exposure increases the risk of contracting HCV. A Japanese study of 154 spouses of probands with HCV-associated liver disease noted a 27% prevalence of anti-HCV antibody, increasing to 60% in spouses of more than 50 years of age.[1]

Perinatal transmission initially was reported first only in the context of maternal HIV coinfection. Subsequent studies demonstrate that non-HIV infected women are capable of transmitting HCV to their offspring in a small percentage of cases. In a study of 53 HCV-infected women, 3 of 54 offspring (5.6%) were positive for HCV RNA.[43] Increased risk has been documented for those mothers with higher titers of HCV RNA; 50% of mothers with viral titers greater than 10^7 infectious U/mL transmitted the infection to their infants.[43] Another study of 17 pregnant HCV-infected women showed that all 18 offspring were positive for anti-HCV by ELISA and RIBA at birth but were negative at 6 months of age. The serologic results of the neonates may simply represent passive maternal antibody transfer; no infant was positive for HCV RNA.[50] The role of breast-feeding as an independent risk factor for transmission remains unknown.

Diagnostic testing has allowed identification of asymptomatic cases, permitting further elucidation of the natural history of HCV. The majority of cases become chronic; at least 50% of all HCV infections and 70% of transfusion-acquired infections persist for more than 6 months. Most acute and chronic HCV infections are clinically silent. ALT and aspartate aminotransferase values are usually 1.5 to 10.0 times normal, but may fluctuate for an extended time. Normal serum aminotransferase values do not necessarily indicate absence of infection. Despite the insidious clinical course, HCV may progress to cirrhosis. In 83 HCV-infected transfusion-dependent thalassemic children followed up for 8 years, resolution was observed in 20%, recurrent or chronic hepatitis in 80%, and cirrhosis in 11%.[27] Less is known about children who acquire HCV by other means.

Hepatocellular carcinoma is associated with chronic HCV infection.[53] In Japan and Western countries, HCC is associated more frequently with HCV than with HBV. The mechanism by which HCV contributes to oncogenesis is unknown. HCV-associated cancer almost always is found in the context of cirrhosis in older patients. Thus, cell damage and accelerated cell turnover are assumed to contribute to oncogenesis. Unlike pediatric HBV-associated HCC, in which direct mechanisms of viral oncogenesis may be invoked, a direct role for HCV is unlikely. The genome of HCV is RNA, precluding integration into the host genome.

Recombinant interferon alfa-2b is licensed for the treatment of chronic HCV infection in adults. The drug is administered as 3 million U given subcutaneously three times per week for 6 months. As detailed earlier, side effects include fatigue, headache, fever, myelosuppression, and depression. Because autoimmune disease is exacerbated by IFN therapy, and autoimmune hepatitis can cause false-positive HCV ELISA results, the distinction between HCV and autoimmune hepatitis is difficult to distinguish in some patients.

Response to treatment is usually defined as normalization of ALT levels; however, owing to fluctuation of ALT values in chronic HCV infection, this parameter is an imperfect reflection of viral clearance. Recent studies include direct evaluation of HCV RNA. A typical response rate judged by normalization of ALT is 50%, with 50% of responders relapsing after the end of treatment. Repeated courses of IFN, using higher dosages or longer durations of treatment, do not produce significant improvement in nonresponders. Factors associated with response include mild liver histopathologic abnormalities, low viral titers, and certain HCV genotypes.

The limited clinical trials of IFN-alfa in children suggest a response rate similar to that of adult trials. An uncontrolled pilot study of 12 children with chronic HCV infection, 10 of whom contracted the infection from unknown sources, used 3 million U of IFN/m^2 thrice weekly for 6 months. At the end of therapy, 36% had normal ALT levels. This percentage climbed to 90% at 15 months of follow-up but fell to 45% by 24 months. All children were HCV-RNA–positive at the outset of the study, and at the conclusion of treatment, only 3 still had detectable HCV RNA.[52] The largest pediatric study examined 51 thalassemic children with HCV infection treated for 15 months. In 21 patients (41%), the ALT levels returned to normal within 6 months, and HCV RNA was no longer detectable. Two children relapsed during the 3-year follow-up time period.[12]

Results of studies in multiply transfused patients may not extend to other children who are infected with HCV. Iron deposition in the liver, often pronounced in these children, adversely affects response to IFN.[12] In addition, multiple parenteral exposures may result in a larger viral inoculum. Further studies are needed to determine response rates and prognostic indicators in various HCV-infected pediatric populations.

Passive prophylaxis against HCV infection does not seem feasible. ISG now contains minimal anti-HCV because contributions from donors with anti-HCV are excluded. Antibodies against HCV, taken from individuals with resolved infections, do not prevent infection in chimpanzees when injected with the virus. In addition, anti-HCV and HCV are present in serum of infected individuals simultaneously, demonstrating that the humoral response is non-neutralizing. Furthermore, rapid evolution of the viral envelope in response to immune pressure selects for viral variants that escape neutralization. Indirect evidence for this is provided by the observation that viral mutations emerge at a reduced rate in HCV-infected agammaglobulinemic patients.

Vaccine development has been impeded by HCV genotypic variation and potential for continued change. The hypervariable region on one envelope protein undergoes constant evolution in response to host immunity. The continual appearance of "quasispecies" makes HCV a moving target. Because antibodies to HCV are not protective, as noted earlier, the creation of HCV vaccines may require a novel approach in priming cell-mediated clearance mechanisms along the lines being pursued for human immunodeficiency virus.

HEPATITIS D

Hepatitis D is a defective virus requiring HBV infection for its propagation. HDV produces a single protein product, called *delta antigen*, which associates with the viral genome to form an amorphous core structure. HBV surface antigens form the outer coat. Although HDV can replicate independently once inside of a cell, HBV surface antigens are required for hepatocyte binding and uptake.

In the United States, an estimated 70,000 people are chronic carriers of HDV and 7500 new cases occur each year. The modes of transmission parallel HBV; HDV can be acquired through parenteral drug use or exposure to blood products. Sexual transmission does occur, although less efficiently than for HBV. Perinatal transmission is rare. The prevalence of HDV in individuals with chronic HBV infection is low in the general population, ranging from 2% to 8%, but higher in populations subject to repeated parenteral exposure; the rate of HDV in HBV-infected intravenous drug abusers ranges from 20% to 53%, and in hemophiliacs, 48% to 80%.[2] In populations in which the majority of HBV infections are acquired through perinatal transmission, such as Native Americans and Native Alaskans, HDV infection is nearly absent.

Hepatitis D virus infection may be acquired by simultaneous HBV coinfection, or by superinfection of a chronic HBV carrier. Coinfection causes more severe acute disease and carries a higher risk of fulminant hepatitis than HBV infection alone; coinfection mortality rates range from 2% to 20%, whereas acute HBV has a mortality rate of less than 1%.[18] Hepatitis D virus superinfection becomes chronic in 90% of cases in the United States and Europe.[49] In these situations, accelerated liver damage is observed; 70% to 80% of HBV-infected patients with superinfection progress to chronic liver disease with cirrhosis, compared with 15% to 30% of patients with HBV only. Superinfection can also cause exacerbation of previously stable HBV disease. These trends hold true for children infected with HDV.[14]

All patients with chronic HBV infection, especially those with severe disease or in high-risk groups, should be tested for HDV, because clinical features are indistinguishable. In coinfection, delta antigen parallels the time course of HBsAg and anti-HDV seroconversion follows the disappearance of the antigen. In superinfection, HBsAg and delta antigen are both found, often at the same time as anti-HDV (see Table 3).

HDV infection cannot be prevented once an individual is infected with HBV except through avoidance of high-risk behavior and exposure. Antibody to HDV is not neutralizing and does not prevent infection, precluding use of ISG. Prevention of HBV infection through universal vaccination is the most important means for controlling HDV infection.

HEPATITIS E

Hepatitis E virus was recently identified as the major agent of enterically transmitted non-A, non-B hepatitis. The viral agent was first visualized by immune electron microscopy in the stool of patients stricken with acute hepatitis associated with waterborne non-A, non-B epidemics. Subsequent purification and passage of purified virus in primates led to success in cloning the viral genome from bile and identifying the viral gene products.[48] This novel enveloped RNA virus seems to be a unique member of the calicivirus family.[46]

Hepatitis E is an important cause of hepatitis in developing countries. It is endemic in central and southeast Asia, India, China, and Africa. In these regions, HEV accounts for more than 50% of acute hepatitis cases and is the most common cause of symptomatic hepatitis in children. Confirmed cases of HEV have occurred only in the United States and Europe in travelers returning from endemic areas.

Transmission of HEV is primarily through contaminated drinking water and fecal-oral spread in epidemics. Outbreaks often occur in the context of rainy seasons, monsoons, or flooding. In sporadic cases, person-to-person transmission may be responsible.

Hepatitis E is an acute self-limited disease. The incubation period ranges from 2 to 9 weeks. Symptoms include jaundice, anorexia, hepatomegaly, and malaise. Subclinical infections occur to an unknown extent. Mortality is low in endemic populations, ranging from 0.5% to 4.0%. The striking exception is in pregnant women, in whom, for unknown reasons, the mortality rate reaches 20%.

A presumptive diagnosis of hepatitis E is often made in endemic areas by clinical symptoms and the exclusion of other infectious agents, such as hepatitis A, B, C, Epstein-Barr virus, and cytomegalovirus; however, diagnosis of HEV infection now can be made definitively with anti-HEV immunoassays against recombinant HEV proteins. Anti-HEV IgM and IgG assays can distinguish between resolved and current infection but have limited utility in the United States. Research settings use RT-PCR to detect the viral RNA, and immunofluorescent probes to detect HEV antigens.

No effective therapy currently exists. Immune serum globulin from developed countries does not prevent or mitigate symptoms of HEV infection. Appropriate sanitary practices, drinking safe water, avoiding uncooked fruits and vegetables, and practicing vigorous hand-washing diminish the risk of infection during travel to endemic areas. Vaccine development seems promising because HEV is limited to one serotype.

SUMMARY

Molecular biology has provided techniques by which two new types of hepatitis, the enterically transmitted HEV and the parenterally transmitted HCV, have been identified. Diagnostic capabilities allow screening of blood products for HCV, increasing the safety of the blood supply, and detection of asymptomatic cases, permitting further delineation of the natural history of this infection. Progress has been made in understanding the sequelae of chronic infection by exploring the mechanisms of tolerance and oncogenesis. Interferon treatment of HBV and HCV shows some efficacy; further exploration of this therapy continues in children. Safe and effective vaccines now exist for HAV and HBV, promising an avenue for the eventual elimination of these infections.

References

1. Akahane Y, Kojima M, Sugai Y, et al: Hepatitis C virus infection in spouses of patients with type C chronic liver disease. Ann Intern Med 120:748–752, 1994
2. Alter MJ, Hadler SC: Delta hepatitis and infection in North America. Prog Clin Biol Res 382:243–250, 1993
3. Alter MJ, Mast EE: The epidemiology of viral hepatitis in the United States. Gastroenterol Clin North Am 23:437–455, 1994
4. Alter MJ, Hadler SC, Judson FN, et al: Risk factors for acute non-A, non-B hepatitis in the United States and association with hepatitis C virus infection. JAMA 264:2231–2235, 1990
5. Barbera C, Bortoletti F, Crivellaro C, et al: Recombinant interferon-alpha 2a hastens the rate of HBeAg clearance in children with chronic hepatitis B. Hepatology 20:287–290, 1994
6. Bortolotti F, Cadrobbi P, Crivellaro C, et al: Long-term outcome of chronic type B hepatitis in patients who acquire hepatitis B virus infection in childhood. Gastroenterology 99:805–810, 1990
7. Brechot C: Polymerase chain reaction for the diagnosis of viral hepatitis B and C. Gut 34(suppl 2):39–44, 1993
8. Brunetto MR, Giarin MM, Oliveri F, et al: Wild-type and e antigen hepatitis B viruses and course of chronic hepatitis. Proc Natl Acad Sci USA 88:4186–4190, 1991
9. Centers for Disease Control: Hepatitis Surveillance Report. 53:Dec 23, 1990
10. Centers for Disease Control: Hepatitis surveillance report no. 54. Atlanta, Centers for Disease Control, 1992, p 1
11. Centers for Disease Control Immunization Practices Advisory Committee: Hepatitis B virus: A comprehensive strategy for eliminating transmission in the United States through universal childhood vaccination. MMWR 40:1–25, 1991
12. Clemente MG, Congia M, Lai ME, et al: Effect of iron overload on the response to recombinant interferon alpha treatment in transfusion-dependent patients with thalassemia major and chronic hepatitis C. J Pediatr 125:123–128, 1994

13. Ebeling F, Naukkarinen R, Leikola J: Recombinant immunoblot assay for hepatitis C antibody as a predictor of infectivity. Lancet 335:982–983, 1990
14. Farci P, Barbera C, Navone C, et al: Infection with the delta agent in children. Gut 26:4–7, 1985
15. Francis DP, Hadler SC, Thompson SE, et al: Prevention of hepatitis B with vaccine: Report from the Centers for Disease Control multicenter efficacy trial among homosexual men. Ann Intern Med 97:362–366, 1982
16. Fried MW, Shindo M, Fong TL, et al: Absence of hepatitis C viral RNA from saliva and semen of patients with chronic hepatitis C. Gastroenterology 102:1306–1308, 1992
17. Gupta S, Shafritz DA: Viral mechanisms in hepatic oncogenesis. In Arias IM (ed): The Liver: Biology and Pathobiology. New York, Raven Press, 1994, pp 1429–1454
18. Hadler SC, DeMonzon M, Ponzetto A, et al: Delta virus infection and severe hepatitis: An epidemic in Yupca Indians of Venezuela. Ann Intern Med 100:339–340, 1984
19. Hadler SC, Francis DP, Maynard JE, et al: Long-term immunogenicity and efficacy of hepatitis B vaccine in homosexual men. N Engl J Med 315:209–214, 1986
20. Hamasaki K, Nakata K, Nagayama Y, et al: Changes in the prevalence of HBeAg-negative mutant hepatitis B virus during the course of chronic hepatitis B. Hepatology 20:8–14, 1994
21. Hsu HH, Wright TL, Luba D, et al: Failure to detect hepatitis C virus genome in human secretions with the polymerase chain reaction. Hepatology 14:763–767, 1991
22. Immunization Advisory Committee: Recommendations for protection against viral hepatitis. MMWR 39:1–26, 1990
23. Jilg W, Schmidt M, Dienhardt F: Vaccination against hepatitis B: Comparison of three different vaccination schedules. J Infect Dis 160:766–769, 1989
24. Korenman J, Baker B, Waggoner J, et al: Long-term remission outcome of chronic type B hepatitis in patients who acquire hepatitis B virus infection in childhood. Gastroenterology 99:805–810, 1990
25. Kuo G, Choo QL, Alter HJ, et al: An assay for circulating antibodies to a major etiologic virus of human non-A, non-B hepatitis. Science 244:362–364, 1989
26. Lai CL, Lin HJ, Lau JN, et al: Effect of recombinant alpha2 interferon with or without prednisone in Chinese HBsAg carrier children. Quarterly J Med 78:155–163, 1991
27. Lai ME, DeVirgilis S, Argiolu F, et al: Evaluation of antibodies to hepatitis C virus in a long-term prospective study of posttransfusion hepatitis among thalassemic children: comparison between first- and second-generation assay. J Pediatr Gastroenterol Nutr 16:458–464, 1993
28. Lau JYN, Davis GL, Kniffen J, et al: Significance of serum hepatitis C virus RNA levels in chronic hepatitis C. Lancet 341:1501–1504, 1993
29. Lever AML, Webster ADB, Brown D, et al: Non-A, non-B hepatitis occurring in agammaglobulinemia patients after intravenous immunoglobulin. Lancet 2:1062–1064, 1984
30. Liang TJ, Hasegawa K, Rimon N, et al: A hepatitis B virus mutant associated with an epidemic of fulminant hepatitis. N Engl J Med 324:1705–1709, 1991
31. Lo KJ, Lee SD, Tsay YT, et al: Long-term immunogenicity and efficacy of hepatitis B vaccine in infants born to HBeAg-positive HBsAg-carrier mothers. Hepatology 8:1647–1650, 1988
32. Lok ASF, Lai CL: A longitudinal follow-up of asymptomatic hepatitis B surface antigen-positive Chinese children. Hepatology 8:1130–1133, 1988
33. Mannucci PM, Santagostino E, DiBona E, et al: The outbreak of hepatitis A in Italian patients with hemophilia: Facts and fancies. Vox Sang 67(suppl):31–35, 1994
34. Margolis HS, Alter MJ, Hadler SC: Hepatitis B: Evolving epidemiology and implications for control. Semin Liv Dis 11:84–92, 1991
35. Marwick C: Hepatitis A vaccine set for 2-year-olds to adults. JAMA 273:906–907, 1995
36. McMahon BJ, Alward WLM, Hall DB, et al: Acute hepatitis B virus infection: Relation of age to the clinical expression of disease and subsequent development of the carrier state. J Infect Dis 151:599–603, 1985
37. Milich DR, Jones JE, Hughes JL, et al: Is a function of the secreted hepatitis B e antigen to induce immunologic tolerance in utero? Proc Natl Acad Sci USA 87:6599–6603, 1990

38. Milich DR, Jones JE, Hughes JL, et al: Role of T-cell tolerance in the persistence of hepatitis B virus infection. J Immunother 14:226–233, 1993
39. Nakatsuji Y, Matsumoto A, Tanaka E, et al: Detection of chronic hepatitis C virus infection by four diagnostic systems: First-generation and second-generation enzyme-linked immunosorbent assay, second-generation recombinant immunoblot assay and nested polymerase chain reaction analysis. Hepatology 16:300–305, 1992
40. Ngatchu T, Stroffolini T, Rapicetta M, et al: Seroprevalence of anti-HCV in an urban child population: a pilot survey in a developing area, Cameroon. J Trop Med Hyg 95:57–61, 1992
41. Noble RC, Kane MA, Reeves SA, et al: Post-transfusion hepatitis A in a neonatal intensive care unit. JAMA 252:2711–2715, 1984
42. Nowicki MJ, Balistreri WF: The hepatitis C virus: Identification, epidemiology and clinical controversies. J Pediatr Gastroenterol Nutr 20:248–274, 1995
43. Ohto H, Terazawa S, Sasaki N, et al: Transmission of hepatitis C virus from mothers to infants. N Engl J Med 330:744–750, 1994
44. Perillo RP, Schiff ER, Davis GL, et al: A randomized, controlled trial of interferon alfa-2b alone and after prednisone withdrawal for the treatment of chronic hepatitis B. N Engl J Med 323:295–301, 1990
45. Poovorawan Y, Sanpavat S, Pongpunlert W, et al: Protective efficacy of a recombinant DNA hepatitis B vaccine in neonates of HBe antigen-positive mothers. JAMA 261:3278–3281, 1989
46. Purdy MA, Krawczynski K: Hepatitis E. Gastroenterol Clin North Am 23:537–546, 1994
47. Resti M, Azzari C, Rossi ME, et al: Prevalence of hepatitis C virus antibody in beta-thalassemic polytransfused children in a long-term follow-up. Vox Sang 60:246–247, 1991
48. Reyes G, Purdy MA, Kim JP, et al: Isolation of a cDNA from the virus responsible for enterically transmitted non-A, non-B hepatitis. Science 247:1335–1339, 1990
49. Rizzetto M: Hepatitis delta virus disease: An overview. Prog Clin Biol Res 382:425–430, 1993
50. Roudot-Thoraval F, Pawlotsky JM, Thiers V, et al: Lack of mother-to-infant transmission of hepatitis C virus in human immunodeficiency virus-seronegative women: A prospective study with hepatitis C virus RNA testing. Hepatology 17:772–777, 1993
51. Ruiz-Moreno M, Rua MJ, Castillo I, et al: Treatment of children with chronic hepatitis C with recombinant interferon-alfa: A pilot study. Hepatology 16:882–885, 1992
52. Ruiz-Moreno M, Rua MJ, Molina J, et al: Prospective, randomized trial of interferon-alpha in children with chronic hepatitis B. Hepatology 13:1035–1039, 1991
53. Simonetti RG, Camma C, Fiorello F, et al: Hepatitis C virus infection as a risk factor for hepatocellular carcinoma in patients with cirrhosis. Ann Intern Med 116:97–102, 1992
54. Sokal EM, Wirth S, Goyers S, et al: Interferon alpha-2b therapy in children with chronic hepatitis B. Gut 34:s87–s90, 1993
55. Steffen R, Kane MA, Shapiro CN, et al: Epidemiology and prevention of hepatitis A in travelers. JAMA 272:885–889, 1994
56. Stevens CE, Taylor PE, Tong MJ, et al: Yeast recombinant hepatitis B vaccine: Efficacy with hepatitis B immune globulin in prevention of perinatal hepatitis B virus transmission. JAMA 257:2612–2616, 1987
57. Tanaka E, Kiyosawa K, Soeyama T, et al: Prevalence of antibody to hepatitis C virus in Japanese schoolchildren: comparison with adult blood donors. Am J Trop Med Hyg 46:460–464, 1992
58. Troisi CL, Hollinger B, Hoots WK, et al: A multicenter study of viral hepatitis in a United States hemophilic population. Blood 81:412–418, 1993
59. Utili R, Sagnelli E, Baeta GB, et al: Treatment of chronic hepatitis B in children with prednisone followed by alfa-interferon: A controlled randomized study. J Hepatol 20:163–167, 1994
60. Van der Poel CL, Cuypers HTM, Reesink HW, et al: Confirmation of hepatitis C virus infection by new four-antigen recombinant immunoblot assay. Lancet 337:317–319, 1991
61. Wainwright RB, McMahon BJ, Bulkow LR, et al: Duration of immunogenicity and

efficacy of hepatitis B vaccine in a Yupik Eskimo population. JAMA 261:2362–2366, 1989
62. Watson JC, Fleming DW, Borella AJ, et al: Vertical transmission of hepatitis A resulting in an outbreak in a neonatal intensive care unit. J Infect Dis 167:567–571, 1993
63. Werzberger A, Mensch B, Kuter B, et al: A controlled trial of a formalin-inactivated hepatitis A vaccine in healthy children. N Engl J Med 327:453–457, 1992

Address reprint requests to

Joel E. Lavine, MD, PhD
UCSD Medical Center
Joint Program in Pediatric Gastroenterology and Nutrition
200 West Arbor Drive
San Diego, CA 92103-8450

0031–3955/96 $0.00 + .20

BILIARY TRACT DISEASE IN CHILDREN

Colston F. McEvoy, MD, and Frederick J. Suchy, MD

This article considers the more common neonatal cholangiopathies and unique aspects of biliary disorders in older children. Table 1 outlines various disorders of the bile ducts that are encountered during infancy and childhood. Hepatobiliary disease in the fetus and neonate presents an important challenge in that not only is hepatic structure and function disturbed but also normal development may be retarded or altered by the disease process. The discussion of some disorders, such as bile duct lesions in allograft rejection and graft versus host disease, is beyond the scope of this article.

DISEASES OF THE BILE DUCTS

Extrahepatic Biliary Atresia

Extrahepatic biliary atresia is a disease of the infant in which all or part of the extrahepatic bile ducts is destroyed or absent, leading to profound cholestasis and progressive biliary cirrhosis.[8, 50] Although the diagnosis is relatively uncommon, occurring in 1:10,000 to 1:15,000 live births, it accounts for approximately one third of neonates referred for evaluation of cholestasis and is the most frequent cause of death from liver disease and indication for liver transplantation (~50% of all cases) in children.[113]

Extrahepatic biliary atresia is not inherited in the majority of cases. HLA identical twins discordant for biliary atresia have been described

From the Pediatric Gastroenterology/Hepatology Section, Department of Pediatrics, Yale University School of Medicine, New Haven, Connecticut

TABLE 1. DISORDERS OF THE BILE DUCTS IN INFANTS AND CHILDREN

Extrahepatic biliary atresia
Choledochal cysts
Spontaneous perforation of the common bile duct
Mucous plug syndrome
Sclerosing cholangitis (neonatal, IBD-associated, immune deficiency)
Paucity of the intrahepatic bile ducts (syndromatic and non-syndromatic)
Caroli's disease
Cystic fibrosis
Biliary helminthiasis
Idiopathic bile duct stricture (? congenital)
Post-traumatic common duct stricture
Bile duct tumors (intrinsic and extrinsic)
Bile duct obstruction of pancreatic disease (inflammatory or neoplastic)
Graft-versus-host disease
Allograft rejection

in several reports; however, more than 32 cases of the disorder have been reported in 14 families.[100] Cases in stillbirths or in premature infants are very rare. A significant increase in HLA B12 antigen has been found among patients with biliary atresia without associated anomalies (23 of 47); a rate 3.23 times that seen in controls. The haplotypes A9-B5 and A28-B35 were also found more frequently.[93, 98]

Biliary atresia occurs more commonly in females than in males.[8, 43, 50] Most infants are full term and of normal birth weight. The perinatal course is typically unremarkable. Postnatal weight gain and development are initially normal. Jaundice is observed by parents or the physician after a period of physiologic hyperbilirubinemia. The possibility of hepatobiliary disease must be considered in any neonate jaundiced beyond 14 days of age.[71] Stools are acholic at presentation but may contain a variable amount of bile pigment in the first weeks of life with evolving bile duct obstruction.[62, 71]

Laboratory studies are not diagnostic. Values in biliary atresia often overlap with those found in patients with intrahepatic cholestasis.[8, 50] Serum bilirubin levels range between 6 and 12 mg/dL with approximately 50% of the total being conjugated. Serum aminotransferase levels are slightly to moderately elevated. Serum alkaline phosphatase, γ-glutamyltranspeptidase and 5' nucleotidase levels are also increased.

The etiology of extrahepatic biliary atresia has not been established despite considerable investigation. There is no evidence, even in cases with other congenital anomalies, that biliary atresia results from a failure in morphogenesis or recanalization of the common bile duct during embryonic development. In the majority of infants, obstructive obliteration of the biliary tract occurs postnatally.[62] Extrahepatic anomalies are present in 10% to 25% of patients and include cardiovascular defects, polysplenia, preduodenal or absent portal vein, malrotation, situs inversus, and bowel atresias.[15, 29] A rare fetal type of biliary atresia has also been described in which congenital malformations occur more commonly and cholestatic jaundice is present from birth. A bile duct remnant cannot be identified at the time of exploratory laparotomy.[95]

Numerous mechanisms have been proposed to account for the progressive obliteration of the extrahepatic biliary tree.[62] An ischemic or toxic origin of extrahepatic bile duct injury is unlikely. Abnormal toxic bile acid metabolites specific for the disorder have not been identified. Congenital infections with cytomegalovirus, Epstein-Barr virus, or rubella virus have been found occasionally but the presence of these common agents may be coincidental.[8, 43, 50] A possible role for reovirus type 3 has been proposed based on serologic evaluation of patients and from immunolocalization of reovirus 3 antigens in a bile duct remnant of a patient with biliary atresia[75, 76]; however, these serologic data have not been confirmed by other workers.[12] In a recent study, reovirus 3 RNA could not be detected in biliary tissue removed from 33 infants with biliary atresia using the polymerase chain reaction.[101]

On liver biopsy, the hepatic architecture is well preserved early in the course of the disease. Bile ductular proliferation is an important but variable finding indicative of large duct obstruction. Bile plugs in the ducts of portal triads strongly suggest biliary obstruction. Canalicular and cellular bile stasis reflect the severity of the cholestasis. Portal tract fibrosis and edema are often present.[8, 44, 61, 62] Swelling, vacuolization, and even sloughing of the biliary epithelium into the duct lumen may be observed. Portal tracts may be infiltrated with inflammatory cells. In approximately 25% of patients, giant cell transformation of hepatocytes may be present. Bile ductules may be arrayed in a ductal plate pattern, suggesting that the disease has altered with the normal process of ductular remodeling and development. Biliary fibrosis or even cirrhosis may be found on presentation or can develop during the first year of life with or without the successful restoration of bile flow.

The pathology of the extrahepatic bile ducts is variable.[50, 73] A useful classification of the anatomic variants is based on the predominant site of the atresia. Type I atresia involves obliteration of the common bile duct, but the proximal ducts are patent. In patients with type II atresia, the hepatic duct is obstructed, but cystically dilated bile ducts are found at the porta hepatis. In patients with type IIa atresia, the cystic and common ducts remain patent, whereas in patients with type IIb atresia, these structures are also obliterated. These forms of biliary atresia have been referred to as "surgically correctable" but comprise less than 10% of all patients with the disorder. Ninety percent or more of patients have type III atresia with obstruction of ducts at or above the porta hepatis. A cone of dense fibrous tissue envelopes the entire perihilar area. The gallbladder is fibrotic in 80% of cases. The type III variant has been referred to as "noncorrectable" because no patent hepatic or dilated hilar ducts can be found for a simple biliary-enteric anastomosis.

The fibrous remnant on microscopic examination shows complete fibrous obliteration of at least a portion of the extrahepatic bile ducts.[39] Bile ducts within the liver extending to the porta hepatis are initially patent during the first weeks of life but are progressively destroyed. The same process that damaged the extrahepatic ducts may be causal; the noxious effect of biliary obstruction is a contributing factor.[86]

When imaging and liver histology are unable to exclude biliary atresia, exploratory laparotomy and operative cholangiography are necessary to document the site of obstruction and properly guide attempts at surgical treatment.[69, 95] A simple anastomosis between patent proximal portions of the biliary system or cystic structures in the porta hepatis and a segment of bowel may be possible in approximately 10% of patients with the so-called "correctable" form of biliary atresia.[69, 95] However, the hepatoportoenterostomy procedure developed by Kasai is necessary in the majority of cases with obliteration of the proximal extrahepatic biliary tree.[73] The fibrous common bile duct is resected above the bifurcation of the portal vein. The fibrous cone of tissue at the porta hepatis is excised flush with the liver surface in an effort to expose an area that may contain residual, microscopic bile ducts; however, transsection of a biliary tree that is patent but small because of biliary hypoplasia or severe intrahepatic cholestasis should be avoided. A Roux-en-Y loop of jejunum is anastomosed to the bare edge of the transsected porta hepatis to serve as a conduit for biliary drainage. Many modifications of the original operation, most involving exteriorization of the Roux-en-Y loop with cutaneous bile diversion, have largely been abandoned. They were developed to decrease the high incidence of postoperative ascending cholangitis, but no evidence shows that the procedures are effective. Severe fluid and electrolyte losses from the stoma and massive bleeding from peristomal varices are frequent complications.[42] The original Kasai operation is now used by most pediatric surgeons to avoid these problems. Multiple attempts at revision of a nonfunctional hepatoportoenterostomy should also be avoided because subsequent adhesions resulting from multiple operations may make liver transplantation more difficult if required at a later date.

The prognosis of untreated biliary atresia is extremely poor, with death from liver failure usually occurring within 2 years. The hepatoportoenterostomy procedure can restore bile flow in most infants who undergo the procedure, but is often not curative.[33, 41, 42, 56, 82] In a nationwide survey of major pediatric centers in Japan, only 325 of 2013 patients survived for more than 10 years, and only 157 (7.8%) remained jaundice-free with normal liver function.[73] Many factors influence the outcome following hepatoportoenterostomy. First, the age at which the operation is performed has been found to be most critical.[33, 41, 42, 56, 82] Bile flow has been re-established in recent series from the United States, Japan, and Europe in 80% to 90% of infants who were referred for surgery within 60 days after birth.[53, 56, 82] In contrast, a success rate of less than 20% can be expected in infants who are 90 days of age or older at the time of surgery. Predictors of a poor outcome were caucasian race, operative age greater than 60 days, the presence of cirrhosis on initial biopsy, totally nonpatent extrahepatic ducts, and absence of ducts at the level of the liver hilus.[53] Bile duct profiles of 150 mm or greater, lined with columnar epithelium, have been associated by some workers with a good surgical result.[39] Schweizer recently found that prehilar bile duct structures of more than 400 microns were associated with a favorable prognosis.[94]

The severity of intrahepatic biliary cholangiopathy and the extent of hepatocyte injury are also important determinants of prognosis.[33, 53, 94, 107] Significant hepatocyte injury as indicated by lobular disarray, and giant cell transformation has been also associated with a poor outcome.[107] Recurrent bouts of ascending bacterial cholangitis, which are most frequent during the first 2 years after operation, can contribute to the ongoing bile duct injury and can even lead to reobstruction.[33] Infection is thought to spread by contiguous invasion of organisms from the intestinal tract into patent biliary radicles.

Liver transplantation is now an essential component in the management of extrahepatic biliary atresia, and should be performed in patients whose operation fails to restore bile flow, who are referred late (probably at 120 days of age or later), and who evolve to end-stage liver disease despite bile drainage.[28, 55, 70, 90] A previous portoenterostomy may make liver transplantation more difficult technically, owing to intra-abdominal adhesions and the various enteric conduits that sometimes are encountered; however, despite increased blood loss and operative time, survival is comparable with children transplanted for other liver diseases. With use of reduced-size allografts and living-related donors, rates of survival at 1 year have exceeded 90% in several series.[90]

Primary Sclerosing Cholangitis

Sclerosing cholangitis is an uncommon, chronic, progressive disease of the biliary tract characterized by inflammation and fibrosis of the intrahepatic and extrahepatic biliary ductal systems, leading to eventual biliary cirrhosis. Primary sclerosing cholangitis (PSC) refers to this pathologic process in the absence of choledocholithiasis or a history of bile duct surgery. In adults, carcinoma of the bile ducts must also be excluded; however, this has not been reported in children. PSC is associated with inflammatory bowel disease (IBD), most commonly ulcerative colitis, in 70% of adult patients.[63] This association is seen less frequently in children than in adults. The sex distribution of PSC in children does not show the apparent male preponderance observed in adult cases. Approximately 160 cases of sclerosing cholangitis have been reported in children, and most of these have been in the last 8 years, presumably owing to improvements in pediatric cholangiography.[19, 31, 34, 99] In addition to inflammatory bowel disease, other diseases commonly are associated with PSC, such as histiocytosis X and immunodeficiency. Many cases of PSC in children are idiopathic with a subset presenting in the neonatal period.

A neonatal form of PSC presents as jaundice within the first 2 weeks of age that resolves by 1 year of age, usually by 4 to 6 months. Despite clearing of jaundice, these children eventually develop cirrhosis diagnosed between 1 and 10 years of age.[5, 7, 31] Interestingly, more consanguinity is noted in this subset of patients with PSC.

IBD-associated PSC is usually observed with ulcerative colitis, although a few cases have been reported with Crohn's disease. Bowel symptoms can precede, present simultaneously, or occur years after the diagnosis of hepatic disease. Treatment of bowel disease, including colectomy, does not influence the progression of PSC.[19, 31, 34]

In histiocytosis X, the cholestasis can occur before, but most commonly is found after, diagnosis. These children can have multiple organ involvement with histiocytosis X, including diabetes insipidus, bone lesions, skin lesions, lymphadenopathy, or exopthalmos. Chemotherapy does not affect the course of PSC.[31, 64]

Children with various immunodeficiencies, both cellular and humoral, seem to develop sclerosing cholangitis. Cryptosporidia and CMV have been found concurrently in some of these patients and in adults with AIDS. Treatment for these infections has no proven effect on the biliary tract disease.[31, 40, 99]

No definitive diagnostic test exists for PSC. The diagnosis is based on a combination of biochemical, histologic, and radiologic data. Typically, adult patients present with fatigue, weight loss, pruritus, right upper quadrant pain, and intermittent jaundice.[63, 112] In children, the clinical presentation is more variable, with the most common symptoms being abdominal pain, jaundice, or chronic diarrhea. On physical examination, hepatomegaly is sometimes present and may be associated with splenomegaly, scleral icterus, or, rarely, ascites. Although there are no specific laboratory abnormalities in patients with PSC, the alkaline phosphatase level is commonly elevated, and the transaminases may be mildly elevated. Hyperbilirubinemia is seen in fewer than half of pediatric patients. Autoantibodies, including antinuclear antibody (ANA) and anti-smooth muscle antibody (SMA) may be found in some patients.[19, 31, 34, 99]

On liver biopsy, the histologic findings may be suggestive of PSC but again are not diagnostic. Four histologic stages have been described: stage 1 includes cholangitis or hepatitis confined to the portal tract; stage 2 inflammation extends out into the periportal area, producing hepatitis or fibrosis (piecemeal necrosis); stage 3 shows septal fibrosis or bridging necrosis; and stage 4 is cirrhosis.[68] Other common histologic features include a reduction of bile ducts, ductular proliferation, and copper deposition. The characteristic "onion skin" fibrosis that is classically described in PSC is uncommonly seen. This lesion is the result of fibrous-obliterative cholangitis early in the disease process that produces concentric fibrosis and edema around an intralobular duct.

Differentiation of PSC from autoimmune hepatitis, particularly in the presence of circulating non–organ-specific autoantibodies and hepatitic features on liver biopsy, may be difficult.[68] Given the clinical, laboratory, and histologic findings described, the diagnosis of PSC must be established by cholangiography. Now that endoscopic retrograde cholangiopancreatography (ERCP) has become feasible in children, it is often the method of choice for visualizing the intra- and extrahepatic bile ducts. Percutaneous transhepatic cholangiography is another option. The cholangiographic findings demonstrate alternating strictures and areas of dilation producing a beaded appearance of the intrahepatic and often extrahepatic ducts. Occasionally, a dominant stricture of the extrahepatic ducts or papillary stenosis is found. A distinct pattern, noted in the neonatal form, consists of thin, irregular intrahepatic ducts with rarefaction of peripheral branches and diffuse narrowing of the extrahepatic ducts.[31, 40]

The etiology of primary sclerosing cholangitis is unknown. An immunologic mechanism is suspected, given evidence that many patients with PSC have circulating immune complexes, hypergammaglobulinemia, and autoantibodies such as antinuclear and antismooth muscle antibodies.[11, 67, 72] A high incidence of circulating anticolon, antineutrophil nuclear antibodies, and antineutrophil cytoplasmic antibodies (ANCAs) has been found in patients with ulcerative colitis and PSC.[112] Also, genetic factors may be involved because PSC is associated with several HLA haplotypes, including HLA-B8, HLA-DR3, and HLA-DRw52a, which are associated with other autoimmune diseases.[17, 85] Other potential causes have been postulated, such as portal bacteremia, the absorption of toxic bile acids, and proinflammatory bacterial products from the inflamed colon in IBD. The presence of PSC in patients without bowel disease and the fact that PSC can precede colitis or occur after colectomy does not support these theories. Copper has been proposed as a potential toxin because it is found in excess on liver biopsies. However, chelation with D-penicillamine has had no beneficial effect in patients with PSC. No evidence implicates any viral cause. Cytomegalovirus (CMV), despite its presence in some immune deficient patients, does not characteristically produce a fibrous-obliterative cholangitis or disease of the large bile ducts such as that seen in PSC. Typical CMV viral inclusions have not been demonstrated in liver biopsies of PSC patients.[112]

The prognosis of PSC in children is guarded. The clinical course of the disorder is variable but usually progressive. The median survival time from onset of symptoms in a recent series of 56 children was approximately 10 years, similar to that reported in adults. The occurrence of jaundice after the neonatal period with a persisting serum bilirubin more than five times the normal value was associated with a poor outcome. Hepatocellular carcinoma may also occur, but cholangiocarcinoma, an important complication of adult PSC, has not yet been reported in children.[31]

The treatment of PSC is unsatisfactory. No published reports of controlled trials convincingly demonstrate a medical therapy that improves histology and prolongs survival. Uncontrolled experience has suggested a benefit from immunosuppressive therapy with prednisone and azathioprine. Ursodeoxycholic acid therapy in adults and in a limited number of children has led to an improvement in clinical symptoms and a reduction in liver test abnormalities.[112] Some patients may benefit from percutaneous or endoscopic balloon dilatation of a focal dominant stricture,[40] but attempts at surgical relief of obstruction and biliary reconstruction should be avoided. Liver transplantation is an important option for patients progressing to end-stage liver disease. Long-term results seem excellent, with no recurrence of PSC in the transplanted organs of children. The recurrence of PSC in adults after liver transplantation has been reported.[112]

Choledochal Cyst

Choledochal cysts are congenital anomalies of the biliary tract manifested by cystic dilatation of the extrahepatic biliary tree; intrahepatic bile ducts also may be involved.[27, 91] The incidence is 1 in 13,000 to 15,000 population in Western countries, but rates as high as 1 per 1000 have been described in Japan. The condition is not familial, and females are more commonly affected. Cases have been described in all age groups, but approximately two thirds of patients present before the age of 10 years. Owing to the frequent use of fetal ultrasonography, there is increasing antenatal diagnosis of choledochal cysts.[9]

Segmental or diffuse fusiform dilatation of the common bile duct is considered type I cysts and accounts for 60% to 90% of cases.[92] The type II cyst is a choledochal diverticulum. A choledochocele (type III), dilatation of the intraduodenal portion of the common bile duct, may be a variant of the type II cyst. Type IV cysts are subdivided into type IVa with multiple intrahepatic and extrahepatic cysts, and type IVb, with multiple extrahepatic cysts. The type IVb variant is uncommon and may overlap with type I. Type V cysts, or Caroli's disease, consisting of single or multiple dilatations of the intrahepatic ductal system, probably should not be viewed as a form of choledochal cyst.

The etiology of choledochal cysts is unknown. Congenital weakness of the bile duct wall, a primary abnormality of epithelial proliferation during embryologic ductal development, and congenital obstruction are possible causes.[91] A high incidence (~ 40%) of an anomalous junction of the pancreatic and common bile ducts has been described that could potentially allow reflux of pancreatic secretions into the biliary tree, producing subsequent weakness and dilatation.

The cyst wall is fibrous, often without an epithelial lining. The tissue may be chronically inflamed. Inflammatory obstruction of the terminal portion of the common bile duct is commonly found in infants with a choledochal cyst. Carcinoma of the cyst wall may develop by adolescence, even after internal drainage and relief of obstruction.[60, 91]

Many patients present during the first months of life with cholestatic jaundice and acholic stools.[60, 91] In patients detected antenatally, 8 of 12 (67%) developed jaundice in the first days of life. Vomiting, irritability, and failure to thrive may occur. Hepatomegaly is present, but less than one third of patients have a palpable abdominal mass. Features of portal hypertension and ascites may be present. Progressive hepatic injury can occur during the first months of life as a result of biliary obstruction.[27, 91]

Epigastric pain is the most common symptom in older patients, often resulting from pancreatitis.[60, 91] Intermittent jaundice and fever may result from recurrent bouts of cholangitis. Less than 20% of patients manifest the classic triad of pain, jaundice, and a palpable abdominal mass.

Ultrasonography is the most useful initial study to diagnose a choledochal cyst.[60, 91, 92] In the infant, the operative cholangiogram is essential in defining the extent of intrahepatic and extrahepatic disease. Percutaneous transhepatic cholangiography or endoscopic retrograde cholangiography may be of value in the older child to define the cyst anatomy, the site of biliary origin, and the extent of both extrahepatic and intrahepatic disease (including the presence of intraductal strictures and calculi).

Surgical excision of the cyst with Roux-en-Y hepaticojejunostomy gives excellent long-term results.[18] Excision of the cyst reduces bile stasis and the risk for subsequent cholangitis and malignancy. Simple decompression and internal drainage should be done only when the complicated anatomy, usually with extensive extrahepatic and intrahepatic involvement, does not allow complete excision. Long-term follow-up is essential, particularly after cyst enterostomy, because there is a continued risk of recurrent cholangitis, lithiasis, pancreatitis, and cancer.[18, 91]

Caroli's Disease

Caroli's disease is a segmental, saccular dilatation of the intrahepatic bile ducts.[78, 106] This rare disorder is congenital and can occur with ectasia of the hepatic bile ducts and can be associated with congenital hepatic fibrosis (CHF). Dilatation of the extrahepatic bile ducts similar to a choledochal cyst can be present. Renal disease is common, ranging from renal tubular ectasia to infantile polycystic disease. About 75% of patients are male. The mode of inheritance of the simple type is not resolved. The form associated with CHF seems to be inherited as an autosomal recessive trait.

Liver biopsy often demonstrates features of acute or chronic cholangitis with portal tract edema and fibrosis.[4, 78, 106] In cases associated with CHF, the so-called *ductal plate malformation* is found. The bile duct lumen forms an epithelium-lined circular cleft encircling a central core of vascularized connective tissue. Alternatively, a series of bile duct lumina are arranged circumferentially around a central fibrous core. The cystically dilated intrahepatic bile ducts are lined by epithelium that may be ulcerated and hyperplastic. The cysts may contain biliary sludge, calculi, and purulent material.[4, 78]

Hepatomegaly and abdominal pain may be first observed during infancy or childhood.[4, 78, 106] The patient may present with bacterial cholangitis.[78] Fever and intermittent jaundice may occur during episodes of biliary sepsis. Hepatosplenomegaly and polycystic kidneys are prominent in cases associated with CHF; these patients may present with bleeding esophageal varices.

Liver biochemical tests may show mild to moderate elevations of serum bilirubin, alkaline phosphatase, and aminotransferase levels, particularly during episodes of cholangitis.[4, 78, 106] Liver synthetic function is well preserved during early life but may be compromised by repeated episodes of infection and biliary obstruction within the cystic bile ducts. Variable elevations of the blood urea nitrogen and serum creatinine reflect the severity of the underlying kidney disease.

The cystic dilatation of the intrahepatic bile ducts is well demonstrated on ultrasonography and computerized tomography.[14] The process may rarely be limited to one lobe. Polycystic kidneys or hyperechogenicity of papillae may be detected. A normal common duct with segmental, saccular dilatations of the intrahepatic bile ducts is found on percutaneous or endoscopic cholangiography.

Recurrent cholangitis is the most significant problem and can result in sepsis and liver abscess.[14, 91] Eradication of infection with antibiotics can be extremely difficult, particularly in the presence of calculi that can develop within the cystically dilated bile ducts. The prognosis in the setting of persistent or recurrent infection is poor. Removal of stones by surgery, endoscopic methods, or lithotripsy usually is not feasible. Surgical drainage procedures generally are not effective and can make eventual liver transplantation more difficult. In 12 patients, ursodeoxycholic acid therapy led to partial (nine patients) or complete (three patients) dissolution of intrahepatic stones.[88] Cholangiocarcinoma may develop within the abnormal bile ducts. Portal hypertension and variceal bleeding may predominate in patients with CHF and Caroli's disease. Patients with extensive calculi may develop intractable abdominal pain. Polycystic kidney disease often leads to chronic renal failure. Liver transplantation has been successfully performed in patients with extensive disease and frequent complications.

Paucity of the Interlobular Bile Ducts

A paucity of interlobolar bile ducts may be an isolated finding in neonates with idiopathic cholestasis or a feature of a wide spectrum of known disorders. These include intrauterine infections with rubella and cytomegalovirus, genetic disorders such as alpha-1-antitrypsin deficiency, and inborn errors of bile acid metabolism.[8, 51, 52] Bile duct paucity may occur without associated developmental anomalies and without a documented intrauterine infection or genetic disorder; however, this idiopathic form of nonsyndromatic bile duct paucity is likely to be heterogeneous in etiology and has been extremely variable in clinical features and prognosis. Cholestasis typically develops early in infancy and may be associated with progressive liver injury.[45]

Syndromatic Paucity of Intralobular Bile Ducts

Syndromatic paucity of intralobular bile ducts (also known as *Alagille's syndrome* or *arteriohepatic dysplasia*) is the most common form of familial intrahepatic cholestasis.[2, 3] Chronic cholestasis related to a decreased number of interlobular bile ducts and a variety of other congenital malformations are characteristic features.[2, 77, 97] Analysis of familial pedigrees indicates an autosomal dominant mode of transmission with reduced penetrance and variable expressivity,[2] but the syndrome occurs commonly in the absence of other affected family members. Cytogenetic and molecular studies have localized the gene for the disorder to the short arm of chromosome 20 on the basis of deletions of 20p in some patients.[6, 104]

Chronic cholestasis of varying severity affects 90% to 95% of patients and becomes apparent in most patients during the first 2 years of life.[2, 3] Jaundice and clay-colored stools are often observed during the neonatal period. In contrast with extrahepatic biliary atresia, the liver may be normal in size or minimally enlarged, and splenomegaly is not common early in the course. Intense pruritus may be present by 6 months of age. Cutaneous xanthomas often develop on the extensor surfaces of the fingers and in creases of the palms and popliteal areas.

Dysmorphic facies may be overlooked in the neonate and become more characteristic with age.[2, 3] The forehead is typically broad and the eyes deeply set and widely spaced. A triangular appearance to the face results from a somewhat small and pointed mandible. The malar eminence is flattened and the ears prominent. The specificity of these facial features compared with those of other cholestatic patients has been questioned.[102]

Phenotypic expression of extrahepatic anomalies varies considerably.[3, 51] Short stature is a regular feature but can be only partially attributed to the severity of chronic cholestasis. Growth hormone insensitivity associated with elevated circulating growth hormone-binding protein has recently been described in these patients.[13] Fifteen percent to 20% of patients are mildly to moderately retarded. Congenital heart disease, particularly peripheral pulmonic stenosis, occurs in approximately 90% of cases.[3, 45] Systemic vascular malformations also have been described. Variable shortening of the distal phalanges and vertebral arch defects (butterfly vertebrae, hemivertebrae, and a decrease in the interpedicular distance) are common. Eye anomalies include posterior embryotoxon (mesodermal dysgenesis of the iris and cornea), retinal pigmentation, and iris strands. Renal abnormalities and hypogonadism may occur.

Liver biochemical tests reveal a hyperbilirubinemia between 2 and 8 mg/dL (with ~ 50% of the total being conjugated) during infancy and intermittently later in life.[2, 3, 77] Serum alkaline phosphatase, γ-glutamyltranspeptidase, 5' nucleotidase levels are moderately to markedly elevated. Serum aminotransferase levels are mildly to moderately increased. Serum triglyceride levels may be extremely high (500 to

> 1000 mg/dL). Serum cholesterol levels may be 200 mg/dL or higher. Total serum bile acid concentrations can be markedly elevated, even in the absence of jaundice. The bile acid species in serum, urine, and bile do not differ qualitatively from other cholestatic patients.

A paucity of interlobular bile ducts is defined as a significantly decreased ratio of the number of interlobular bile ducts to the number of portal areas (less than 0.4).[3, 51, 52] Giant cell transformation of hepatocytes, variable cholestasis, bile ductular proliferation, and portal inflammation may be prominent in the neonate. The number of interlobular bile ducts is often not decreased on initial liver biopsy, but progressive bile duct loss may be demonstrated after 3 months of age. Bile ductular injury may consist of cellular infiltration of portal triads contiguous to interlobular bile ducts, lymphocytic infiltration and pyknosis of biliary epithelium and periductal fibrosis. Mild periportal fibrosis may be present in older patients but progression to cirrhosis occurs uncommonly. The extrahepatic bile ducts are often narrowed or hypoplastic. A block in bile secretion at the level of the Golgi apparatus or in the pericanalicular cytoplasm has been suggested by electron microscopic studies.[111]

The mechanisms leading to bile duct paucity are undefined.[51] There has been little support for a developmental malformation of bile ducts in syndromatic bile duct paucity. Duct destruction is the only established mechanism for duct paucity. How the hepatobiliary disease relates to the congenital malformations in other organ systems is unknown also.

The clinical course is marked by varying degrees of cholestasis, which is often exacerbated during intercurrent viral infections.[1-3] Pruritus, cutaneous xanthomata, and neuromuscular symptoms related to vitamin E deficiency can cause significant morbidity. Treatment should focus on nutritional support, the prevention or correction of fat soluble vitamin deficiencies, and measures to relieve pruritus and xanthomas.

The long-term prognosis has been considered relatively good. Death occurred in 21 of 80 patients with this disorder followed by Alagille and associates, but only four patients died from liver disease.[3] However, in a recent series of children followed for 10 years, 8 of 21 patients required liver transplantation.[47] Hepatocellular carcinoma has been a complication.[57] Survival and candidacy for liver transplantation may be limited by the severity of the associated cardiovascular anomalies.[3, 47] The survival rate in 23 patients 2 to 9 years after liver transplantation was 57%. The higher than expected mortality was attributed to cardiac disease or a previous Kasai procedure.[110]

Cystic Fibrosis

Symptomatic liver disease in cystic fibrosis has been observed in 2% to 18% of patients and can be the presenting or predominant feature of the disorder.[83, 84, 89] With 60% of patients surviving into adulthood, hepatobiliary complications are being increasingly recognized. A unique form of focal biliary cirrhosis in these patients may progress to multilobular cirrhosis.[83, 89] In a study of 1100 patients with cystic fibrosis across a wide age range, a progressive rise occurred in the prevalence of clinically apparent liver disease from 0.3% in the 0- to 5-year-old age group to a peak of 8.7% among those aged 16 to 20 years.[96] There was a prevalence of 4.1% in patients more than 20 years of age. The mean age of presentation in this series was 9.8 years. Biochemical abnormalities without clinical signs were detected in 5.6% of the 0- to 5-year-old group and 16.0% of the 16- to 20-year-olds. In another series of patients followed over three decades, the average age of onset of liver disease in patients in whom cirrhosis developed was 7 years. The incidence of multilobular cirrhosis was 7% (31/450 patients).[35] Liver disease is more common in male patients than in female patients, with a ratio of 3:1 among adolescents. No strong evidence exists for the familial concordance of liver disease. Several studies have been unable to find mutations in the cystic fibrosis gene, which occur more frequently in patients with liver disease.[21, 32]

Patients may rarely present in the neonatal period with cholestatic jaundice.[84, 89] Meconium ileus occurs in approximately half of cases. Liver biopsy shows bile plugging in portal tracts, bile ductular proliferation, and portal fibrosis. If laparotomy is done to differentiate the disorder from biliary atresia, the extrahepatic bile ducts may seem small or obstructed by thick, tenacious mucous. It is thought to be of value to remove the inspissated material by irrigation, but a hepatoportoenterostomy should be avoided.[84] The liver disease often improves spontaneously but portends a severe course.[21]

Hepatobiliary disease in children may be asymptomatic for many years.[84, 89] Recurrent abdominal pain localized to the right upper quadrant may occur. Patients also can present with bleeding esophageal varices.

The liver is variably enlarged with a hard, nodular edge. Marked splenomegaly can be observed as a result of portal hypertension. Jaundice and ascites are an indication of advanced liver disease.

Liver tests may be normal initially, even with hepatomegaly, but with progression mild to moderate elevations of serum aminotransferase levels, and moderate to marked elevations of serum alkaline phosphatase and 5' nucleotidase can be expected.[84, 89] Conjugated hyperbilirubinemia occurs in older patients with more advanced disease.

Delayed clearance of isotope and either a nonvisualized or poorly emptying gallbladder are often found on hepatobiliary scintigraphy.[38] Strictures of the common bile duct occur in some patients on cholangiography. Variable dilatation, narrowing, and beading of the intrahepatic ducts simulating primary sclerosing cholangitis also have been observed.[79]

Liver biopsy may show inspissated granular material within portal bile ductules, ductular proliferation, a chronic inflammatory infiltrate, and variable fibrosis. The pathognomonic lesion of cystic fibrosis, focal biliary cirrhosis, was present at postmortem examination in approximately 10% of infants during the first 3 months of life and in approximately 27% of children more than 1 year of age.[79] Progression to a multilobular cirrhosis occurs in approximately 10% of patients with increasing age.

Obstruction produced by abnormal viscous secretions and mucous plugs may underlie the hepatobiliary disease in cystic fibrosis.[83, 84, 89] Biliary sludge resulting from lithogenic bile and an increase in the ratio of hydrophobic to hydrophilic bile acids may contribute.[80] Cytotoxic bile acids, stasis, infection, and the abnormal secretory properties of biliary epithelium may predispose to progressive bile duct injury and the formation of strictures of the common and intrahepatic bile ducts. Obstruction of the intrapancreatic portion of the common bile duct may contribute to the development of biliary cirrhosis in some patients.[81]

The pattern of hepatic injury in cystic fibrosis and the propensity to develop biliary cirrhosis has long suggested the bile ducts were central to the pathophysiology of liver disease.[66] Several recent advances, particularly the cloning of the cystic fibrosis gene and the ability to isolate bile duct cells, has supported this notion.[59] Specific antibody and molecular probes for the cystic fibrosis gene product, the so-called *cystic fibrosis transmembrane regulator* (CFTR), have convincingly localized expression of CFTR protein and mRNA to bile duct epithelial cells but not to hepatocytes.[20] Moreover, electrophysiologic studies have verified that bile duct cells demonstrate cAMP-stimulated chloride channel activity with the same properties as CFTR.[37]

The use of the hydrophilic bile acid, ursodeoxycholic acid, is under study as an option for the treatment and possible prevention of liver disease. This tertiary bile acid has potent choleretic and cytoprotective properties and has had a beneficial effect on cholestasis in conditions such as primary biliary cirrhosis. In several studies, the administration of ursodeoxycholic acid in a dose of 10 to 20 mg/kg/d for 6 months led to a modest (~30–60%) decrease in serum aminotransferase and alkaline phosphatase levels and an improvement in nutritional status.[23–25] In one study, duct dilatation decreased substantially in 8 of 9 treated patients, and there was decreased intrahepatic retention and more rapid biliary outflow of tracer on hepatic scintigraphy.[23] Side effects were minimal. The effect of these changes on the progression of the liver disease and survival is uncertain. The efficacy of earlier treatment and higher doses of ursodeoxycholic acid is under study.

Orthotopic liver transplantation has been performed successfully in patients with cystic fibrosis.[26] In one series, 62% of these carefully selected recipients have survived, one for 5 years. Pulmonary function has remained stable or even improved in most patients. Multiorgan transplantation of lungs, heart, and liver has also been successfully performed in several patients.[35]

Pilot experiments are underway to develop strategies to treat the hepatobiliary disease of cystic fibrosis by somatic gene transfer. Thus far, only animal studies have been completed, but the results seem promising. To specifically target recombinant genes to the biliary epithelium, recombinant adenoviruses expressing human CFTR were infused retrograde into the biliary tree of the rat through the common bile duct. Conditions were established for achieving recombinant gene expression in virtually all cells of the intrahepatic bile ducts in vivo.[115]

DISEASES OF THE GALLBLADDER

Cholelithiasis

Cholelithiasis occurs most often in children in association with a variety of predisposing conditions.[30, 36] Gallstones are uncommon in otherwise healthy children, but in two recent series, no known predisposing condition was found in 7 of 13 (54%) and 17 of 40 (42%) infants fewer than 12 months of age.[30, 87] Pigmented gallstones predominate in infants and children.[48, 105] Gallstones have been reported at any age, including during fetal life, but the majority of cases present near the time of puberty.[30, 36, 105] The conditions associated with an increased risk of cholelithiasis are listed in Table 2.

Certain factors may be particularly important in the pathogenesis of gallstones during infancy and childhood. Cholecystitis occurs in sick, premature infants who often undergo a period of prolonged fasting without frequent stimulation of gallbladder contraction and require periods of prolonged parenteral nutrition. Bouts of sepsis, abdominal surgery, frequent blood transfusions, and the use of diuretics and narcotic analgesics are associated.[30, 36] Children with ileal disease or resection suffer an increased incidence of gallstones.[46] Children who have been treated for cancer have an increased incidence of gallstones. An enlarged, distended gallbladder filled with sludge may develop, particularly in the critically ill infant, before the evolution to cholelithiasis. Analysis of gallstones has been limited but has generally shown them to be pigmented stones composed of cholesterol-calcium bilirubinate.

Chronic hemolytic disorders are commonly associated with black

TABLE 2. CONDITIONS ASSOCIATED WITH CHOLELITHIASIS IN CHILDREN

0–12 Mo. (%)	1–5 Yrs. (%)	6–21 Yrs. (%)
None (36.4)	Hepatobiliary disease (28.6)	Pregnancy (37.2)
TPN (29.1)	Abdominal surgery (21.4)	Hemolytic disease (22.5)
Abdominal surgery (29.1)	Artificial heart valve (14.3)	Obesity (8.1)
Sepsis (14.8)	None (14.3)	Abdominal surgery (5.1)
Bronchopulmonary dysplasia (12.7)	Malabsorption (7.1)	None (3.4)
Hemolytic disease (5.5)		Hepatobiliary disease (2.7)
Malabsorption (5.5)		TPN (2.7)
Necrotizing enterocolitis (5.5)		Malabsorption (2.8)
Hepatobiliary disease (3.6)		

Data from Freisen and Roberts based on review of 693 reported cases of cholelithiasis.[36]

pigment gallstones. Thirty to sixty percent of patients with sickle cell disease develop pigment stones. These stones are composed predominantly of calcium bilirubinate, with substantial amounts of crystalline calcium carbonate and phosphate. Stone development is age-dependent and progressive during childhood but is stable after 14 years of age.[65]

Obstructive jaundice in infants has also been reported secondary to brown pigment stones, which may be found in the extrahepatic biliary tree and the gallbladder.[65, 109] Brown pigment stones are composed of varying proportions of calcium bilirubinate, calcium phosphate, calcium palmitate, cholesterol, and organic residue. The stones are produced by bacterial hydrolysis of conjugated bilirubin. High β-glucuronidase activity has been detected in biles of affected patients. Culture of bile is frequently positive for *Eschericia coli* and bacteroides.[109]

Older children and adolescents without an identifiable cause for cholelithiasis are more likely to be female and obese. These patients often have a positive family history of gallstones and a greater likelihood of developing adult-like symptoms.[10, 30, 36] Cholesterol gallstones are more commonly found in these patients than in infants. Pima indians who have an extraordinarily high prevalence of cholesterol gallstones have provided important insights into the pathogenesis of gallstones. Bile highly saturated with cholesterol has not been detected among Pimas until pubertal growth and development.[10] A sex-related difference in bile acid pool size and difference in the frequency of gallstones begin during puberty as young men show a significant rise in bile acid pool with age, whereas young women show only a minimal rise. A small bile acid pool is an important risk factor for development of cholesterol gallstones.

Gallstones are often discovered incidentally during the investigation of another problem or during the process of screening a patient at high risk for cholelithiasis. Many patients are asymptomatic. Intermittent abdominal pain of variable severity may occur in older children and may be localized to the right upper quadrant. Infants may present with irritability, cholestatic jaundice, and acholic stools. Tenderness in the right upper quadrant indicates the possibility of cholecystitis. Children have a lower incidence of common duct stones than adults.[48]

Liver biochemical tests are normal in the asymptomatic patient; elevations of aminotransferases, alkaline phosphatase, and conjugated bilirubin occur as a result of cholecystitis or ductal obstruction. Pancreatitis occurs in 5% to 10% of patients.

Plain film radiographs of the abdomen may show calculi, but this is dependent on the calcium content of the stone. Ultrasonography is the most sensitive and specific imaging technique for demonstrating gallstones and dilation of the intrahepatic or extrahepatic bile ducts.[48] Failure to visualize the gallbladder on hepatobiliary scintigraphy is suggestive of acute cholecystitis.

Cholecystectomy is indicated in patients with symptoms or a nonfunctioning gallbladder.[30, 48] Operative cholangiography and exploration of the common duct may be required based on clinical imaging and operative findings. Laparoscopic cholecystectomy now is being frequently used, even in small children and infants.[49] In asymptomatic patients with so-called "silent gallstones," management is controversial because of a lag time of over a decade between initial stone formation and the development of symptoms in adults.[74] In cases associated with hepatic disease, severe obesity, or cystic fibrosis, the operative risk may be substantial, and clinical judgment must be applied as to whether a cholecystectomy should be performed. Spontaneous resolution of cholelithiasis and even common duct stones has been reported in infants.[30, 58] However, patients with obstructive cholestasis must be carefully observed for sepsis and cholangitis. Because recurrence of lithiasis is rare in infants, cholecystectomy may not be required. There is little experience with the use of ursodeoxycholic acid for dissolution of gallstones in children. It would not likely be of value in the predominantly pigmented stones found in this age group. Moreover, ursodeoxycholic acid failed to dissolve radiolucent gallstones in 10 children with cystic fibrosis.[22]

Calculous Cholecystitis

Cholecystitis is an acute or chronic inflammation of the gallbladder.[48, 87] This complication is thought to occur less commonly in children than in adults, but the incidence is probably underestimated. In a recent series, 32 of 50 children presented with right upper quadrant pain without ductal obstruction that was most likely related to chronic cholecystitis.[87] The acute form is usually associated with cholelithiasis and is precipitated by impaction of a stone in the cystic duct. Infarction, gangrene, and perforation can occur as complications. Proliferation of bacteria within the obstructed gallbladder lumen can contribute to the process. Chronic calculous cholecystitis is the more common form and develops insidiously or follows several attacks of acute cholecystitis.

Acute cholecystitis is associated with right upper quadrant pain, often accompanied by nausea and vomiting. The pain may be poorly localized in infants. The patient may seem acutely ill with shallow respirations. Children have a higher incidence of jaundice (approximately 50%).[87] The patient may be febrile, particularly with superimposed bacterial infection. Guarding of the abdomen is commonly observed, with tenderness in the right upper quadrant and a positive Murphy's sign.

Chronic cholecystitis is usually more indolent. Recurrent bouts of upper abdominal discomfort of varying severity are a constant feature. Intolerance to fatty food occurs in older children. Physical examination may elicit local tenderness over the gallbladder or may be negative.

The white blood cell count is often elevated in acute cholecystitis with a predominance of polymorphonuclear leukocytes. Serum bilirubin and alkaline phosphatase levels may be increased. Serum aminotransaminase levels may be normal but significant elevations, suggesting hepatocellular disease, can occur early in the course of the common duct obstruction. The white blood cell count and liver biochemical tests are usually normal in chronic cholecystitis.

The plain film of the abdomen may reveal calcifications in the right upper quadrant in the acute or chronic form of the disease.[30, 48, 87] An abdominal ultrasound is the most useful imaging modality in demonstrating gallstones. Thickening of the gallbladder wall and obstructive dilatation of the biliary tract also may be defined. Hepatobiliary scintigraphy is of value in patients with chronic cholecystitis in demonstrating a nonfunctioning gallbladder.

Cholecystectomy should be performed as soon as fluid deficits are corrected and infection controlled. Percutaneous drainage via a transhepatic cholecystostomy may be required in the high-risk, acutely ill patient. Care should be taken to exclude common duct stones through operative cholangiography and, if necessary, duct exploration.

Cholecystectomy is also the treatment of choice for chronic calculous cholecystitis. Laparoscopic cholecystectomy may be appropriate in selected patients.[49]

Acute Acalculous Cholecystitis

Acute acalculous cholecystitis is an acute inflammation of the gallbladder without gallstones and often is associated with infection or systemic illness.[108] Streptococci (groups A and B); gram-negative organisms, including salmonella, *Shigella,* and *E. coli;* and parasitic infestations with *Ascaris* or *Giardia lamblia* have been associated. Systemic vasculitis from periarteritis nodosa and Kawasaki disease may be causal but are more likely to be associated with acute hydrops of the gallbladder. Congenital narrowing or inflammation of the cystic duct or external compression from enlarged lymph nodes has been found in some children with acute acalculous cholecystitis.

Right upper quadrant or epigastric pain, nausea, vomiting, fever, and jaundice may be present. An enlarged, tender gallbladder is sometimes palpable.

Laboratory evaluation may reveal elevated serum levels of alkaline phosphatase and bilirubin. Leukocytosis may occur. An enlarged, thick-walled gallbladder distended with sludge but without calculi is found on ultrasonography.

Treatment of the systemic infection should be started. Cholecystectomy is usually required. The gallbladder is inflamed on laparotomy, and cultures of bile may be positive for bacteria or contain parasites.

Acute Hydrops of the Gallbladder

Acute distention of the gallbladder occurs in infants and children without gallstones and an inflammatory process.[16] However, there may be a temporal relationship to systemic infections including scarlet fever and leptospirosis. Acute hydrops has also been associated with the mucocutaneous lymph node (Kawasaki) disease.[114] It is being increasingly reported in critically ill patients, particularly infants, on prolonged parenteral nutrition. Prolonged fasting and the use of narcotic analgesics are predisposing factors. In some cases, the cause is not identified. There may be a continuum of disease with noncalculous cholecystitis if hydrops progresses to infection of the biliary tree and gallbladder inflammation.

Hydrops is associated with the acute onset of crampy abdominal pain and, often, nausea and vomiting. Fever and jaundice may be present. The abdomen is usually distended with tenderness in the right upper quadrant. The distended gallbladder may be palpable.

Laboratory studies are not usually helpful. The white blood cell count may be elevated. Liver biochemical tests may be mildly elevated.

Ultrasonography confirms the presence of an enlarged, distended gallbladder without calculi. Serial imaging of the gallbladder may be useful in following the course of the illness and in verifying resolution of hydrops.[103]

Treatment of gallbladder hydrops is usually nonoperative with a focus on supportive care and managing the intercurrent illness. The process subsides spontaneously in most patients. Particularly in children on total parenteral nutrition, enteral feeding has been initiated. Laparotomy may be required if there is a concern about cholecystitis, if the hydrops fails to resolve, or if hydrops leads to compromise of gallbladder perfusion. A generalized mesenteric adenitis of lymph nodes near the cystic duct that does not produce mechanical compression has been associated with the condition. Cholecystectomy may be necessary if the gallbladder becomes gangrenous; however, in most cases, pathologic examination of the gallbladder shows only edema and mild inflammation. Bile cultures are usually sterile. Once viability of the gallbladder has been confirmed, many surgeons treat acute hydrops by a simple cholecystostomy rather than cholecystectomy. Gallbladder function returns to normal in most cases.

References

1. Alagille D: Management of paucity of interlobular bile ducts. J Hepatology 1:561, 1985
2. Alagille D, Estrada A, Hadchouel M, et al: Syndromatic paucity of intrahepatic bile ducts (Alagille syndrome or arteriohepatic dysplasia): Review of 80 cases. J Pediatr 110:195, 1987
3. Alagille D, Odievre M, Gautier M, et al: Hepatic ductular hypoplasia associated with characteristic facies, vertebral malformations, retarded physical, mental, and sexual development, and cardiac murmur. J Pediatr 86:63, 1975
4. Alvarez F, Bernard O, Brunelle F, et al: Congenital hepatic fibrosis in children. J Pediatr 99:370, 1981
5. Amedee-Manesme O, Bernard O, Brunelle F, et al: Sclerosing cholangitis with neonatal onset. J Pediatr 111:225, 1987
6. Anad F, Burn J, Matthews D, et al: Alagille syndrome and deletion of 20p. J Med Genet 27:729, 1990

7. Baker AJ, Portmann B, Westaby D, et al: Neonatal sclerosing cholangitis in two siblings: A category of progressive intrahepatic cholestasis. J Pediatr Gastroenterol Nutr 17:317, 1993
8. Balistreri WF: Neonatal cholestasis-medical progress. J Pediatr 106:171, 1985
9. Bancroft JD, Bucuvalas JC, Ryckman FC, et al: Antenatal diagnosis of choledochal cyst. [review] J Pediatr Gastroenterol Nutr 18:142–145, 1994
10. Bennion LJ, Knowler WC, Mott DM, et al: Development of lithgenic bile during puberty in Pima indians. N Engl J Med 300:874, 1979
11. Bodenheimer HC, LaRusso NF, Thayer WR, et al: Elevated circulating immune complexes in primary sclerosing cholangitis. Hepatology 3:150, 1983
12. Brown WR, Sokol RJ, Levin MJ, et al: Lack of correlation between infection with reovirus 3 and extrahepatic biliary atresia or neonatal hepatitis. J Pediatr 113:670, 1988
13. Bucuvalas JC, Horn JA, Carlsson L, et al: Growth hormone insensitivity associated with elevated circulating growth hormone-binding protein with Alagille syndrome and short stature. J Clin Endocrinol Metab 76:1477–1482, 1993
14. Burt MJ, Chambers ST, Chapman BA, et al: Two cases of Caroli's disease: Diagnosis and management. J Gastroent Hepatol 9:194–197, 1994
15. Carmi R, Magee CA, Neill CA, et al: Extrahepatic biliary atresia and associated anomalies: Etiologic heterogeneity suggested by distinctive patterns of associations. [Review] Am J Med Genet 45:683–693, 1993
16. Chamberlain JW, Hight DW: Acute hydrops of the gallbladder in childhood. Surgery 68:899, 1970
17. Chapman RW, Varghese Z, Gaul R, et al: Association of primary sclerosing cholangitis with HLA-B8. Gut 24:38, 1983
18. Chijiiwa K, Koga A: Surgical management and long-term follow-up of patients with choledochal cysts. Am J Surg 165:238–242, 1993
19. Classen M, Goetze H, Richter H, et al: Primary sclerosing cholangitis in children. J Pediatr Gastroenterol Nutr 6:197, 1987
20. Cohn JA, Strong TV, Picciotto MR, et al: Localization of the cystic fibrosis transmembrane conductance regulator in human bile duct epithelial cells. Gastroenterology 105:1857–1864, 1993
21. Colombo C, Apostolo MG, Ferrari M, et al: Analysis of risk factors for the development of liver disease associated with cystic fibrosis. J Pediatr 124:393–399, 1994
22. Colombo C, Bertolini E, Assaisso ML, et al: Failure of ursodeoxycholic acid to dissolve radiolucent gallstones in patients with cystic fibrosis. Acta Paediatr 82:562–565, 1993
23. Colombo C, Castellani MR, Balistreri WF, et al: Scintigraphic documentation of an improvement in hepatobiliary excretory function after treatment with ursodeoxycholic acid in patients with cystic fibrosis and associated liver disease. Hepatology 15:677–684, 1992
24. Colombo C, Setchell KDR, Podda M, et al: Effects of ursodeoxycholic acid therapy for liver disease associated with cystic fibrosis. J Pediatr 117:482, 1990
25. Cotting J, Lentze MJ, Reichen J: Effects of ursodeoxycholic acid treatment on nutrition and liver function in patients with cystic fibrosis and longstanding cholestasis. Gut 31:918, 1990
26. Cox KL, Ward RE, Furgiuele TL, et al: Orthotopic liver transplantation in patients with cystic fibrosis. Pediatrics 80:571, 1987
27. Crittenden SL, McKinley MJ: Choledochal cysts—clinical features and classification. Am J Gastroenterol 80:643, 1985
28. Cuervas-Mons V, Rimola A, Van Thiel DH, et al: Does previous abdominal surgery alter the outcome of pediatric patients subjected to orthotopic liver transplantation? Gastroenterology 90:853, 1986
29. Davenport M, Savage M, Mowat AP, et al: Biliary atresia splenic malformation syndrome: An etiologic and prognostic subgroup. Surgery 113:662–668, 1993
30. Debray D, Pariente D, Gauthier F, et al: Cholelithiasis in infancy: A study of 40 cases. J Pediatr 122:385–391, 1993
31. Debray D, Pariente D, Urvoas E, et al: Sclerosing cholangitis in children. J Pediatr 124:49, 1994
32. Duthie A, Doherty DG, Williams C, et al: Genotype analysis for delta F508, G551D,

R553X mutations in children and young adults with cystic fibrosis with and without chronic liver disease. Hepatology 15:660–664, 1992

33. Ecoffey C, Rothman E, Bernard O, et al: Bacterial cholangitis after surgery for biliary atresia. J Pediatr 111:824, 1987
34. El-Shabrawi M, Wilkinson ML, Portmann B, et al: Primary sclerosing cholangitis in childhood. Gastroenterology 92:1226, 1987
35. Feigelson J, Anagnostopoulos C, Poquet M, et al: Liver cirrhosis in cystic fibrosis-therapeutic implications and long-term follow-up. Arch Dis Child 68:653–657, 1993
36. Frieson CA, Roberts CC: Cholelithiasis: Clinical characteristics in children. Clin Pediatr 28:294–298, 1989
37. Fitz JG, Basavappa S, McGill J, et al: Regulation of membrane chloride currents in rat bile duct epithelial cells. J Clin Invest 91:319–328, 1993
38. Gaskin JJ, Waters DLM, Howman-Biles R, et al: Liver disease and common-bile-duct stenosis in cystic fibrosis. N Engl J Med 318:340, 1988
39. Gautier M, Elliot N: Extrahepatic biliary atresia: Morphological study of 98 biliary remnants. Arch Pathol Lab Med 105:397, 1981
40. Gremse DA, Bucuvalas JC, Bongiovanni GL: Papillary stenosis and sclerosing cholangitis in an immunodeficient child. Gastroenterology 96:1600, 1989
41. Grosfeld JL, Fitzgerald JF, Predaina R, et al: The efficacy of hepatoportoenterostomy in biliary atresia. Surgery 106:692, 1989
42. Gurevitz M, Weber T, Danis R, et al: Sodium homeostasis in infants with biliary drainage procedures. Am J Dis Child 140:535, 1986
43. Hays DM, Kimura K: Biliary Atresia: Japanese Experience. London, Harvard University Press, 1980
44. Hays DM, Woolley MM, Snyder WH Jr, et al: Diagnosis of biliary atresia: Relative accuracy of percutaneous liver biopsy, open liver biopsy, and operative cholangiography. J Pediatr 71:598, 1967
45. Heathcote J, Deodhar KP, Scheuer PJ, et al: Intrahepatic cholestasis in childhood. N Engl J Med 295:801, 1976
46. Heubi JE, O'Connell NC, Setchell KD: Ileal resection/dysfunction predisposes to lithogenic bile only after puberty. Gastroenterology 103:636–640, 1992
47. Hoffenberg EJ, Schneider J, Narkewicz MJ, et al: Poor outcome of childhood Alagille syndrome (syndromic paucity of interlobular bile ducts). Gastroenterology 106:A907, 1994
48. Holcomb GW Jr, Holcomb GW III: Cholelithiasis in infants, children, and adolescents. Pediatr Rev 11:268–274, 1990
49. Holcomb GW III, Naffis D: Laparoscopic cholecystectomy in infants. J Pediatr Surg 29:86–87, 1994
50. Howard ER: Extrahepatic biliary atresia: A review of current management. Br J Surg 70:193, 1983
51. Kahn E: Paucity of interlobular bile ducts: Arteriohepatic dysplasia and nonsyndromic duct paucity. In Abramowsky CR, Bernstein J, Rosenberg HS (eds): Transplantation Pathology—Hepatic Morphogenesis. Perspect Pediatr Pathol. Basel, Karger, 1991, pp 168–215
52. Kahn E, Daum F, Markowitz J, et al: Nonsyndromatic paucity of interlobular bile ducts: Light and electron microscopic evaluation of sequential liver biopsies in early childhood. Hepatology 6:890, 1986
53. Karrer FM, Lilly JR, Stewart BA, et al: Biliary atresia registry, 1976 to 1989. J Pediatr Surg 254:1076, 1990
54. Kasai M: Treatment of biliary atresia with special reference to hepatic porto-enterostomy and its modifications. Prog Pediatr Surg 6:5, 1974
55. Kasai M, Mochizuk I, Ohkohchi N, et al: Surgical limitation for biliary atresia—indication for liver transplantation. J Pediatr Surg 24:851, 1989
56. Kasai M, Ohi R, Chiba T: Long-term survivors after surgery for biliary atresia. In Ohi R (ed): Biliary Atresia. Tokyo, Professional Postgraduate Service, 1987, pp 277–281
57. Kaufman SS, Wood RP, Shaw BW Jr, et al: Hepatocarcinoma in a child with the Alagille syndrome. Am J Dis Child 141:698, 1987

58. Keller MS, Markle BM, Laffey PA, et al: Spontaneous resolution of cholelithiasis in infants. Radiology 157:345, 1985
59. Kerem B, Rommens JM, Buchman JA, et al: Identification of the cystic fibrosis gene: Genetic analysis. Science 245:1073, 1989
60. Kim S: Choledochal cyst: Survey by the surgical section of The American Academy of Pediatrics. J Pediatr Surg 16:402, 1981
61. Lai MW, Chang MH, Hsu SC, et al: Differential diagnosis of extrahepatic biliary atresia from neonatal hepatitis: A prospective study. J Pediatr Gastroenterol Nutr 18:121–127, 1994
62. Landing BH: Considerations of the pathogenesis of neonatal hepatitis, biliary atresia and choledochal cyst. The concept of infantile obstructive cholangiopathy. Prog Pediatr Surg 6:113, 1975
63. LaRusso NF, Wiesner RH, Ludwig J, et al: Primary sclerosing cholangitis. N Engl J Med 310:899, 1984
64. Leblanc A, Hadchouel M, Jehan P, et al: Obstructive jaundice in children with histiocytosis X. Gastroenterology 80:143, 1981
65. Leuschner U, Güldütuna S, Hellstern A: Pathogenesis of pigment stones and medical treatment. J Gastroenterol Hepatol 9:87–98, 1994
66. Lindblad A, Hultcrantz R, Strandvik B: Bile-duct destruction and collagen deposition: A prominent ultrastructural feature of the liver in cystic fibrosis. Hepatology 16:372–381, 1992
67. Lo SK, Chapman RWG, Cheeseman P, et al: Antineutrophil antibody: A test for autoimmune primary sclerosing cholangitis in childhood? Gut 34:199, 1993
68. Ludwig J, Barham S, LaRusso N, et al: Morphologic features of chronic hepatitis associated with primary sclerosing cholangitis. Hepatology 1:632, 1981
69. Manolaki AG, Larcher VF, Mowat AP, et al: The prelaparotomy diagnosis of extrahepatic biliary atresia. Arch Dis Child 58:591, 1983
70. Meister RK, Esquivel CO, Cox KL, et al: The influence of portoenterostomy with stoma on morbidity in pediatric patients with biliary atresia undergoing orthotopic liver transplantation. J Pediatr Surg 28:387–390, 1993
71. Mieli-Vergani G, Howard ER, Portman B, et al: Late referral for biliary atresia: Missed opportunities for effective surgery. Lancet 2:421, 1989
72. Mieli-Vergani G, Lobo-Yeo A, McFarlane B, et al: Different immune mechanisms leading to autoimmunity in primary sclerosing cholangitis and autoimmune chronic active hepatitis of childhood. Hepatology 9:198, 1989
73. Miyano T, Fujimoto T, Ohya T, et al: Current concept of treatment of biliary atresia. World J Surg 17:332–336, 1993
74. Mok HYI, Druffel ERM, Rampone W: Chronology of cholelithiasis: Dating gallstones from atmosphere rabiocarbon produced by nuclear bomb explosion. N Engl J Med 314:1075, 1986
75. Morecki R, Glaser JH, Cho S, et al: Biliary atresia and reovirus type 3 infection. N Engl J Med 307:481, 1982
76. Morecki R, Glaser JH, Johnson AB, et al: Detection of reovirus type 3 in the porta hepatis of an infant with extrahepatic biliary atresia: ultrastructural and immunocytochemical study. Hepatology 4:1137, 1984
77. Mueller RF, Pagon RA, Pepin MG, et al: Arteriohepatic dysplasia: Phenotypic features and family studies. Clin Genet 25:323, 1984
78. Murray-Lyon IM, Shilkin KB, Laws JW, et al: Non-obstructive dilatation of the intrahepatic biliary tree with cholangitis. Q J Med 164:477, 1972
79. Nagel RA, Javaid A, Meire HB, et al: Liver disease and bile duct abnormalities in adults with cystic fibrosis. Lancet ii:1422, 1989
80. Nakagawa M, Colombo C, Ketchell KDR: Comprehensive study of the biliary bile acid composition of patients with cystic fibrosis and associated liver disease before and after UDCA administration. Hepatology 12:322, 1990
81. O'Brien S, Keogan M, Casey M, et al: Biliary complications of cystic fibrosis. Gut 33:387–391, 1992
82. Ohi R, Nio M, Chiba T, et al: Long-term follow-up after surgery for patients with biliary atresia. J Pediatr Surg 25:442, 1990

83. Oppenheimer EH, Esterly JR: Hepatic changes in young infants with cystic fibrosis: Possible relation to focal biliary cirrhosis. J Pediatr 86:683, 1975
84. Park RW, Grand RJ: Gastrointestinal manifestations of cystic fibrosis: A review. Gastroenterology 81:1143, 1981
85. Prochazka EJ, Terasaki PI, Park MS, et al: Association of primary sclerosing cholangitis with HLA-DRw52a. N Engl J Med 322:1842, 1990
86. Raweily EA, Gibson AAM, Burt AD: Abnormalities of intrahepatic bile ducts in extrahepatic biliary atresia. Histopathology 17:521, 1990
87. Reif S, Sloven DG, Lebenthal E: Gallstones in children. Characterization by age etiology and outcome. Am J Dis Child 145:105–108, 1991
88. Ros E, Navarro S, Bru C, et al: Ursodeoxycholic acid treatment of primary hepatolithiasis in Caroli's syndrome. Lancet 342:404–406, 1993
89. Roy CC, Weber AM, Morin CL, et al: Hepatobiliary disease in cystic fibrosis: A survey of current issues and concepts. J Pediatr Gastroenterol Nutr 1:469, 1982
90. Ryckman F, Fisher J, Pederson S, et al: Improved survival in biliary atresia patients in the era of liver transplantation. J Pediatr Surg 28:382–385, 1993
91. Ryckman FC, Noseworthy J: Neonatal cholestatic conditions requiring surgical reconstruction. Sem Liver Dis 7:134, 1987
92. Savader SJ, Benenati JF, Venbrux AC, et al: Choledochal cyst: Classification and cholangiographic appearance. Am J Roent 156:327, 1991
93. Schreiber RA, Kleinman RE: (editorial) Genetics, immunology, and biliary atresia: An opening or a diversion? J Pediatr Gastroenterol Nutr 16:111–113, 1993
94. Schweizer P: Extrahepatic biliary atresia: An analytic assessment of prognostic factors. Contribution to a rational therapeutic approach. Zeitschrift fur Kinderchirurgie 45:365–370, 1990
95. Schweizer P: Treatment of extrahepatic bile duct atresia: Results and long-term prognosis after hepatic portoenterostomy. Pediatr Surg Int 1:30, 1986
96. Scott-Jupp R, Lama M, Tanner MS: Prevalence of liver disease in cystic fibrosis. Arch Dis Child 66:698, 1991
97. Shulman SA, Hyams JS, Gunta R, et al: Arteriohepatic dysplasia (Alagille Syndrome): Extreme variability among affected family members. Am J Med Genet 19:325, 1984
98. Silveira TR, Salzano FM, Donaldson PT, et al: Association between HLA and extrahepatic biliary atresia. J Pediatr Gastroenterol Nutr 16:114–117, 1993
99. Sisto A, Feldman P, Garel L, et al: Primary sclerosing cholangitis in children: Study of five cases and review of the literature. Pediatrics 80:918, 1987
100. Smith BM, Laberge JM, Schreiber R, et al: Familial biliary atresia in three siblings including twins. J Pediatr Surg 26:1331–1333, 1991
101. Sokol RJ, Endo N, Ohara JI, et al: Reovirus 3 RNA not detected by polymerase chain reaction in tissues from infants with extrahepatic biliary atresia. Hepatology 14:125A, 1991
102. Sokol RJ, Heubi JE, Balistreri WF: Intrahepatic "cholestasis facies": Is it specific for Alagille syndrome? J Pediatr 103:205, 1983
103. Solvis TL, Hight DW, Philippart AI, et al: Sonography in the diagnosis and management of hydrops of the gallbladder in children with mucocutaneous lymph node syndrome. Pediatrics 5:785, 1980
104. Spinner NB, Rand EB, Fortina P, et al: Cytologically balanced t(2:20) in a two-generation family with Alagille syndrome: Cytogenic and molecular studies. Am J Hum Genet 55:238–243, 1994
105. Suchet IB, Labatte MF, Dyck CS, et al: Fetal cholelithiasis: A case report and review of the literature. J Clin Ultrasound 21:198–202, 1993
106. Summerfield JA, Nagafuchi Y, Sherlock S, et al: Hepatobiliary fibropolycystic diseases: A clinical and histological review of 51 patients. J Hepatology 2:141, 1986
107. Tan CEL, Davenport M, Driver M, et al: Does the morphology of the extrahepatic biliary remnants in biliary atresia influence survival? A review of 205 cases. J Pediatr Surg 29:1459–1464, 1994
108. Ternberg JL, Keating JP: Acute acalculous cholecystitis: Complication of other illnesses in childhood. Arch Surg 110:543, 1978

109. Treem WR, Malet PF, Gourley GR, et al: Bile and stone analysis in two infants with brown pigment gallstones and infected bile. Gastroenterology 96:519, 1989
110. Tzakis AG, Reyes J, Tepetes K, et al: Liver transplantation for Alagille's syndrome. Arch Surg 128:337–339, 1993
111. Valencia-Mayoral P, Weber J, Cutz E, et al: Possible defect in the bile secretory apparatus in arteriohepatic dysplasia (Alagille's syndrome): A review with observations on the ultrastructure of liver. Hepatology 4:691, 1984
112. Weisner RH: Current concepts in primary sclerosing cholangitis. Mayo Clin Proc 69:969, 1994
113. Whitington PF, Balistreri WF: Liver transplantation in pediatrics: Indications, contraindications, and pretransplant management. J Pediatr 118:169, 1991
114. Wirth S, Baumann W, Keller KM, et al: Kawasaki's disease with acute hydrops of the gallbladder. Report of a case and review of the literature. Klin Paediatr 197:68, 1985
115. Yang Y, Raper SE, Cohn JA, et al: An approach for treating the hepatobiliary disease of cystic fibrosis by somatic gene transfer. Proc Natl Acad Sci USA 90:4601–4605, 1993

Address reprint requests to

Colston F. McEvoy, MD
Department of Pediatrics
Yale University School of Medicine
333 Cedar Street
New Haven, CT 06520

LIVER TRANSPLANTATION AND ITS LONG-TERM MANAGEMENT IN CHILDREN

Hanmin Lee, MD, and Joseph P. Vacanti, MD

Liver transplantation is an effective treatment for a variety of acute and chronic diseases of the liver in the pediatric population. Of the 3442 liver transplantations performed in the United States in 1993, 524 (15%) were in patients fewer than 18 years of age.[5] The success rate has risen dramatically in the past 12 years since liver transplantation was considered to be a therapeutic, rather than an experimental, treatment for liver disease.[65]

Despite the improvements in liver transplantation, many pitfalls remain. The complications of rejection, opportunistic infection, and adverse side effects of medications are common to all liver transplantation patients. The ever-worsening donor-organ shortage remains the major barrier to effective therapy for children who need hepatic replacement. Growth and development specific to pediatric liver transplant patients are issues also. To optimize care to the pediatric patient who has undergone liver transplantation, a coordinated effort is undertaken between the surgeon and the pediatrician and involves the family and the nursing, psychiatric, social work, and nutritional staffs.

This article outlines the history of pediatric liver transplantation. The indications for pediatric liver transplantation and the preoperative, intraoperative, and postoperative management of transplanted children are then discussed. In addition, current areas of research in the field of end-stage pediatric liver disease are reviewed.

From the Divisions of Surgical Research (HL) and Organ Transplantation (JPV), Department of Surgery, The Children's Hospital; and the Department of Surgery, Harvard Medical School (JPV), Boston, Massachusetts

HISTORY

The first human liver transplantation was performed by Starzl in 1963[86] based largely on experimental work done by Starzl's group in Denver[83, 84] and Moore's group in Boston.[63] The first long-term survivor, reported in 1968 by Starzl, was a 1.5-year-old child who underwent liver transplantation in 1967 for a large hepatoma.[80] She survived for 13 months before dying from metastatic hepatoma. The clinical introduction of cyclosporine as an immunosuppressant by Calne and colleagues of England in 1979 led to a marked improvement in 1-year survival rates.[23] Groups using immunosuppressive therapy of cyclosporine in combination with corticosteroids were able to demonstrate 1-year survival rates of 65%.[81, 85, 100] Prior to this time, 1-year survival rates reported by Starzl's group ranged from 29% to 50%.[82] The improved survival rate led to the National Institutes of Health Consensus Conference on liver transplantation in 1983 that concluded that liver transplantation should be considered an accepted treatment for liver disease.[65]

Since 1980, continued improvements have led to an overall 1-year survival rate of 78.6% in the United States from 1987 to 1992, including 79.7% in the pediatric population during this same period.[5] Several recent series report 1-year survival rates of 85% to 90% after liver transplantation in pediatric patients.[54, 76, 96] In addition to cyclosporine, other newly developed immunosuppressants, such as FK506 and OKT3, have been shown by some groups to increase graft and patient survival.[36, 96] FK506 has replaced cyclosporine in the immunosuppressant regimen in some transplantation centers.

Another important advance was the development of University of Wisconsin (UW) solution for prolonged organ preservation.[51] This allowed transport of donor organs across greater distances and operations to be performed during regularly staffed operating hours. Veno-veno bypass, introduced by Starzl's group in Pittsburgh in 1983, decreased the cardiovascular instability that complicated many of the earlier transplants.[30] In addition, prophylaxis and treatment for opportunistic infections secondary to the immunosuppressants have improved. One of the more important advances is the use of antiviral agents, especially those targeted against cytomegalovirus (CMV), which has been the most devastating pathogen in immunosuppressed patients after transplantation.

INDICATIONS FOR TRANSPLANTATION

A consensus conference was held in 1993 in Paris to determine the indications and contraindications for liver transplantation.[24] Absolute contraindications were concluded to be as follows: (1) extrahepatic organ failure unless the failing organ could be cotransplanted; (2) uncontrolled immune deficiency; and (3) uncontrolled extrahepatic infection.[22] Situations in which liver transplantation are clearly indicated in childhood liver diseases were concluded to be extrahepatic biliary atresia after failure of a Kasai portoenterostomy, other cholestatic diseases including Byler's disease, cirrhosis secondary to α_1-antitrypsin deficiency or interlobular bile duct paucity, and inborn errors of metabolism. In addition, fulminant hepatitis and subfulminant hepatitis were concluded to be conditions in which liver transplantation could significantly alter prognosis.

Because the conference considered only the diseases that make up 90% to 95% of the common indications for liver transplantation, no comment was made on other pediatric liver diseases regarding possible transplantation. Table 1 provides a comprehensive list of childhood diseases in which liver transplantation has been performed. The catego-

Table 1. PEDIATRIC DISEASES THAT HAVE LED TO LIVER TRANSPLANTATION

I. Extrahepatic biliary obstruction
    Extrahepatic biliary atresia
    Traumatic biliary obstruction
II. Cholestatic diseases
    Parenteral nutrition related cholestastasis
    Alagille syndrome
    Nonsyndromic bile duct paucity
    Byler's disease
III. Metabolic diseases
    Wilson's disease
    Tyrosinemia
    Glycogen storage diseases, types I, III, IV
    Niemann-Pick disease
    Crigler-Najjar disease
    Hyperoxaluria
    Familial hypercholesterolemia
    Cystic fibrosis
    Hemophilia A, B
    Erythropoietic protoporphyria
    Sea-blue histiocyte syndrome
    Urea cycle enzyme deficiency
    α_1-Antitrypsin deficiency
    Perinatal hemochromatosis–iron storage deficiency
IV. Hepatitis, acute or chronic
    Hepatitis A
    Hepatitis B
    Non-A, non-B hepatitis
    Drug-induced hepatitis
    Autoimmune hepatitis
    Idiopathic neonatal hepatitis
V. Malignant tumors
    Hepatocellular carcinoma
    Fibrolamellar carcinoma
    Hepatoblastoma
    Sarcoma
    Hemangioendothelioma
VI. Benign tumors
    Hemangioma
    Inflammatory pseudotumor
VII. Miscellaneous
    Cryptogenic cirrhosis
    Budd-Chiari syndrome

ries are not mutually exclusive, and some of the diseases fit into more than one category. Generally, liver transplantation is indicated for end-stage liver disease from any etiology in the absence of the previously mentioned contraindications. End-stage liver disease is evidenced by irreversible, progressive liver dysfunction, variceal bleeding, encephalopathy, synthetic dysfunction, poor growth, or poor nutritional status.[101] In addition, unresectable tumors and liver-based metabolic deficiencies may be indications for liver transplantation. Some of the common specific indications for pediatric liver transplantation are discussed later.

Biliary Atresia

Biliary atresia is a disease of unknown etiology in which progressive destruction of extrahepatic bile ducts takes place. The incidence is approximately 1 in 15,000 live births, with a slight predominance in girls.[60] Once the diagnosis of biliary atresia has been made, prompt surgical intervention is warranted. Without surgical therapy, the average survival in infants with biliary atresia is 12 months.[1]

Liver failure secondary to biliary atresia is the most common indication for pediatric liver transplantation. Groups have reported that between 46% and 63% of their pediatric liver transplant series are comprised of children with biliary atresia.[4, 18, 21, 50, 54, 76] The experience at The Children's Hospital in Boston has been consistent with these numbers, with 54% of the liver transplant series being from biliary atresia.[98]

Surgical intervention with Kasai's portoenterostomy and liver transplantation have dramatically improved the prognosis.[37, 55, 56] Most groups advocate first performing a Kasai portoenterostomy and subsequently transplanting those children with deteriorating liver function.[68, 98, 104] Initially performing a Kasai portoenterostomy as compared with immediate transplantation has several benefits. First, a significant portion of patients achieve successful long-term biliary drainage. These patients are spared taking lifelong immunosuppressants. Many more patients achieve variable success with the Kasai operation, delaying a liver transplantation and immunosuppression until they are older. Transplantation is more likely to be successful in older children. In addition, a successful Kasai operation alleviates some of the problem of donor-organ shortage; however, the 5-year survival rate in patients who undergo the Kasai operation without transplantation is only 30% to 60%, and, thus, liver transplantation is important in increasing long-term survival of patients with biliary atresia.[61]

In the authors' experience, during a follow-up period of 1 to 8 years, combining Kasai operation with liver transplantation produced an 89% survival rate in 28 children.[99] One third of the patients required liver transplantation. Although a previous Kasai operation may increase blood loss and technical difficulty for subsequent liver transplantation, no increased mortality occurred in this series. Recent studies suggest that approximately one third of patients who undergo a Kasai operation achieve successful long-term biliary drainage.[61] Of the remaining children, 25% have poor initial results from a Kasai operation and require early transplantation, whereas the remaining children have fair results but eventually may require transplantation.[99]

Cholestatic Diseases

Byler's disease, also known as familial intrahepatic cholestasis, is a poorly understood disease that leads to cholestasis and cirrhosis. Results with liver transplantation have been good.[31] Alagille syndrome, also known as *arteriohepatic dysplasia,* is characterized by a paucity of interlobular bile ducts, characteristic facies, cardiovascular abnormalities, vertebral anomalies, and posterior embryotoxon.[32] The paucity of interlobular bile ducts leads to cholestasis and liver disease. Byler's disease and Alagille syndrome are sometimes collectively referred to as familial cholestatic disease. Paucity of interlobular bile ducts also may present in a nonsyndromic form without the other manifestations of Alagille syndrome.[31] Chronically ill patients that require parenteral nutrition may develop fatty infiltration of the liver and cholestasis resulting in liver failure. The liver disease may become sufficiently severe enough to warrant liver transplantation.

Metabolic Disorders

Metabolic disorders as a whole make up the second most common indication for pediatric liver transplantation at approximately 19% of the total.[50] α1-Antitrypsin disease is the most common of the metabolic disorders.[76, 89] α1-Antitrypsin disease is caused by the alteration of a single amino acid in the α1-antitrypsin protein.[40] This defect leads to progressive liver disease and may require transplantation. A predisposition to hepatocellular carcinoma may be present also. Results with liver transplantation for α1-antitrypsin disease have been excellent.

Tyrosinemia is an autosomal recessive disease in which an enzyme deficiency leads to elevated blood concentrations of tryosine and methionine.[39] The age of onset is variable. In the acute form, patients develop symptoms of liver failure within the first year of life and have a fulminant course. Patients with the chronic form develop symptoms later and develop cirrhosis. They have a strong predisposition to developing hepatocellular carcinoma.

Wilson's disease is caused by defective copper metabolism due to deficient levels of ceruloplasmin.[41] Liver disease secondary to Wilson's disease may be acute or chronic in nature and may be difficult to differentiate from hepatitis or cirrhosis of other causes. Neurologic manifestations, ophthalmic manifestations (Kayser-Fleischer rings), a low plasma level of ceruloplasmin, and an elevated plasma level of copper may be helpful in making the diagnosis.

Crigler-Najjar syndrome involves a complete (type I) or partial (type II) deficiency in bilirubin UDPglucuronyl transferase.[70] Type II usually can be treated successfully with phenobarbital. Type I is poorly responsive to any medical treatment and requires transplantation.

Hepatitis

Acute fulminant hepatitis carries greater than a 70% mortality rate without transplantation.[74] Although various treatments have been attempted, liver transplantation offers the best chance for survival.[102] The most common causes are viral hepatitis (A, B, and C) and drug-induced (paracetamol and halothane). Survival rates with liver transplantation range from 40% to 80% depending on the severity of liver failure.[102]

Treatment for cirrhosis due to chronic infection with hepatitis B is controversial.[24] A high risk for reinfection exists, and long-term survival is poor. The use of antihepatitis B immunoglobulins may protect against reinfection and recently has been advocated for use in transplantation for hepatitis B. Long-term follow-up is not yet available.

Hepatitis C also carries a risk of reinfection, although it is less than that with hepatitis B. The long-term efficacy of transplantation for patients with hepatitis C is not yet known.[24]

Tumors

Liver transplantation for unresectable nonmetastatic hepatocellular carcinoma has a lower success rate than that for liver transplantation for other reasons. Because of the lower success rate, liver transplantation for hepatocellular carcinoma is now being combined with perioperative chemotherapy, including intraoperative chemoembolization in the hopes of gaining better results.[71]

Cholangiocellular carcinomas, hemangiosarcomas, and nonendocrine liver metastases respond poorly to liver transplantation, and patients with these diseases are not considered for transplantation. Alternatively, fibrolamellar carcinoma, epithelioid hemangioendothelioma, hepatoblastoma, and metastases from endocrine tumors respond relatively well to transplantation.[71]

Symptomatic, unresectable benign liver tumors, such as hemangioma and inflammatory pseudotumor, respond well to transplantation. In the absence of any other effective treatment modality, liver transplantation is considered.

PREOPERATIVE EVALUATION

The patient and family must undergo a thorough multidisciplinary preoperative evaluation to ensure the best outcome from a liver transplantation. The transplant surgeon, primary pediatrician, hepatologist, transplant coordinator, nutritionist, psychologist, social worker, anesthesiologist, respiratory therapist, radiologist, pathologist, immunologist, hematologist, and infectious disease expert are all involved not only in the postoperative care but also in the preoperative care.

Initial evaluation includes a thorough review of past medical history and a complete physical examination. The cause of the liver disease should be confirmed. Blood tests should include a complete blood count, electrolytes, coagulation studies, liver function tests, total protein and albumin levels, blood type, and viral serologies. Each organ system is evaluated and consultations made as indicated. In addition, the patient's immunization record is reviewed. Live vaccines are avoided when possible to prevent complications with immunosuppressants after the transplantation.

In-depth psychosocial assessment is performed. Counseling is available from psychologists and social work staffs. The family is emotionally prepared for the length of the patient's operation, and postoperative hospitalization, and the reality of lifelong postoperative care. In addition, any questions the family has regarding financial considerations are addressed.

Nutritional evaluation is important to identify any nutritional deficiencies. Many patients with liver disease have nutritional deficiencies. Specifically, patients may be in negative nitrogen balance with decreased stores of protein, including deficient levels of branched chain and essential amino acids.[43] Poor nutritional status is correlated with poor surgical outcome.[64] Important factors to measure are serum albumin level, height, weight, triceps skin thickness, and midarm muscle area.[43] If supplementation is needed, enteral feedings are the preferred route, and oral feedings are used when tolerated by the patient. Some children may require tube feedings to meet nutritional requirements. If supplementation by the gastrointestinal tract is impossible, parental nutrition can effectively deliver calories but has increased morbidity over enteral supplementation.

To evaluate the surgical anatomy, an abdominal Doppler ultrasound is performed. Other imaging modalities, such as angiography, venography, computed tomography scanning, and magnetic resonance imaging, may be useful in delineating abnormalities.

Prior to operation, any coagulation disorders are corrected and the blood bank is notified well in advance to prepare units of packed cells, platelets, and fresh frozen plasma for the operation.

DONOR LIVER PROCUREMENT

Although a few patients undergo living-related liver transplants, the vast majority of patients require cadaveric liver transplant. Allocation of donor livers is determined by multifactorial criteria as determined by the United Network for Organs Sharing.[5] These patients are placed on the transplant waiting list and are stratified into a priority list of four groups to minimize deaths of those on the list (Table 2). Status 4 patients have the highest priority for an organ, whereas status I patients have the lowest. Within each status, patients who have been on the list longer have higher priority for a given organ. Priority is given to patients who are at centers within the same region in which the organ was procured.

In addition, ABO blood group match is taken into consideration. Priority is given to patients who have blood types that match the donor organ over patients who have blood groups that are compatible with the potential organ. ABO-incompatible organs generally are used only in emergent cases. Transplantation of ABO incompatible livers is more successful in the infant, but the risk of graft failure increases with age. The results with ABO-incompatible donor livers has been mixed, with some centers reporting poor results, whereas others report good results.[58, 98] Unlike kidney transplants, histocompatibility matching has not proven to be a factor in organ or patient survival and is not used as a factor in determining liver allocation.

Size-matched organs are given preference in organ allocation; however, because of the severe scarcity of pediatric donor livers, techniques are used to reduce the size of adult donor livers to fit pediatric recipients. Reduced-size liver grafting was first introduced in 1984 by Bismuth and Houssin.[9] The donor liver is excised and then reduced ex vivo on the back table. Portions of the liver that have been used include the left lobe, the left lateral segment, the right lobe, and the extended right lobe (right lobe and medial segment of left lobe).[7, 14] Frequently, interposition grafts are required to complete vascular anastomoses. Although initial reports showed poor results from reduced-sized liver grafting, recent reports have shown results equaling those of full-sized liver grafts.[16, 28, 53]

Split-liver transplantation is a variation of the reduced-sized grafting technique.[33] The liver is divided into right and left lobes, and then both are used for transplantation. The obvious advantage of this technique is a doubling of the potential donor liver pool. Initial reports of this technique showed results inferior to those of reduced-sized or whole-organ liver transplantation.[33, 93]

Living-related liver transplantation was first performed in 1988 in Brazil by Raia and coworkers.[73] The first series was reported by Broelsch and coworkers in Chicago.[15] The technique has been used predominantly

Table 2. UNOS CATEGORIES FOR LIVER WAITING LIST PATIENTS

Status	Description
Status I	End-stage liver disease, but at home and functioning normally
Status II	Requires continuous medical care but not continuous hospitalization
Status III	Continuously hospitalized, but not in the intensive care unit
Status IV	In the intensive care unit with a life expectancy of less than 7 days unless transplanted

for pediatric liver transplantation and has found particular utility in Japan, where cadaveric liver transplantation is not performed. Series from Chicago; Kyoto, Japan; and Hamburg, Germany show results comparable with cadaveric liver transplantation.[13, 15, 69] The benefits of living-related liver transplantation include increasing the donor pool and timing of the surgery to maximize the recipient's preoperative condition. These benefits are weighed against the risk to the donor.

The segment of the donor's liver that is excised for transplantation is either the left lobe or the left lateral segment of the left lobe, depending on size requirements. Immediately after the segment has been excised, it is flushed through with UW preservation solution. Frequently, interposition grafts are required to complete the vascular anastomoses. Saphenous vein from the donor is harvested for this purpose. Figure 1 shows the implanted liver.

OPERATIVE PROCEDURE

For whole-organ transplantation, operative techniques are based on those originally formulated by Starzl and colleagues.[86] The patient is brought to the operating room and anesthetized. Antibiotic prophylaxis

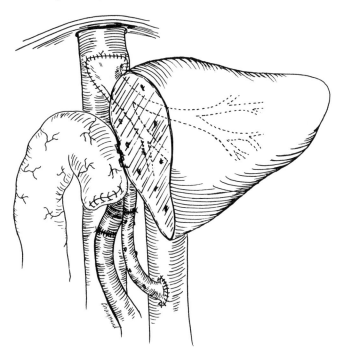

Figure 1. Living-related liver transplantation of left lateral segment with Roux-en-Y biliary conduit.

is given. Multiple large bore intravenous lines for rapid fluid infusion and a central venous line for monitoring central pressures and for giving medications are placed. The patient is widely prepped and draped. The abdomen is then entered through a bilateral subcostal incision with a superior extension of this incision in the midline to the xyphoid process. Several factors may complicate the initial part of the operation. Excessive bleeding may occur owing to inadequate clotting factors and varicosities of the abdominal wall and abdominal viscera due to portal hypertension. Secondly, many children needing a liver transplantation have undergone a previous abdominal operation, such as a Kasai portoenterostomy, and may have adhesions. Careful hemostasis is achieved to prevent blood loss and further consumption of clotting factors.

Once the abdomen has been entered, the porta hepatis is dissected free. The hepatic artery must be dissected and its origin noted, because anatomic variations are common. The common bile duct and portal vein are dissected and identified also. The common bile duct is divided at this point. If the patient has had a previous Kasai portoenterostomy, the Roux-en-Y limb must be dissected free and taken down. The Roux-en-Y limb may be used for the biliary anastomosis to the new liver, or a new one created if the prior reconstruction is damaged or inadequate.

The liver is then mobilized by dividing the left and right triangular ligaments. Retroperitoneal dissection is then performed. The infrahepatic and suprahepatic vena cava are identified and vascular control is achieved. In older children, veno-veno bypass may be used to minimize hemodynamic instability. In cases in which reduced-size or living-related donors are used, the inferior vena cava is not divided. Rather, the hepatic veins are dissected free and ligated, leaving the vena cava intact.

Because clamping of the vena cava may cause hypotension by decreasing venous return, the vena cava is test-clamped. If the patient becomes hypotensive, fluid is given until the patient can tolerate the clamping. The portal vein, hepatic artery, and infrahepatic and suprahepatic vena cava are then clamped and divided. The diseased liver is excised. Any bleeding caused by the retroperitoneal dissection is then easily exposed and controlled.

The donor liver is then placed. The superior and inferior caval anastomoses are performed first. In the case of living-related or reduced-size grafts, an end-to-side anastomosis from the origin of the hepatic veins is performed. The graft is flushed with a cold saline solution from the portal vein to wash out UW solution that is high in potassium and lactic acid from ischemia. After flushing, the portal anastomosis is completed, re-establishing perfusion through the liver. Arterial reconstruction can be achieved with either a Carrel patch of donor aorta or celiac axis to hepatic artery or as an aortic conduit to the infrarenal aorta of the recipient.

The method of biliary reconstruction is variable and depends on the existing anatomy. A primary duct-to-duct anastomosis sometimes is possible and is performed over a T-tube stent. Frequently in children, this is not possible because of the small size of the common bile duct.

In these cases, a Roux-en-Y loop of jejunum is used for the biliary anastomosis. If present, the gallbladder is routinely removed to prevent stone formation.

Once again, careful hemostasis is achieved. The area is widely drained with closed-suction catheters, and the abdomen closed in layers. Figure 2 shows the implanted liver with a Roux-en-Y biliary reconstruction.

POSTOPERATIVE CARE

After the transplantation, patients are taken to the intensive care unit. Respiratory and hemodynamic status is continuously monitored. Antibiotic prophylaxis is continued. Intravenous cyclosporine and methylprednisolone are given as immunosuppressive agents. Many groups also use azathioprine as a third agent. Success with FK506 as the primary

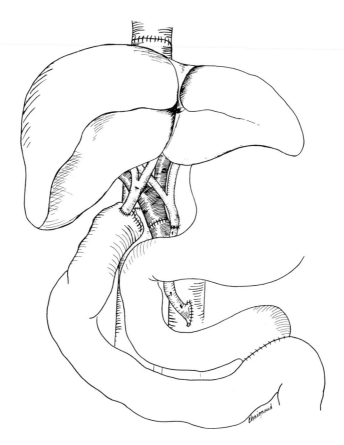

Figure 2. Whole-organ liver transplantation with Roux-en-Y biliary conduit.

immunosuppressant in pediatric patients with liver transplantation has also been reported.[95] Serial examinations of the complete blood count, chemistries, coagulation factors, and liver function tests are performed. If the patient has external biliary drainage, bile production is monitored. Good bile flow is another indicator for graft function.

The patient is extubated the following day if standard extubation criteria are met. An abdominal Doppler ultrasound is performed to assess patency of the portal vein and hepatic artery on postoperative day 1. Surgical wounds and catheter sites are observed on a daily basis to monitor for signs of possible infection. Medications are changed to the oral form when the patient is able to tolerate them. Approximately 1 week after transplantation, if a T tube is present, a cholangiogram is performed to determine whether the bile duct is patent and has no leakage. The T tube is then clamped if the cholangiogram is satisfactory. Cyclosporine doses are adjusted according to the level and hepatic and renal function. Optimal cyclosporine levels vary from center to center. The average hospitalization after transplantation in one series was reported at 37.6 days.[54]

IMMUNOSUPPRESSANTS

Immunosuppressant regimens have improved since the early days of liver transplantation. In particular, the use of cyclosporine and FK506 has greatly increased graft and patient survival rates. Cyclosporine and FK506 allow the use of lower doses of corticosteroids, which is of particular importance in the pediatric population. Cyclosporine or FK506, moderate doses of corticosteroids, and, in some centers, azathioprine comprise the usual maintenance immunosuppressants for liver transplant recipients. FK506, steroid pulses, antilymphocyte globulin (ALG), antithymocyte globulin (ATG), and OKT3 frequently are used during rejection. The standard regimen used at The Children's Hospital in Boston is cyclosporine and steroids with azathioprine, which are added after an episode of rejection. Steroid pulse therapy and OKT3 are used to treat rejection. Descriptions of the most common immunosuppressants used today follows.

Cyclosporine

The discovery of cyclosporine in Switzerland from the fungus *Tolypocladium inflatum Gams* in 1972 and its subsequent clinical use in 1979 were among the most important advances in transplantation.[10, 23] Cyclosporine is used effectively in kidney, heart, lung, liver, and bone marrow transplantation. Cyclosporine is an 11 amino acid, cyclic peptide that selectively inhibits interleukin (IL)-2 production by T helper cells.[52] IL-2 causes the proliferation and differentiation of T helper and T cytotoxic and suppresser cells. IL-2 also has stimulatory effects on macrophages, B lymphocytes, NK, and LAK cells. The immunosuppressive effects seem to be specific for lymphocytes and seem to have minimal effect on granulocytes.

Cyclosporine is given both orally and intravenously. The relative bioequivalence of the oral form to the intravenous form is 1:3.[52] It is poorly soluble in water and is usually given as a suspension or dissolved in oil. Of note, cyclosporine is given in a glass cup and not a plastic cup because it binds to plastic. Its absorption from the gastrointestinal tract is often unpredictable. It is metabolized in the liver by the cytochrome P-450 system and excreted through the bile. Significant reabsorption occurs in the intestine, leading to an enterohepatic cycle. Its absorption is affected by gastrointestinal disorders, such as diarrhea, that decrease absorption. In addition, increased bile flow leads to increased excretion of cyclosporine, especially when bile is drained externally. Typically, as bile output via the T tube increases in the immediate postoperative period, the cyclosporine dosage required to maintain the same level is increased. Many drugs affect cyclosporine levels by altering its metabolism by the cytochrome P-450 system. Some drugs, such as phenytoin and phenobarbital, induce this system, increase excretion, and decrease cyclosporine levels.[52] Other drugs, most notably the calcium channel blockers diltiazem and verapamil, compete with cyclosporine for excretion and increase levels.[52] The calcium channel blockers are helpful also in decreasing the hypertensive effects often seen with cyclosporine. Some of these drugs are used to decrease the amount of cyclosporine needed to attain a given therapeutic level. Table 3 provides drugs that affect cyclosporine levels.

Adverse effects include nephrotoxicity, hepatotoxicity, hyperkalemia, hirsutism, neurotoxicities, and hypertension.[52] The most common side effect is nephrotoxicity, which is observed in as many as 80% to 90% of patients.[49] If renal function is severely compromised, it may become necessary to reduce the dose of cyclosporine or even discontinue it. Neurologic toxicity also is commonly observed and is manifested by tremulousness, headaches, and, rarely, seizures. Cyclosporine trough levels in the blood are checked 12 or 24 hours after dosing to maintain therapeutic levels and to monitor for toxic levels.[35] Cyclosporine hepatotoxicity may be difficult to differentiate from rejection.

Table 3. COMMONLY USED DRUGS THAT AFFECT CYCLOSPORINE LEVELS

Drugs that Increase Levels	Drugs that Decrease Levels
Diltiazem	Rifampin
Ketoconazole	Phenytoin
Erythromycin	Phenobarbital
Verapamil	Carbamazepine
Metoclopramide	Isoniazid

FK506

FK506, a macrolide antibiotic, was discovered in 1987 in Japan from the fungus *Streptomyces tsukubaensis*.[57] Although structurally different, its mechanism of action is similar to that of cyclosporine in vitro and in vivo.[17] Like cyclosporine, IL-2 production is inhibited as is T lymphocyte stimulation and proliferation. Compared with cyclosporine, it is approximately 100 times more potent.[17]

FK506 can be given both orally and intravenously. It is well absorbed orally. It is metabolized in the liver by the cytochrome P-450 system and is excreted in the bile and urine. Drugs that increase FK506 levels include cimetidine, cyclosporine, fluconazole, ketoconazole, verapamil, doxycycline, and erythromycin. Drugs that reduce FK506 levels include carbamazepine, corticosteroids, isoniazid, phenobarbital, and phenytoin.[29] Adverse side effects are nephrotoxicity, neurotoxicity, hypertension, diabetes, and hyperkalemia.[17]

The early data from Starzl's group in Pittsburgh showed increased survival in adult and pediatric populations when cyclosporine was replaced with FK506 in the immunosuppressive regimen.[96] In addition, FK506 was able to reverse rejection in some cases in which cyclosporine was being used as the primary immunosuppressant.[95] They also showed lower rates of side effects, including infection.[2, 44, 94] Other centers have not shown similar beneficial effects of FK506 over cyclosporine, and its superiority in liver transplantation remains controversial.

Corticosteroids

Corticosteroids were among the first immunosuppressants successfully used in allograft transplantation and continue to be used today. Although corticosteroids rarely are effective alone in preventing rejection, as seen by early transplant experiences, they act synergistically with other immunosuppressive agents. In addition, high-dose steroids are effective in reversing rejection and are frequently given as a first-line drug for rejection.

Corticosteroids act by suppressing the immune response by multiple mechanisms. IL-1 and IL-2 production is inhibited as is the expression of histocompatibility antigens, decreasing the T-cell–mediated immune response.[32, 42, 48] Steroids also inhibit differentiation of monocytes into macrophages and exert anti-inflammatory effects by inhibiting arachidonic acid metabolism.[32]

Complications of corticosteroid use include growth retardation, cushingoid habitus, hypertension, hyperglycemia, weight gain, peptic ulceration, intestinal perforation, psychosis, pancreatitis, delayed wound healing, and osteoporosis. The use of multiple-drug immunosuppressant regimens in organ transplantation allows use of relatively small doses of corticosteroids and, thus, minimizes the adverse side effects.

Corticosteroids can be given intravenously (i.e., methylprednisolone or hydrocortisone) or orally (prednisone, prednisolone). They are given intravenously until the patient can take oral medications.

Azathioprine

Azathioprine was used in the first human liver transplantation in 1963.[86] It was the cornerstone, together with corticosteroids, for most immunosuppressive regimens for liver transplantation until cyclosporine became widely used. It is still frequently used as part of triple-therapy regimens together with prednisone and either cyclosporine or FK506.

Azathioprine is a purine analog that interferes with nucleic acid synthesis. As such, its effect is greatest on cells that are rapidly dividing. Its main immunosuppressive effect is the inhibition of T-cell activation and proliferation.[29] The major toxicity is bone-marrow suppression, in particular, neutropenia.[29] The complete blood count must be carefully monitored and the dose of azathioprine adjusted according to the white blood cell count. Other side effects include pruritus, hepatitis, pancreatitis, and gastrointestinal upset. Allopurinol inhibits metabolism of azathioprine, and, to prevent toxicity, the two drugs should not be given together.

Antilymphocyte Globulin and Antithymocyte Globulin

Antilymphocyte globulin and ATG are polyclonal antibody preparations derived from animals immunized against human lymphocytes or thymocytes, respectively.[72] Antilymphocyte globulin and ATG have been used as part of multidrug maintenance regimens, as replacement for cyclosporine during cyclosporine toxicity, and to reverse rejection. When injected, they cause a sharp decrease in the white blood cell count and the function and number of T cells.[45] Side effects associated with the injection include fever, chills, rashes, and, occasionally, anaphylaxis. Adverse effects of the drugs are neutropenia, thrombocytopenia, and severe opportunistic viral infections.[29]

OKT3

OKT3 is a monoclonal antibody preparation made against the CD3 antigen, which is expressed on all T cells. Injection of OKT3 causes a rapid and severe decrease in the number of circulating T cells. Side effects include fever, pulmonary edema with respiratory failure, and neutropenia.[25, 34] OKT3 has been shown to be highly effective in treating rejection.[26]

At The Children's Hospital in Boston, a skin test is performed prior to the first dose of OKT3 to test for an allergic response. If this test is negative, the patient is premedicated with acetaminophen, diphenhydra-mine, and methylprednisolone. The dose given is 2.5 mg IV for patients weighing fewer than 30 kg and 5.0 mg for patients weighing more than 30 kg. Patients are closely monitored for signs of an allergic response or anaphylaxis. Treatment with OKT3 is continued for 7 to 14 days.

COMPLICATIONS

Primary Graft Nonfunction

One of the more serious early complications of pediatric liver trans-plantation is primary graft nonfunction. Patients may have hemody-namic instability, renal failure, increasing encephalophathy, acidosis, coagulopathy, and worsening liver-function tests. Primary graft non-function may be secondary to poor graft preservation, reperfusion injury, humoral rejection, or thrombosis of the portal vein or hepatic artery. The incidence of primary graft nonfunction varies in series from 5% to 38%.[70, 98] The incidence of hepatic artery thrombosis has been reported at 7% to 33%.[20, 54, 76] Smaller patients seem to be at higher risk for thrombosis of the hepatic artery.[98] Some of the grafts recover; how-ever, the prognosis is poor in severe cases unless retransplantation is performed. Some have advocated total hepatectomy in the most severe cases to improve the patient's hemodynamic status while waiting for a new donor organ.

Hypertension

The most common complication after liver transplantation is hyper-tension. The etiology is not completely understood, but the use of cyclosporine and corticosteroids or represents two of the causes. The use of such antihypertensive agents as thiazide diuretics, calcium channel blockers, beta-blockers, or ACE inhibitors may be necessary to control blood pressure.

Rejection

Although the use of cyclosporine dramatically decreases episodes of rejection, acute and chronic rejection is relatively common. Hyperacute rejection, thought to be caused by preformed antibodies, is rare in liver transplantation. Acute rejection occurs in 40% to 90% of patients following transplantation and is mediated by T cells.[8, 20, 54, 89] Signs and symptoms may include fever, an elevation in the bilirubin, transami-nases, alkaline phosphatase, and an increased prothrombin time. Bile production may decrease, and the bile may become thinner and lighter. Rejection may be difficult to differentiate from other causes of worsening hepatic function, such as bacterial, viral, or fungal infection, or cyclosporine toxicity. In addition, many cases of rejection are associated with infection. If no clear cause is evident, a biopsy of the liver usually is helpful.[29] Histologically, invasion of lymphocytes and mononuclear cells occurs, and infiltration of and damage to the bile ducts with vasculitis is present. Acute rejection is graded into mild, moderate, and severe categories based on the degree of inflammation and damage. Acute rejection becomes less frequent and milder as the time from transplantation increases.

The treatment of acute rejection usually begins with a bolus or recycling of high-dose corticosteroids. Corticosteroids can reverse rejection in 50% to 75% of cases.[26] Rejection refractory to treatment with corticosteroids is treated with OKT3, ALG, ATG, or FK506. OKT3 reverses rejection in more than 90% of cases.[26]

Chronic rejection is manifested by gradual destruction of bile ducts and obliterative arteriopathy. A gradual rise in liver function tests indicative of biliary obstruction occurs. Histologically, the degree of inflammatory cell infiltration is less than that seen with acute rejection. Progressive destruction of the bile ducts leads to the term *vanishing bile duct syndrome*. In addition, arteries may become narrowed by the presence of subendothelial foam cells. The treatment is to control the rejection by increasing or adding immunosuppressants. Severe chronic rejection is difficult to treat and may necessitate retransplantation.

Infection

Viral, fungal, and bacterial infections are a major cause of morbidity and mortality after liver transplantation. The use of immunosuppressants, chronic malnutrition, indwelling catheters, and transfusions are all reasons for the increased risk of infection. The incidence of infection varies in pediatric series from 40% to 73%, and many children suffer from more than one episode.[38, 46, 54] Although the risk decreases over time, opportunistic infections remain a lifelong hazard for liver transplantation patients.

Bacterial sources are the most common cause for infection in pediatric liver transplantation.[38] The most commonly infected sites are the abdomen, the bloodstream, the surgical wound, and the lung. Bacterial infections commonly are associated with problems with the biliary or vascular anastomoses. In addition, cholangitis from the biliary reconstruction may be a source of infection. The most common organisms are gram-negative bacilli, enterococci, and staphylococci.

Treatment consists of appropriate antibiotic coverage and drainage of an abscess if it exists. If any underlying cause, such as an anastomotic stricture or thrombosis, is found, it is treated also.

Viral infection is second to bacterial infection in incidence in the pediatric population.[38] Cytomegalovirus and Epstein-Barr virus (EBV) are the two most common viral pathogens after liver transplantation.

Many normal children and even more normal adults are seropositive with CMV and EBV and are asymptomatic. Although some patients who have undergone liver transplantation may also remain asymptomatic on seroconversion to CMV and EBV, in others, symptomatic infection develops. Other less common viral pathogens include herpes simplex, varicella, adenovirus, and respiratory syncytial virus.

Cytomegalovirus is one of the more significant pathogens in liver transplantation.[12] In patients who are seropositive, inection may develop owing to reactivation of latent CMV. In patients who are seronegative, infection may develop secondarily owing to a seropositive organ or blood from a seropositive donor. The incidence rate of developing a CMV infection after transplantation is higher in seropositive patients. Because of the lower incidence rate of CMV seropositivity in the pediatric population compared with the adult population, the incidence rate of CMV infection after liver transplantation in children is lower. However, CMV infection in patients who are initially seronegative is more severe than in patients who are initially seropositive.[38]

Common sites of CMV infection in liver transplant recipients are the lungs, the gastrointestinal tract, and the liver and biliary tree.[38] Clinically, the diagnosis may be difficult to make. Symptoms range from a mild viral syndrome to fulminant disseminated CMV infection. Fever, malaise, abdominal pain, worsening liver function tests, diarrhea, cough, and neutropenia may be seen. If the infection is in the liver, the symptoms may be difficult to differentiate from rejection. Definitive diagnosis can be made by bronchoscopy and bronchoalveolar lavage, endoscopy and biopsy, or liver biopsy, depending on the site of infection. Histologic specimens show inclusion bodies. The detection of an early antigen from blood samples also may be helpful in the diagnosis.[77]

The most effective treatment of CMV is ganciclovir, which inhibits CMV DNA polymerase. It is effective in treating 72% to 85% of CMV infections.[90] The principal toxicity is neutropenia, which is reversible after stopping the drug.[90] Attempts at prophylaxis have included acyclovir and CMV immune globulin. The results of prophylaxis remain unclear.

Epstein-Barr virus is another major viral pathogen in liver transplantation.[12] Like CMV, EBV may reactivate after liver transplantation. Also, EBV seropositivity is much higher in the adult population. Primary infection, however, is more common in the pediatric population, whereas reactivation is more common in adults.[38] Epstein-Barr virus predisposes to lymphoproliferative disorders. Clinically, lymphoproliferative disorders may manifest as a benign mononucleosis syndrome or may present as a monoclonal lymphoma. It may also present as a polyclonal B-cell proliferation that may progress to lymphoma. The incidence of lymphoproliferative disorders in children is 4%.[47] In addition, EBV may cause hepatitis.

Diagnosis of EBV infection is made by confirming EBV seropositivity in the serum and by staining tissue for special markers. Primary infection seems to carry a greater incidence of lymphoproliferative disorders than does reactivation, predisposing the pediatric liver transplantation patient to a higher rate of lymphoproliferative disorders.

The treatment for EBV-related lymphoproliferative disorders is limited. Antiviral agents, such as acyclovir and ganciclovir, seem to have little efficacy. The lymphoproliferative disorders may respond to a reduction in the immunosuppressive regimen.

Fungal infections are less common than either bacterial or viral infections.[38] The great majority of fungal infections are caused by *Candida albicans*. *Candida* may reside as normal inhabitants of bowel flora, and this serves as a source of infection in liver transplantation recipients. The use of antibacterials increases the incidence of candidal infection. The most common site of infection is intra-abdominal. The morbidity and mortality rates associated with candidal infections are high but are at least partially attributable to the high association of candidal infections with bacterial and viral infections and other intra-abdominal complications. The most effective treatment is with intravenous amphotericin B.

Malignancy

Various tumors have an increased incidence in patients with liver transplantation due to the use of immunosuppressants. Skin cancer is the most common neoplasm after transplantation, and patients on immunosuppression should avoid excess sun exposure.[11] Squamous cell carcinoma is more common than basal cell carcinoma. Genitourinary carcinomas and carcinoma of the digestive tract are among the most common types of cancers seen after transplantation. Lymphoproliferative disorders may be the most well-studied tumors after transplantation and were discussed earlier with EBV. Kaposi's sarcoma, rarely observed in immunocompetent patients, has a greatly increased rate in patients after transplantation.

QUALITY OF LIFE

The prognosis for end-stage liver disease in children has been greatly improved with liver transplantation. Liver transplantation increases survival and decreases both the number of hospitalizations and the total number of days spent hospitalized when compared with pretransplantation periods.[107] In addition, children take fewer medications postoperatively than preoperatively.[107]

Liver transplantation has had a successful impact on growth also.[78, 106] Studies have shown that most children show a period of accelerated growth after transplantation and that most children are able to attain height within the normal range.[78] In addition, one study showed that nutritional status is greatly improved by transplantation, as evidenced by an increase in the mean serum albumin level from 3.1 g/dL pretransplantation to 4.4 g/dL post-transplantation.[78]

Cognitive and developmental skills seem to be improved also. Motor, behavioral, and social skills have been shown to improve post-transplantation. More than 75% of children in one study were within one grade or in grades appropriate to their age.[106]

Neuropsychological deficits have been recorded in children after liver transplantation, however. One study compared children after liver transplantation with children with cystic fibrosis to control for some of the effects of chronic disease.[87] Children in the liver transplantation group scored lower in most parameters, including learning and memory, academic achievement, abstraction and concept formation, visual–spatial function, and motor function. The two groups scored equally in the areas of verbal intelligence, alertness and concentration, motor perception, and sensory perception. Some of these deficits have been theorized to be the effects of toxins from liver disease on the developing brain. Children in whom liver disease presented at an earlier age have poorer mental function than those in whom liver disease presented later.[88] Decreasing cerebral perfusion pressure during the operation is theorized to contribute to some of the cognitive deficits. In addition, medications such as corticosteroids and cyclosporine are thought to contribute to growth and developmental deficiencies.

The child and family also may suffer psychological difficulties. After an initial period of euphoria, the family may become disillusioned and suffer feelings of hopelessness when the patient suffers postoperative complications and the reality of lifelong immunosuppression becomes apparent. The child may suffer from bouts of anxiety and depression.[103]

Thus, although liver transplantation greatly improves the quality of life in most children, and most children are able to attain a normal level of function, cognitive, social, and physical development remain deficient. Although the long-term effects are difficult to measure as yet, they will become more apparent as the number of children growing into adulthood after liver transplantation increases.

EXPERIMENTAL TREATMENT

To address the limited number of donor organs, researchers are investigating a variety of temporary and permanent treatments for liver disease. Many groups have attempted to produce a bioartificial liver that could treat liver disease similar to the way a dialysis machine treats renal disease.[67, 92, 105] Most of the groups use porcine hepatocytes or a transformed line of hepatocytes housed in a bioreactor allowing plasma from patients with liver failure to perfuse through it. Several groups have taken their bioartificial liver into clinical trials to treat severe acute liver failure.[75, 91] They can be used either as a bridge to liver transplantation or to allow recovery of the native liver. Other approaches to temporarily treating severe liver disease have included cross-circulation of plasma with other humans and ex vivo perfusion with porcine livers.[19, 66]

The use of xenografts was attempted by Starzl's group in Pittsburgh.[79] Two patients with end-stage liver disease had liver xenografts from baboons. Baboons were chosen as donors partially because they are believed to be immune to hepatitis B. The cause of one of the patient's liver disease was hepatitis B. That patient survived for 70 days postoperatively. Both patients were given an extra immunosuppressive agent, cyclophosphamide, which was thought to decrease the humoral component for rejection. Humoral mediated rejection is thought to be important in xenograft transplantation.

Hepatocellular transplantation has long been investigated as a method of either temporary or permanent replacement of diseased liver. Many groups have attempted hepatocellular injection into the spleens or livers of experimental animals. A novel approach to hepatocellular transplantation has been the application of tissue engineering techniques.[59] Hepatocytes are seeded onto biodegradable polymer that serves as a temporary extracellular matrix and to induce vascular in-growth.[62] The seeded polymer is then implanted into a vascular-rich area, such as the mesentery of small intestine. This model has been shown to partially correct liver enzyme deficiencies in experimental animal models.[6] Hepatocellular transplantation is a particularly attractive potential procedure in the pediatric population in which many transplants are performed for a single enzyme deficiency.[97]

Continued research in experimental treatments is important as donor scarcity worsens. Despite expanding the donor pool by such means as living-related liver transplants or split-liver grafting, more than 500 people died in 1993 while awaiting liver transplantation, 88 of whom were in the pediatric population.[5] A total of 30,000 patients die each year of liver disease.[3] In addition, the median number of days that patients await a transplantation has gradually increased. In 1993, the median number of days liver transplant candidates waited for an organ was 142 days.[5] The lengthy wait often causes increased preoperative and postoperative morbidity and mortality.

SUMMARY

Since the advent of the use of cyclosporine in the immunosuppressant regimen, liver transplantation has been proven to be a safe and effective treatment for a variety of childhood liver diseases. The 1-year survival rate for liver transplants in patients fewer than 18 years of age is 80% and in some recent series approaches 90%. The quality of life of most children who undergo liver transplantation is greatly improved, and most children go on to lead productive, normal lives; however, liver transplantation and postoperative immunosuppression are associated with significant attendant morbidity. Together with treating possible complications common to all liver transplant patients, the issue of attaining normal growth and development is critical to a successful outcome. With this regard, careful long-term management of the immunosuppressive regimen and maintaining adequate nutritional status are especially important. The patient must be closely followed postoperatively by the transplant coordinator with the pediatrician and the transplant team.

To ensure more effective treatment of liver diseases in the future, research must be continued in the areas of operative and perioperative management, immunosuppressive drugs, and the treatment of opportunistic infections. In addition, research into new treatments offers hope for cure with less morbidity and mortality.

References

1. Adelman S: Prognosis of uncorrected biliary atresia: an update. J Pediatr Surg 13:389–391, 1978
2. Alessiani M, Kusne S, Fung JJ: CMV infection in liver transplantation under cyclosporine or FK 506 immunosuppression. Transplant Proc 23:3035–3037, 1991
3. American Liver Foundation, Vital Statistics of the United States, vol 2, part A, 1988
4. Andrews WS, Wanek E, Fyock B, et al: Pediatric liver transplantation: A 3-year experience. J Pediatr Surg 24:77–82, 1989
5. Annual Report of the US Scientific Registry of Transplant Recipients and the Organ Procurement and Transplantation Network. 1994
6. Asonuma K, Gilbert JC, Stein JE, et al: Quantitation of transplanted hepatic mass necessary to cure the Gunn rat model of hyperbilirubinemia. J Pediatr Surg 27:298–301, 1992
7. Badger IL, Czerniak A, Beath S, et al: Hepatic transplantation in children using reduced size allografts. Br J Surg 79:47–49, 1992
8. Becht MB, Pedersen SH, Ryckman FC, et al: Growth and nutritional management of pediatric patients after orthotopic liver transplantation. Gastroenertol Clin North Am 22:367–380, 1993
9. Bismuth H, Houssin D: Reduced-size orthotopic liver transplantation in children. Surgery 95:36–72, 1984
10. Borel JF: Comparative study of in vitro and in vivo drug effects on cell-mediated cytotoxicity. Immunology 31:631–641, 1976
11. Braun DK, Davies M, Lowes JR, et al: Medical Complications. In Neuberger J, Lucey MR (eds): Liver transplantation: Practice and management. London, BMJ Publishing Group, 1994, pp 227–278
12. Breinig MK, Zitelli B, Starzl TE, et al: Epstein-Barr virus, cytomegalovirus, and other viral infections in children after liver transplantation. J Infect Dis 156:273–279, 1987
13. Broelsch CE, Burdelski M, Rogiers X, et al: Living donor for liver transplantation. Hepatology 20:49S–55S, 1994
14. Broelsch CE, Emond JC, Thistlethwaite JR, et al: Liver transplantation with reduced-size donor organs. Transplantation 45:519–523, 1988
15. Broelsch CE, Emond JC, Whitington PF, et al: Application of reduced-size liver transplants as split grafts, auxiliary orthotopic grafts, and living related segmental transplants. Ann Surg 212:368–377, 1990
16. Broelsch CE, Whitington PF, Emond JC: Evolution and future perspectives for reduced-size hepatic transplantation. Surg Gynecol Obstet 171:353–359, 1990
17. Bumgardner GL, Roberts JP: New immunosuppressive agents. Gastroenterol Clin North Am 22:421–449, 1993
18. Burdelski M, Schmidt K, Hoyer PF, et al: Liver transplantation in children: The Hannover experience. Transplant Proc 19:3277–3281, 1987
19. Burnell JM, Dawborn JK, Epstein RB, et al: Acute hepatic coma treated by cross-circulation or exchange transfusion. N Engl J Med 276:935–943, 1967

20. Busuttil RW, Seu P, Millis JM, et al: Liver transplantation in children. Ann Surg 213:48–57, 1991
21. Busuttil RW, Shaked A, Millis JM, et al: One thousand liver transplants. Ann Surg 219:490–499, 1994
22. Calne R: Contraindications to liver transplantation. Hepatology 20:3–4S, 1994
23. Calne RY, Rolles K, White DJG, et al: Cyclosporin A initially as the only immunosuppressant in 34 recipients of cadaveric organs: 32 kidneys, 2 pancreases, and 2 livers. Lancet 2:1033–1036, 1979
24. Consensus statement on indication for liver transplantation: Paris, June 22-23, 1993. Hepatology 20:639–685, 1994
25. Cosimi AB: Clinical development of orthoclone OKT3. Transplant Proc 19:7–16, 1987
26. Cosimi AB, Cho SI, Delmonico FL, et al: A randomized clinical trial comparing OKT3 and steroids for treatment of hepatic allograft rejection. Transplant Proc 19:2431–2433, 1987
27. Davies M: Immunosuppressive drugs. In Neuberger J, Lucey MR (eds): Liver transplantation: Practice and management. London, BMJ Publishing Group, 1994, pp 190–209
28. de Hemptinne B, de Ville de Goyet J, Kestens PJ, et al: Volume reduction of the liver graft before orthotopic transplantation: Report of a clinical experience in 11 cases. Transplant Proc 19:3317–3322, 1987
29. de Ville de Goyet J: Monitoring of orthotopic liver transplantation in children by means of serial graft biopsies. Transplant Proc 19:3323–3326, 1987
30. Denmark SW, Shaw BW Jr, Starzl TE, et al: Veno-venous bypass without systemic anticoagulation in canine and human liver transplantation. Surgical Forum 31:380–382, 1983
31. Desmet VJ, Callea F: Cholestatic syndromes of infancy and childhood. In Zakim D, Boyer TD (eds): Hepatology, vol 2. Philadelphia, WB Saunders, 1990, pp 1355–1395
32. Dupont E, Wybran J, Toussaint C: Glucocorticosteroids and organ transplantation. Transplantation 37:331–335, 1984
33. Emond JC, Whitington PF, Thistlethwaite JR, et al: Transplantation of two patients with one liver. Ann Surg 212:14–22, 1990
34. Esquivel CO, Fung JJ, Markus B, et al: OKT3 in the reversal of acute hepatic allograft rejection. Transplant Proc 19:2443–2446, 1987
35. Freese D, Snover D, Ascher N, et al: Cyclosporin-A in prevention of rejection for long-term liver transplants. Hepatology 5:1020, 1985
36. Fung JJ, Markus BH, Gordon CO, et al: Impact of orthoclone OKT3 on liver transplantation. Transplant Proc 19:37–44, 1987
37. Gartner JC, Zitelli BJ, Malatack JJ, et al: Orthotopic liver transplantation in children: Two-year experience with 47 patients. Pediatrics 74:140–145, 1984
38. George DL, Arnow PM, Fox A, et al: Patterns of infection after pediatric liver transplantation. Am J Dis Child 146:924–929, 1992
39. Ghisham FK, Greene HL: Alpha 1-antitrypsin deficiency. In Zakim D, Boyer TD (eds): Hepatology, vol 2. Philadelphia, WB Saunders, 1990, pp 1349–1355
40. Ghisham FK, Greene HL: Inborn errors of metabolism that lead to permanent liver injury. In Zakim D, Boyer TD (eds): Hepatology, vol 2. Philadelphia, WB Saunders, 1990, pp 1301–1348
41. Gollan JL: Copper metabolism, Wilson's disease and hepatic copper toxicosis. In Zakim D, Boyer TD (eds): Hepatology, vol 2. Philadelphia, WB Saunders, 1990, pp 1249–1272
42. Goodwin JS, Durgaprasadarao A, Sierakowski S, et al: Mechanism of action of glucocorticosteroids. J Clin Invest 77:1244–1250, 1986
43. Goulet OJ, de Ville de Goyet J, Otte JB, et al: Preoperative nutritional evaluation and support for liver transplantation in children. Transplant Proc 19:3249–3255, 1987
44. Green M, Tzakis A, Reyes J, et al: Infectious complications of pediatric liver transplantation under FK 506. Transplant Proc 23:3038–3039, 1991
45. Heyworth M: Clinical experience with antilymphocyte serum. Immunol Rev 65:79–97, 1982

46. Hiatt JR, Ament ME, Berquist WJ, et al: Pediatric liver transplantation at UCLA. Transplant Proc 19:3282–3288, 1987
47. Ho M, Jaffe R, Miller G, et al: The frequency of Epstein-Barr virus infection and associated lymphoproliferative syndrome after transplantation and its manifestations in children. Transplantation 45:719–727, 1988
48. Hokland M, Larsen B, Heron I, et al: Corticosteroids decrease the expression of B2-microglobulin and histocompatibility antigens on human peripheral blood lymphocytes in vitro. Clin Exp Immunol 44:239–246, 1981
49. Iwatsuki S, Starzl TE, Shaw BW, et al: Long-term use of cyclosporine in liver recipients. Transplantation 36:641–643, 1983
50. Iwatsuki S, Starzl TE, Todo S, et al: Experience in 1000 liver transplants under cyclosporine-steroid therapy: A survival report. Transplant Proc 20:498–504, 1988
51. Jamieson NV, Sundberg R, Lindell S, et al: Successful 24- to 30-hour preservation of the canine liver: A preliminary report. Transplant Proc 23:210–216, 1988
52. Kahan BD: Cyclosporine. N Engl J Med 321:1725–1738, 1989
53. Kalayoglu M, D'Allessandro AM, Sollinger HW, et al: Experience with reduced-size liver transplantation in infants and children. Transplant Proc 22:1489–1491, 1990
54. Kalayoglu M, Stratta RJ, Sollinger HW, et al: Liver transplantation in infants and children. J Pediatr Surg 24:70–76, 1989
55. Kasai M, Kimura S, Asakura Y, et al: Surgical treatment of biliary atresia. J Pediatr Surg 3:665–675, 1968
56. Kasai M, Ohi R, Chiba T, et al: A patient with biliary atresia who died 28 years after hepatic portojejunostomy. J Pediatr Surg 23:430–431, 1988
57. Kino T, Hatanaka H, Hashmoto M, et al: FK 506, a novel immunosuppressant isolated from streptomyces, I. Termination, isolation and physico-chemical and biological characteristics. J Antibiot 40:1249–1255, 1987
58. Krom RAF, Wiesner RH, Rettke SR, et al: The first 100 liver transplantations at the Mayo Clinic. Mayo Clin Proc 64:84–94, 1989
59. Langer R, Vacanti JP: Tissue Engineering. Science 260:920–926, 1993
60. Lilly JR: Biliary atresia: The jaundiced infant. In Welch KJ, Randolph JG, Ravitch MM, et al (eds): Pediatric Surgery. Chicago, Year Book Publishers, 1986, pp 1047–1056
61. Lin J, Wang K, Chuang J: The efficacy of Kasai operation for biliary atresia: A single institutional experience. J Pediatr Surg 27:704–706, 1992
62. Mooney DJ, Kaufmann PM, Sano K, et al: Transplantation of hepatocytes using porous, biodegradable sponges. Transplant Proc 26:3425, 1994
63. Moore FD, Wheeler HB, Demissianos HV, et al: Experimental whole-organ transplantation of the liver and of the spleen. Ann Surg 152:374–381, 1960
64. Moukarzel AA, Najm I, Vargas J, et al: Effect of nutritional status on outcome of orthotopic liver transplantation in pediatric patients. Transplant Proc 22:1560–1563, 1990
65. National Institutes of Health Consensus Conference, June 20–23, 1983. Hepatology 4:1075–1095, 1984
66. Norman JC, Brown ME, Saravis CA, et al: Perfusion techniques in temporary human-isolated ex vivo porcine liver cross circulation. J Surg Res 6:121–165, 1966
67. Olumide F, Eliashiv A, Kralios N, et al: Hepatic support with hepatocyte suspensions in a permeable membrane dialyzer. Surgery 82:599–606, 1977
68. Otte JB, de Ville de Goyet J, Reding R, et al: Sequential treatment of biliary atresia with Kasai portenterostomy and liver transplantation: A review. Hepatology 20:41S–48S, 1994
69. Ozawa K, Uemoto S, Tanaka K, et al: An appraisal of pediatric liver transplantation from living relatives. Ann Surg 216:547–553, 1992
70. Paradis KJG, Freese DK, Sharp HL: A pediatric perspective on liver transplantation. Pediatr Clin North Am 35:409–433, 1988
71. Pichlmayr R, Weimann A, Burckhardt R: Indications for liver transplantation in hepatobiliary malignancy. Hepatology 20:33S–40S, 1994
72. Raefsky EL, Gascon P, Gratwohl A, et al: Biological and immunological characterization of ATG and ALG. Blood 68:712–719, 1986
73. Raia S, Nervy JR, Mies S: Liver transplantation from live donors. Lancet II:497, 1989

74. Rakela J, Lange S, Ludwig J, et al: Fulminant hepatitis: The Mayo Clinic experience with 34 cases. Mayo Clin Proc 60:348, 1985
75. Rozga J, Podesta L, LePage E, et al: A bioartificial liver to treat severe acute liver failure. Ann Surg 219:538–546, 1994
76. Salt A, Noble-Jamieson G, Barnes ND, et al: Liver transplantation in 100 children: Cambridge and King's College Hospital series. Br Med J 304:416–421, 1992
77. Sano K, Tanaka K, Uemoto S, et al: Cytomegalovirus infection in living related liver transplantation: Rapid diagnosis by human monoclonal antibody staining of blood leucocytes. Transplantation Science 4:105–111, 1994
78. Spolidoro JVNS, Berquist WE, Pehlivanoglu E, et al: Growth acceleration in children after orthotopic liver transplantation. Clinical and Laboratory Observations 112:41–44, 1988
79. Starzl TE, Fung J, Tzakis A, et al: Baboon-to-human liver transplantation. Lancet 341:65–71, 1993
80. Starzl TE, Groth CG, Brettschneider L, et al: Orthotopic homotransplantation of the human liver. Ann Surg 168:392–415, 1968
81. Starzl TE, Iwatsuki S, Klintmalm G, et al: Liver transplantation, 1980, with particular reference to cyclosporin-A. Transplant Proc 13:281–285, 1981
82. Starzl TE, Iwatsuki S, Van Thiel DH, et al: Evolution of liver transplantation. Hepatology 2:614–636, 1982
83. Starzl TE, Kaupp HA Jr., Brock DR, et al: Studies on the rejection of the transplanted homologous dog liver. Surg Gynecol Obstet 112:135–144, 1961
84. Starzl TE, Kaupp Jr HA, Brock DR, et al: Reconstructive problems in canine liver homotransplantation with special reference to the postoperative role of hepatic venous flow. Surg Gynecol Obstet 111:733–743, 1960
85. Starzl TE, Klintmalm GBG, Porter KA, et al: Liver transplantation with use of cyclosporin A and prednisone. N Engl J Med 305:266–269, 1981
86. Starzl TE, Marchioro TL, von Kaulla KN, et al: Homotransplantation of the liver in humans. Surg Gynecol Obstet 117:659–676, 1963
87. Stewart SM, Hiltebeitel C, Nici J, et al: Neuropsychological outcome of pediatric liver transplantation. Pediatrics 87:368–376, 1991
88. Stewart SM, Uauy R, Kennard BD, et al: Mental development and growth in children with chronic liver disease of early and late onset. Pediatrics 82:167–172, 1987
89. Stock PG, Ascher NL, Najarian JS: Pediatric liver transplantation using combination immunosuppressive therapy. Transplant Proc 19:3303–3308, 1987
90. Stratta RJ, Shaefer MS, Markin RS, et al: Gancyclovir therapy for viral disease in liver transplant recipients. Clin Transplant 5:287–293, 1991
91. Sussman NL, Kelly JH: Improved liver function following treatment with an extracorporeal liver assist device. Artif Organs 17:27–30, 1993
92. Sussman NL, Chong MG, Koussayer T, et al: Reversal of fulminant hepatic failure using an extracorporeal liver assist device. Hepatology 16:60–65, 1992
93. Thistlethwaite JR Jr: Increased utilization of organ donors: Transplantation of two recipients from single donor livers. Transplant Proc 22:1485–1486, 1990
94. Torre-Cisneros J, Manez R, Kusne S, et al: The spectrum of aspergillosis in liver transplant patients: Comparison of FK 506 and cyclosporine immunosuppresion. Transplant Proc 23:3040–3041, 1991
95. Tzakis AG, Fung JJ, Todo S, et al: Use of FK 506 in pediatric patients. Transplant Proc 23:924–927, 1991
96. Tzakis AG, Reyes J, Todo M, et al: FK 506 versus cyclosporine in pediatric liver transplantation. Transplant Proc 23:3010–3015, 1991
97. Uyama S, Kaufmann PM, Takeda T, et al: Delivery of whole liver-equivalent hepatocyte mass using polymer devices and hepatotrophic stimulation. Transplantation 55:932–935, 1993
98. Vacanti JP, Lillehei CW, Jenkins RL, et al: Liver transplantation in children: the Boston Center experience in the first 30 months. Transplant Proc 19:3261–3266, 1987
99. Vacanti JP, Shamberger RC, Eraklis A, et al: The therapy of biliary atresia combining the Kasai portenterostomy with liver transplantation: A single center experience. J Pediatr Surg 25:149–152, 1990

100. Van Thiel DH, Schade RR, Starzl TE, et al: Liver transplantation in adults. Hepatology 2:637–640, 1982
101. Whitington PF, Balisteri WF: Liver transplantation in pediatrics: Indications, contraindications, and pretransplant management. J Pediatr 118:169–177, 1991
102. Williams R, Wendon J: Indications for orthotopic liver transplantation in fulminant liver failure. Hepatology 20:5S–10S, 1994
103. Windsorova D, Stewart SM, Lovitt R, et al: Emotional adaptation in children after liver transplantation. J Pediatr 119:880–887, 1991
104. Wood RP, Langnas AN, Stratta RJ, et al: Optimal therapy for patients with biliary atresia: Portoenterostomy ("Kasai" procedures) versus primary transplantation. J Pediatr Surg 25:153–162, 1990
105. Yarmush ML, Dunn JCY, Tompkins RG: Assessment of artificial liver support technology. Cell Transplant 1:323–341, 1992
106. Zitelli BJ, Gartner JC, Malatack JJ, et al: Pediatric liver transplantation: Patient evaluation and selection, infectious complications, and life-style after transplantation. Transplant Proc 19:3309–3316, 1987
107. Zitelli BJ, Miller JW, Gartner JC Jr, et al: Changes in life-style after liver transplantation. Pediatrics 82:173–180, 1988

Address reprint requests to

Joseph P. Vacanti, MD
Department of Surgery
Children's Hospital
300 Longwood Avenue
Boston, MA 02115

0031–3955/96 $0.00 + .20

PANCREATIC DISEASES IN CHILDREN

Aaron Lerner, MD, David Branski, MD, and Emanuel Lebenthal, MD

Pancreatic diseases are relatively uncommon in the pediatric age group, and there must be a high index of suspicion to reveal their occurrence. The three major exocrine pancreatic diseases in childhood that are presented are congenital anomalies, pancreatic insufficiency, and pancreatitis. Pancreatic anomalies are considered early in life in infants with high intestinal obstruction, severe intrauterine retardation, neonatal hyperglycemia, failure to thrive, and maldigestion. On the other hand, pancreas divisum anomaly, which exists in 7.5% of patients undergoing endoscopic retrograde cholangiopancreatography (ERCP), is considered an important risk factor in developing pancreatitis later in life.

Pancreatic insufficiency should be considered in children with maldigestion, malabsorption, and steatorrhea. The main cause is cystic fibrosis. Other diseases are presented that are associated with pancreatic insufficiency, including Schwachman-Diamond syndrome, isolated exocrine pancreatic enzyme deficiencies, and Johanson-Blizzard syndrome. The difficulties in the use of pancreatic extracts for providing sufficient caloric intake are discussed.

In contrast with adults, the three leading causes of acute pancreatitis in children are viral infections, drugs, and trauma. Difficulties in the diagnosis, treatment, and complications are presented. Hereditary pancreatitis, as a form of chronic debilitating pancreatitis, is discussed with emphasis on new developments.

From the Pediatric Gastroenterology and Nutrition Unit, Department of Pediatrics, Carmel Medical Center, B. Rappaport Faculty of Medicine, Technion-Israel Institute of Technology, Haifa (AL); the Department of Pediatrics, Shaare Zedek Medical Center, Hebrew University Medical Center (DB); and the Department of Pediatrics, Mount Scopus, Hadassah-Hebrew University Hospital, Jerusalem, Israel (EL)

CONGENITAL ABNORMALITIES OF THE EXOCRINE PANCREAS

Congenital abnormalities of the pancreas are uncommon and usually asymptomatic. Most congenital anomalies of the pancreas are related to the two critical events during morphologic development, rotation and fusion.[56, 67, 100] A brief review of the embryology of the pancreas will help in the understanding of the origin and pathogenesis of the congenital abnormalities.

The pancreas first appears in the fourth-week embryo as two outpouches originating from the primitive foregut just distal to the stomach. The dorsal bud elongates rapidly to eventually form the tail, body, and part of the head of the pancreas. The ventral bud is connected to the primitive bile duct. In the ensuing weeks, it rotates about the duodenum as the biliary tree and duodenum elongate and become positioned posterior and dorsal to the lower portion of the dorsal anlage. At approximately the end of the sixth week of gestation, the two parts fuse and the ventral primordium forms the remainder of the head and uncinate process of the pancreas. Similarly, the axial duct of each primordium has a different origin. The ventral duct originates from the common bile duct, whereas the dorsal one has its origin in the duodenal wall. The two duct systems fuse to form the main pancreatic duct. The ventral duct opens at the ampulla of Vater together with the common bile duct and represents the major duct of the exocrine pancreas. The dorsal duct (i.e., duct of Santorini) is an accessory duct and remains patent in as many as 70% of adults.[77] The following abnormalities are discussed later:

Aplasia
Hypoplasia
Dysplasia
Ductal anomalies
  Pancreas divisum
  Choledochal cyst
Heterotopic pancreas
Annular pancreas

APLASIA, HYPOPLASIA, AND DYSPLASIA

Complete agenesis of the pancreas is rare and probably incompatible with life. In partial agenesis, the pancreas is defective in size and shape, usually involving an abnormal development of the dorsal bud. Although in hypoplasia the pancreas is normal in size and shape, the normal epithelial cells are replaced by fatty tissue, and the duct system is reduced in number of ducts and their terminal differentiation. Dysplasia involves disorganized parenchyma, duct dilatation, and fibromuscular abundance.

The clinical presentation is variable and can include severe intra-uterine retardation, insulin-responsive hyperglycemia and neonatal death, failure to thrive, and pancreatic origin malabsorption. The definitive diagnosis can be made at surgery or autopsy. Other diagnostic modalities, such as angiography, ERCP, abdominal ultrasound, computed tomography (CT), and cholecystokinin (CCK)-secretin stimulation, are helpful.

Sometimes, the pancreatic anomalies go unrecognized because of their sufficient residual pancreatic capacity. Several additional congenital anomalies may be associated, including Johanson-Blizzard syndrome, chromosomal anomalies, hepatic and renal dysplasia, and sideroblastic bone marrow dysfunction.[56, 57]

Pancreatic enzyme replacement therapy and nutritional supplementation are needed for those patients with documented malabsorption, and insulin for those presenting with pancreatic endocrine insufficiency.

DUCTAL ANOMALIES

The normal ductal architecture of main pancreatic duct of Wirsung and accessory duct of Santorini exists in 60% to 70% of individuals.[126] In the rest of the population, numerous variations exist.[56] Pancreas divisum is implicated as a possible important contributing factor to acute pancreatitis in patients of all ages. In addition, the association of choledochal cyst, pancreatic duct changes, and pancreatitis is presented.

Pancreas Divisum

Pancreas divisum results from incomplete fusion of the dorsal and ventral pancreatic ductal systems and their respective pancreatic tissues. In this anatomic aberration, the major part of the pancreas is drained by the accessory papilla, which may be too small to drain the secretions.[77] The associated anatomic or functional stenosis, at the accessory papilla, may account for the increased incidence of acute or recurrent pancreatitis in these patients who lack an alternate pancreatic outflow. Pancreatic divisum is the most common congenital anomaly of the pancreas, existing in as many as 7.5% of patients undergoing ERCP or 50% among individuals undergoing ERCP for pancreatitis.[12] Although the cause-and-effect relationship between pancreatitis and pancreas divisum is not well established, their association was frequently described in adults and children.[18, 27, 83, 112, 148]

The diagnosis is made by an ERCP team experienced with children.[33] A short duct of Wirsung confined to the head of the pancreas and a full length duct of Santorini is visualized. The management of recurrent pancreatitis in patients with pancreas divisum is controversial. In more severe instances, ERCP balloon dilatation, papillotomy, or stenting have been performed with variable success.

Choledochal Cyst

Three major types of choledochal cyst are classified by Alonso-Lej and colleagues[4]: (1) cystic dilatation of the entire extrahepatic duct; (2) saccular dilatation of portion of the duct; and (3) choledochocele, cystic dilatation of the intraduodenal duct. Abnormal length and aberrant position of the pancreaticobiliary junction have been associated with development of pancreatitis and pathogenesis of choledochal cyst. Reflux of pancreatic fluid into the biliary tree induced ductal dilatation in animal models, and human choledochal cyst fluid is rich in amylase. Both findings support the association of choledocal cyst and pancreatitis. Most patients are diagnosed before 10 years of age. Right upper quadrant abdominal pain, jaundice, and a palpable right upper quadrant abdominal mass are found in 60% to 70% of cases.[4] The mode of diagnosis of choice is abdominal ultrasonography. Sometimes CT scanning, nuclear study of the biliary tree, ERCP, or upper gastrointestinal contrast study is added. Complete surgical resection and creation of a Roux-en-Y hepatojejunostomy are the best treatment. If impossible, partial resection with complete mucosal excision is performed owing to the increased risk of carcinoma in the unresected cyst mucosa.

HETEROTOPIC PANCREAS

Heterotopic pancreas is synonymous to ectopic, aberrant, or accessory pancreas. It is defined as pancreatic tissue lacking anatomic and vascular continuity with the main body of the pancreas.[56] Heterotopic pancreas is found in 0.55% to 15% of autopsies in different localizations. In 70% of instances, the ectopic pancreas is found in the upper gastrointestinal tract; antrum, 25% within 5 cm of the pylorus; duodenum, 30%; and jejunum, 15%.[101] It was reported in abdominal organs such as colon, appendix, ileum, rectum, omentum, liver, gallbladder, cystic duct, Meckel's diverticula, or in extra-abdominal sites, such as bronchogenic cyst, pulmonary sequestration, and umbilicus.[46, 56, 58, 102] Recently, ectopic pancreas was reported to be localized inside other gastrointestinal abnormalities, such as hiatal hernia, ileal duplication cyst, and gastric duplication.[47, 54, 121]

Usually, the ectopic pancreatic tissue is presented as a firm, irregular, yellow nodule of 2 mm to 4 cm in diameter. The most frequent location is submucosal, and, histologically, the ductal and the acinar components are presented. The endocrine part exists in only one third of cases. In most cases, the congenital anomaly is an incidental finding during a gastrointestinal work-up. Symptoms that have been attributed to aberrant pancreas include abdominal pain (mainly epigastric), gastrointestinal bleeding, dyspepsia, abdominal distension, nausea, and vomiting. Complications are gastrointestinal bleeding, biliary and intestinal obstruction, intussusception, cholecystitis, and jejunal atresia.[56, 147] Several cases of carcinoma arising from ectopic pancreas were reported.[47]

Incidental ectopic pancreas should be left alone.[29] In only a complicated situation or symptomatic association is excision indicated.

ANNULAR PANCREAS

Annular pancreas consists of a flat band of pancreatic tissue encircling the second portion of the duodenum. The incidence is not known, but the Mayo Clinic revealed 15 cases observed during a 20-year period.[65] Pathogenically, three main theories are favored, including[56]: (1) hypertrophy of both the ventral and dorsal anlagen, resulting in complete constriction around the duodenum; (2) persistence and enlargement of the left bud of the paired ventral primordium; and (3) fixation of the tip of the ventral bud prior to rotation. The failure of free rotation of pancreatic tissue of the right ventral outpouching is the most widely accepted theory. Several congenital anomalies are associated with annular pancreas, including Down's syndrome, intestinal malrotation, duodenal obstruction, cardiac anomalies, Meckel's diverticulum, imperforated anus, duodenal bands, spinal defects, and cryptorchidism.[65]

The clinical presentation may occur at any age. Fifty percent of cases present in the pediatric age group, 86% of whom present in the neonatal period.[65] In the neonate, polyhydramnios, feeding difficulties, bile-stained vomiting, and upper abdominal distension are present. Later in life and during adulthood, upper abdominal pain, nausea, vomiting, postprandial fullness, weight loss, and gastrointestinal bleeding may occur.

In the neonate, plain film radiography of the abdomen demonstrates the classic "double bubble," which is diagnostic to duodenal obstruction. The definitive diagnosis is confirmed at laparotomy. In children and adults, barium studies reveal a smooth symmetric filling defect with prestenotic dilatation of the duodenum. The recommended surgical approach is a bypass operation, preferably duodenoduodenostomy or duodenojejunostomy as a second alternative.

PANCREATIC INSUFFICIENCY

Several hereditary disorders of the exocrine pancreas, which have been described as causes for pancreatic insufficiency, maldigestion, and steatorrhea, are as follows:

Cystic fibrosis
Schwachman-Diamond syndrome
Johanson-Blizzard syndrome
Exocrine pancreatic dysfunction with refractory sideroblastic anemia
Pancreatic aplasia/hypoplasia

Isolated exocrine pancreatic enzyme deficiencies
  Lipase
  Lipase-colipase
  Colipase
  Amylase
  Trypsinogen

Cystic fibrosis is, by far, the most common. The ensuing exocrine pancreatic insufficiency can be primary or developmental and may include all of the exocrine pancreatic enzymes or only isolated enzyme deficiency.[38, 75, 78]

Schwachman-Diamond Syndrome

The Schwachman-Diamond syndrome was first described in 1964 and represents the second most common cause of pancreatic insufficiency.[14, 124] Its main features are pancreatic insufficiency, cyclic neutropenia, metaphyseal dysostosis, and growth retardation. Associated manifestations include dental abnormalities, renal dysfunction, hepatomegaly, abnormal lung function, delayed puberty, and ichthyosis. The estimated incidence is 1 in 10,000 to 20,000 live births, with no sex predominance, and the suggested mode of inheritance is autosomal recessive.[16, 128]

Stunted growth is the most constant clinical feature of the syndrome. These patients are usually below the third percentile for height, but linear growth is maintained.

Most often, the malabsorption is manifested during infancy with steatorrhea. Stools are greasy, pale, and foul-smelling. A negative sweat test excludes cystic fibrosis. An increased stool fat excretion or pancreozymin/secretin stimulation test that reveals very low or nonexistent pancreatic zymogen enzymes confirms the diagnosis. Patients with steatorrhea have less than 1% of normal colipase and less than 2% of normal lipase secretion. Patients without steatorrhea have diminished lipase activity that is more than 10% of normal. In contrast with cystic fibrosis, the volume and bicarbonate content of the stimulated pancreatic fluid are usually normal, and its viscosity is normal also.[78] In some patients, spontaneous improvement occurs with disappearance of steatorrhea, whereas in others, steatorrhea persists into adulthood.

Pathologically, the pancreatic size is normal to small, with evidence of fatty infiltration. The ductal and the islet compartments are preserved with only residual acinar tissue left.

The hematologic manifestations in Schwachman-Diamond syndrome are variable. Neutropenia, thrombocytopenia, and anemia are present in 95%, 70%, and 50%, respectively.[1] The neutropenia ($< 1500/mm^3$) is usually intermittent and occurs as often as every 1 to 2 days. To confirm the diagnosis, blood counts are performed twice weekly during a 3-week period. Although the quantitative neutrophil response to infection is appropriate, several qualitative neutrophilic anomalies are described, including defective motility,[2, 116] and unusual surface distribution of concanavalin A receptors that might contribute to abnormal chemotaxis of neutrophils.[114] Impaired neutrophil chemotaxis can be improved with lithium therapy.[7] These neutrophil abnormalities may explain the susceptibility of the patients to infection. Bone marrow examination reveals hypoplasia, fat infiltration, and myeloid maturation arrest.[1]

Several skeletal abnormalities are discribed, including genu and cubitus valgus, thoracic dystrophy, clinoductyly, delayed bone age, short or flared ribs, and long-bone tubulation. The most typical change, however, is metaphyseal dysplasia, which appears in 10% to 60% of the patients, usually in the femur, tibia, or ribs. It is generally symmetric and progressive, appearing after infancy and possibly resolving during puberty.[38, 78]

Other clinical features described in Schwachman-Diamond syndrome are impaired lung functions, developmental retardation, decreased cognitive capacity, dental abnormalities, renal dysfunction, delayed puberty, ichthyotic maculopapular rash, cardiac lesions, associated diabetes mellitus, and Hirschsprung's disease.[1] Hepatomegaly or hepatosplenomegaly may be present. The liver may be infiltrated with fat and may exhibit periportal fibrosis and inflammatory infiltrate.[1, 151]

Malnutrition and growth failure are the results of pancreatic insufficiency. The patients are susceptible to bacterial infections and predisposed to orthopedic complications. They are at risk for aplastic anemia and leukemia, which contribute further to their morbidity and mortality.[122, 153] The association of pancreatic insufficiency with hematopoietic manifestations and leukemia is enigmatic.

The treatment is symptomatic and supportive. Pancreatic enzyme replacement therapy is required for patients with pancreatic insufficiency. Fat-soluble vitamins may be necessary in the few instances with severe maldigestion. Owing to the increased susceptibility to infection, increased awareness of the clinician and appropriate antibiotic coverage are mandatory. Orthopedic intervention is carefully timed, and leukemia or aplastic anemia appropriately treated. Cyclosporin A may be successful for aplastic anemia, and bone marrow transplantation is an alternative therapy in selected patients.[122, 153]

Johanson-Blizzard Syndrome

Johanson-Blizzard syndrome was described in 1971.[60] Its main features are pancreatic insufficiency, nasal alar hypoplasia, absence of permanent teeth, short stature, congenital deafness, psychomotor retardation, ectodermal scalp defects, rectourogenital malformations, imperforated anus, and hypothyroidism (Table 1). The mode of inheritance is autosomal recessive with no sex predilection. Until now, fewer than 40 patients were described.[40, 61, 75, 78, 98] The clinical picture is dominated by the typical dysmorphism, malabsorption, failure to thrive, and, occasion-

Table 1. INCIDENCE OF CLINICAL FEATURES REPORTED IN JOHANSON-BLIZZARD SYNDROME

Clinical Feature	Incidence	Percentage
Pancreatic insufficiency	36/37	97.3
Nasal alar hypoplasia	35/36	97.2
Teeth abnormalities	22/25	88.0
Short stature	27/31	87.1
Congenital deafness	25/31	80.6
Psychomotor retardation	24/31	77.4
Ectodermal scalp defects	26/36	72.2
Rectourogenital malformations	14/38	36.8
Imperforate anus	13/37	35.1
Hypothyroidism	10/30	33.3

ally, clinical hypothyroidism. Recently, several associated diseases were reported, including hypopituitarism and growth hormone insufficiency,[68, 117] diabetes mellitus,[98, 117, 144] and cystic fibrosis in siblings.[78] Although the genetic defect is unknown, most recently the pathophysiology of the pancreatic defect was elucidated.[61] Patients with the syndrome have preservation of ductular output of fluid and electrolytes but a decreased acinar secretion of trypsin, colipase, and total lipase, consistent with a primary acinar cell defect. The preserved ductular output is similar to Schwachman-Diamond syndrome.

Sideroblastic Anemia and Exocrine Pancreatic Insufficiency

Seven patients have been described with sideroblastic anemia and generalized pancreatic insufficiency.[28, 102, 119, 132] The bone marrow aspirate is characterized by vacuolization of the erythroid and myeloid precursors, hemosiderosis, and the presence of ringed sideroblasts. The pancreas represents acinar cell atrophy associated with fibrosis. Recently, a deletion of 4977 base pairs in mitochondrial DNA was described, spanning some key enzymes in the mitochondrial respiratory enzyme defect.[22, 115]

Pancreatic Aplasia and Hypoplasia

A rare syndrome involving exocrine and endocrine pancreatic insufficiency has been reported in three infants.[57, 152] The disorder usually presents with early-onset diabetes mellitus without ketosis. The malabsorptive features are secondary. In an additional patient, total absence of pancreatic acinar cells was reported, but clinical features may share the Schwachman-Diamond and Johanson-Blizzard syndromes and leprechaunism.[137]

Developmental Pancreatic Deficiency

Term newborns have a transient pancreatic insufficiency that persists for several months. Fetal material studies described the course of maturation in terms of pancreatic contents and duodenal concentrations of the enzymes. In addition, the term and preterm infants are unresponsive to pancreatic secretagogues for the first postnatal months. The full-term newborn in the first 4 to 6 months of life is secreting less than 10% of the specific activity of the enzyme lipase and is lacking the pancreatic enzyme amylase.[71, 155] Furthermore, the response to the secretagogues CCK-pancreozymin and secretin is partial and matures after the first 2 to 3 months of life. Thus, the full-term infant early in life cannot exceed 6 g/kg of fat in his or her diet and is not able to fully digest starches (e.g., amylose and amylopectin).

Congenital Lipase Deficiency

Isolated lipase deficiency was originally described in four patients by Sheldon in 1964.[123] Since then, several others have been described.[35, 36, 96, 109] Lipase gene is situated on chromosome 10, but the genetic defect has not yet been elucidated.

The dominant symptom is steatorrhea, presenting as oily bowel movements with oil separating easily from the rest of the stool. The offensive, foul-smelling, oily, bulky stools appear early in life, and despite fat maldigestion and malabsorption, the patient thrives relatively well. The diagnosis is confirmed by pancreozymin–secretin stimulation test that reveals normal proteolytic and amylolitic enzymes. Patients respond well to pancreatic enzyme replacement therapy.

Combined Lipase–Colipase Deficiency

Combined lipase–colipase deficiency has been described in only three patients.[43, 80] As in isolated lipase deficiency, steatorrhea is the presenting symptom. The coefficient of fat absorption improves with pancreatic enzyme replacement.

Isolated Colipase Deficiency

Isolated colipase deficiency is an extremely rare condition that was first reported in two brothers who presented with steatorrhea at the ages of 5 and 6 years.[55] The steatorrhea responded to pancreatic supplementation and to purified colipase administration. The entity must be differentiated from relative colipase deficiency as a cause of steatorrhea.[39]

Congenital Amylase Deficiency

The existence of a true isolated pancreatic amylase deficiency is questionable because the strict criteria for the diagnosis were not fulfilled by the reported cases.[50, 82, 87, 90] The strict criteria include: age of more than 1 year; clinical intolerance of starch-containing food; peak amylase concentration by pancreozymin stimulation, less than 1 standard deviation below the mean for the patient's age; normal lipase, trypsinogen levels, and pH in the duodenal fluid after pancreozymin-secretin stimulation; normal histology and brush-border enzymes of the intestinal mucosa; abnormal starch-loading test in the presence of a normal glucose tolerance test; symptomatic improvement on starch-free diet; normal sweat test; and no other typical features of known hereditary pancreatic insufficiency syndromes. Several of the described cases may represent developmental delay in amylase secretion, and in some, known pancreatic or small bowel disease was not ruled out.

Congenital Trypsinogen Deficiency

Isolated trypsinogen deficiency is very rare and was first reported in three children[95, 142, 143] who had severe malabsorption associated with hypoproteinemia, edema, and anemia. Associated anomalies include imperforated anus or hair depigmentation in two of the patients. The entity must be differentiated from enterokinase deficiency. Because enterokinase activity was not measured at that time, the relation of isolated trypsinogen dificiency to enterokinase deficiency was not clarified. The patients responded to pancreatic enzyme replacement therapy. The use of an elemental diet containing protein hydrolysate is sometimes beneficial to infants.

Congenital Enterokinase Deficiency

Enterokinase is a small intestinal enzyme that activates the zymogen proenzyme in the small intestine. Congenital enterokinase deficiency is a distinct clinical entity that was described first by Hadorn and coworkers in 1969.[51] Eight additional children have been reported since, including two pairs of siblings.[42, 52, 53, 70, 106, 140] The clinical presentation is dominated by diarrhea, failure to thrive, hypoproteinemia, and edema that start early in life. For diagnosis, pancreatic stimulation tests reveal low or absent trypsin activity, which normalizes after the addition of exogenous enterokinase. Intestinal enterokinase is absent or present in very low concentrations. Active pancreatic enzyme supplementation generates normal proteolytic activity in the duodenum or the problem can be resolved by supplying protein hydrolysate to the infant.

TREATMENT FOR PANCREATIC INSUFFICIENCY

Nutritional Management

The failure to thrive encountered in pancreatic insufficiency is the result of a combination of inadequate caloric intake, maldigestion, malabsorption, abnormal nutrient losses, and increased requirements. Because children with pancreatic insufficiency do not grow until the percentage of energy absorption exceeds 100% to 110% that of the recommended daily allowance (RDA), the current recommended caloric intake is 120% to 150% of RDA.[72, 89] Although low-fat diets were previously used, unrestricted dietary fat is now recommended. The fats are now recognized as an important high-density source of calories that improve the palatability of food and supply essential fatty acids. Fat-soluble vitamin deficiencies occur in pancreatic insufficiency. The daily recommended doses are 5000 to 10,000 IU vitamin A, 400 to 800 IU of vitamin D, 50 to 200 IU of vitamin E, and 5 mg twice weekly of vitamin K.

Pancreatic Enzyme Supplementation

Pancreatic enzyme supplementations are constantly evolving. The coating of the pancreatic extract protects inactivation of the enzymes by gastric acid. A newer development is the presentation of the pancreatic extracts as acid-resistant microspheres and microtablets inside acid-resistant capsules. The most recent generation has an increased pancreatic enzyme activity. The lipase activity in the tablets has been increased from 600 to more than 30,000 units. Concomitantly, amylase and protease activities were increased from 7500 to 97,500 units. These improvements in the enzyme extracts resulted in worthwhile reduction in capsule consumption, improved absorption and weight gain, and alleviated abdominal pain and distal ileal obstruction in cystic fibrosis.

Several problems emerged when the previously mentioned pharmaceutical manipulations were used, however.[69, 73, 74] Pancreatic enzymes are formulated, manufactured, and sold without submitting safety, efficacy, or bioavailability data to the Food and Drug Administration. Currently, there is no US Pharmacopeia reference standard for those preparations, and they cannot be used interchangeably in clinical practice. There is a need to check and control not only the claimed initial enzymatic activity but also its activity after a period of incubation at pathophysiologic pH values that present in the patients.[73] Recently, an association between strictures of the ascending colon and high-strength pancreatic enzyme extracts was described; however, a cause-and-effect relationship remains to be established.[69] The authors recommend tailoring the dose of enzyme according to symptoms, stool type, and weight gain.[72] It would be prudent at this time to curtail the use of high-dosage capsules of pancreatin and pancreolipase, setting the limit at

20,000 U. Doses of 3000 U/kg/dose of lipase and 9000 U/kg/dose of protease should not be exceeded.

ACUTE PANCREATITIS IN CHILDREN

Acute pancreatitis is not a common cause of abdominal pain and represents a diagnostic challenge in the pediatric age group. It has numerous causes, an obscure pathogenesis, few effective remedies, and a sometimes unpredictable outcome.[130] In contrast with adults, trauma, drugs, and viral infections are the three leading causes in children. The most frequently used diagnostic tools are serum and urinary amylase, abdominal ultrasonography, and CT. Lately, ERCP is more frequently used in selected cases. The increased awareness, introduction of newer diagnostic and monitoring modalities, and improved therapy further lower the morbidity and mortality rates of this condition in children. This review is an update based on several extensive summaries on the subject.[30, 49, 76, 130]

Classification

The clinical classification of pancreatitis was redefined at the Second International Symposium in Marseille in 1984.[9, 48] The condition was classified to acute or chronic pancreatitis. Acute pancreatitis is an acute abdominal pain accompanied by increased pancreatic enzymes in blood or urine. Morphologically, the lesions can be graded as mild or severe. In the milder form, peripancreatic fat necrosis and interstitial edema are observed. In the severe form, peripancreatic and intrapancreatic fat, with or without parenchymal necrosis, and hemorrhage are added. The process can be diffused or localized and occasionally etiologic-clinical-pathologic correlation is lacking.

Pathophysiology

The pathogenesis of acute pancreatitis is poorly understood. Several mechanisms can initiate the pancreatic inflammation, including increased permeability of the pancreatic duct, overstimulation of the gland, obstruction to pancreatic flow, overdistention of the pancreatic ductal system, toxin exposure, and metabolic abnormalities (e.g., hypercalcemia and hypertriglyceridemia).

The common channel theory, as the cause for acute pancreatitis, was originally suggested by Opie in 1901.[130] In face of obstruction of the ampulla of Vater, there is a bile reflux into the pancreatic ductal tree which induce pancreatitis. Despite numerous studies with animal models, extensive experimentation failed to prove or disprove Opie's theory conclusively. Because gallstone-induced pancreatitis is rare in children, the theory is applicable only to rare cases of distal ductal obstructive abnormalities. The second theory of the duodenal regurgitation through an incompetent sphincter of Oddi may explain a few pediatric cases of duodenal obstruction and pancreatitis.

Because various factors predispose to acute pancreatitis, a number of inductive mechanisms may operate to induce pancreatic inflammation. Whatever the mechanism of inappropriate zymogen activation, once triggered, the acinar cell follows an unpredictable cascade of events leading to pancreatitis. Edema, necrosis, hemorrhage, thrombosis, ischemia, and inflammation are the results. The local process spreads into the peripancreatic spaces with release of toxic factors into the peritoneal space and systemically, leading to remote complications and multiorgan failure.

Etiology

In contrast with adults, in whom 80% of cases of acute pancreatitis are associated with alcoholism and biliary tract disease, the etiology in children is diverse. The most frequent causes are infections, trauma, and drug use. Several predisposing factors can account for the majority of the episodes of acute pancreatitis in children: (1) congenital or acquired obstruction to pancreatic flow; (2) drugs or toxins; (3) metabolic or systemic disorders; (4) infectious agents; and (5) hereditary or idiopathic conditions. Table 2 lists the different causes that were associated with pancreatitis in children. The prevalence of the major causes of acute pancreatitis in children is variable. Reports from North America showed that the most common causes of this pediatric condition were multiorgan failure (22 of 61 patients[150]), or drug intake (16 of 54 patients[62]). In contrast, a recent European series reported mumps infections (39%) and trauma (14%) as the most prevalent causes.[49] Table 3 summarizes etiologic incidence of acute pancreatitis in 272 children.[17, 49, 62, 139, 150, 154] Idiopathic causes and infection are the leading causes.

Diagnosis

The clinical picture of acute pancreatitis is heterogeneous in children; therefore, a high index of suspicion is required. A history of abdominal trauma, exposure to infectious disease, or drug intake should be looked for. The family history should be screened for metabolic or hereditary conditions associated with pancreatitis. Abdominal pain is the most frequent symptom. The pain is sudden in onset but may be slow or gradual. The intensity and duration are variable. Although the most common location is the epigastrium, other locations exist. The typical radiation of the pain to the back observed in adults is missing in 60% to 90% of children.[49, 150] Other accompanying symptoms are

Table 2. ETIOLOGY OF PANCREATITIS IN CHILDREN

Congenital Obstruction to Flow	Hereditary	Infections	Drug or Toxin
Absence of pancreatic duct	Cystic fibrosis	Mumps	Thiazides
Absence or anomalous insertion of common bile duct	Familial with or without aminoaciduria	*Enterovirus*	Furosemide
Stenosis of the ampulla of Vater	Hyperparathyroidism	Epstein-Barr virus	Sulfonamides
Periampullary diverticulum	Hyperlipoproteinemia (types I, IV, and V)	Hepatitis A, cytomegalovirus	Azathioprine
Choledochal cyst	α_1-Antitrypsin deficiency	Rubella	L-Asparaginase
Choledochocele	Congenital partial lipodystrophy	Coxsackie virus	Estrogen
Pancreas divisum		Echovirus	Tetracycline
Anomalous choledochopancreaticoductal junction		Varicella	Trimethoprim-sulfamethoxazole
Annular pancreas		Rubeola	Erythromycin
Intestinal duplication		Measles	Vitamin D, calcium
		Influenza A and B	Methyldopa
		Campylobacter fetus	Nitrofurantoin
		Escherichia coli	Pentamidine
		Yersiniosis	Cimetidine, ranitidine
		Leptospirosis	Sulindac
		Mycoplasma	Metronidazole
		Legionnaires' disease	Valproic acid
		Typhoid fever	Salicylates
		Septic shock	6-Mercaptopurine
		Ascaris lumbricoides	Sulfasalazine
		Clonorchis sinensis	Hyperalimentation
		Malaria	Boric acid poisoning
			Ethionine, ethyl alcohol
			Methyl alcohol
			Organophosphorus insecticides
			Scorpion bites
			Heroin
			Amphetamines
			Acetaminophen overdose

Systemic Disease

Diabetes mellitus
Periarteritis nodosa
Henoch-Schönlein purpura
Systemic lupus erythematosus
Malnutrition or refeeding
Reye's syndrome
Sarcoidosis
Crohn's disease
Kawasaki disease

Metabolic Disease

Hypercalcemia
Uremia
Hemochromatosis
Hypertriglyceridemia

Obstruction to Flow

Gallstones
Pseudocyst
Tumors
Gastric trichobezoar
Post-traumatic duodenal
  obstruction
Lipid intravenous emulsion

Miscellaneous

Trauma
Juvenile tropical pancreatitis
Perforated duodenal ulcer
Postoperative
Post-transplantation
Anorexia nervosa
Idiopathic

Data from Durie PR: Pancreatitis. In Walker WA, Durie PR, Hamilton JR (eds): Pediatric Gastrointestinal Disease. Pathophysiology, Diagnosis, Management. Philadelphia, BC Decker, 1991, pp 1209–1236; Lerner A: Acute pancreatitis in children and adolescents. In Lebenthal E (ed): Textbook of Gastroenterology and Nutrition in Infancy, ed 2. New York, Raven Press, 1989, pp 897–906; and Steinberg W, Tenner S: Acute pancreatitis. N Engl J Med 330:1198–1210, 1984.

139

Table 3. CAUSES OF ACUTE PANCREATITIS IN 272 CHILDREN

Cause	Incidence (%)
Idiopathic causes	22
Trauma	20
Infections	15
Biliary tract disease	14
Drugs	13
Miscellaneous	11
Congenital anomalies	5

Data from references 17, 49, 62, 139, 150, and 154.

vomiting, anorexia, and nausea. Generally, food is an aggravating factor of pain and vomiting.

The most frequent finding is epigastric tenderness with decreased bowel sound. The child assumes a position with flexed knees and hips. The child may be ill, irritable, or quiet. The abdomen may be distended with rebound tenderness and guarding localized to the upper abdomen. Cullen's sign (i.e., bluish periumbilical discoloration) and Grey Turner's sign (i.e., blue discoloration in the flanks) may be seen in severe hemorrhagic pancreatitis. In cases of systemic presentation or remote complication, the clinical picture may be dominated by fulminant deterioration, such as shock, abdominal mass presenting a pseudocyst, respiratory distress due to pleural effusion, or unexplained jaundice or ascites.

Laboratory Investigations

No single diagnostic test exists for acute pancreatitis and some tests may be misleading because of their lack of specificity.[10, 24, 30, 34, 49, 76, 130, 150] Table 4 summarizes the laboratory tests and imaging techniques that are used in acute pancreatitis.

Serum and Urine Amylase

Serum amylase remains the most widely used test in acute pancreatitis. Its serum level rises within 2 to 12 hours, and in uncomplicated

Table 4. LABORATORY TESTS AND IMAGING TECHNIQUES IN ACUTE PANCREATITIS

Laboratory Tests	Imaging Techniques
Serum amylase	Plain film of abdomen
Urine amylase	Plain film of chest
Amylase creatinine clearance ratio	Upper gastrointestinal barium
Amylase isoenzymes	Pancreatic ultrasonography
Serum lipase	Abdominal computed tomography
Serum proteases	Magnetic resonance imaging
Serum ribonuclease	Endoscopic retrograde cholangiopancreatography

cases, remains elevated for 2 to 5 days. A protracted elevation raises the suspicion of a pseudocyst or macroamylasemia. Serum amylase levels greater than three times normal are considered significant for the diagnosis. Because amylase is cleared by the kidneys, elevated urinary amylase levels may exist 24 hours after normalization of serum levels. The level of serum amylase bears no relationship with the severity of pancreatitis or its clinical course. Although serial determination with a gradual decline usually can indicate improvement, clinical deterioration can parallel amylase level normalization.

The sensitivity of amylase in pediatric acute pancreatitis is less than in adults. Investigators have quoted a 40% incidence in children with normal amylase in face of pancreatitis.[24, 50] It has long been appreciated that many nonpancreatic causes of hyperamylasemia exist.[105] Lipemia may interfere with amylase determination,[6] and total acinar destruction may result in normal serum amylase during acute pancreatitis.

Amylase Creatinine Clearance Ratio

The amylase creatinine clearance ratio is calculated as follows:

$$Cam/Ccr = [(\text{amylase in urine})/(\text{amylase in serum})] \times [(\text{creatinine in serum})/(\text{creatinine in urine})]$$

The normal ratio is 1% to 4%, and a ratio above 6% is considered abnormal. The higher ratio in pancreatitis is due to increased renal clearance of amylase in relation to creatinine due to decreased renal tubular reabsorption of amylase in acute pancreatitis. Subsequently, this test is not specific, and in many other conditions of hyperamylasemia, the ratio is high. It is agreed that the clearance ratio does not add any important diagnostic information to that provided by serum amylase determination.[24, 130]

Amylase Isoenzymes

Normally, 60% of serum amylase is salivary and the rest is pancreatic. Although in acute pancreatitis, the majority of serum amylase is of pancreatic origin, other abdominal conditions increase pancreatic isoamylase.[131] Fractionation of isoamylase isoenzymes to pancreatic amylase generally is not superior to the lipase assay.[130]

Serum Lipase

Serum lipase levels usually are elevated in acute pancreatitis and remain elevated longer than serum amylase levels. Considerable controversy exists concerning lipase superiority compared with amylase determination.[131] Lipase is also found in intestinal mucosa, stomach, adipose tissue, leukocytes, and breast milk and can be elevated in the serum of patients with other abdominal conditions.

Serum Immunoreactive Trypsin

The only source of trypsin in the human body is the pancreas. Total immunoreactive trypsin in the serum increases in acute pancreatitis earlier compared with amylase.[31] Its sensitivity is higher than lipase and pancreatic isoamylase with similar specificity.[131]

Ribonuclease

The concentration of serum ribonuclease is low in serum, and pancreatic ribonuclease can be distinguished immunologically from other sources of ribonuclease. Elevated pancreatic ribonuclease levels in serum have been suggested to be indicative of pancreatic necrosis.[149]

Other Laboratory Assays

Less specific laboratory test results can be observed in acute pancreatitis, including elevated serum glucose, hypocalcemia, hemoconcentration, leukocytosis, high bilirubin, alkaline phosphatase, and γ-glutamyl transpeptidase.

Imaging Procedures

Conventional radiology is of limited value in evaluating acute pancreatitis. The most useful and frequently used is abdominal ultrasonography and CT. A plain film of the abdomen usually is performed on every child suspected to have acute pancreatitis to rule out local complication. Table 5 summarizes the radiologic signs of chest and abdominal plain film in acute pancreatitis.[76]

Upper Gastrointestinal Barium Series

Contrast studies of the upper gastrointestinal tract have been largely abandoned and replaced with ultrasonography and CT. The radio-

Table 5. RADIOLOGIC SIGNS FOUND IN ACUTE PANCREATITIS

Chest Radiograph	Abdominal Plain Film
Platelike atelectasis	Regional small bowel ileus (sentinel loop)
Basilar infiltrates	Dilatation of transverse colon (colon cut-off sign)
Elevation(s) of hemidiaphragm(s)	Absence of air in descending colon
Left pleural effusion	Generalized ileus
Pericardial effusion	Blurring of the left psoas margin
Pulmonary edema	Pancreatic califications
	Diffuse abdominal haziness
	Peripancreatic extraluminal gas bubbles
	Pancreatic pseudocyst

graphic signs are indirect and reflect pancreatic enlargement and peripancreatic edema and inflammation. The duodenal loop is widened with medial spiculations and the mucosal folds may be affected. The major indication for the barium study is to detect disorders that may be associated with acute pancreatitis, such as duodenal anomalies, annular pancreas, intestinal obstruction, and abdominal tumors.

Pancreatic Ultrasonography

Abdominal ultrasound is the most frequently used and useful imaging investigation performed in patients with suspected acute pancreatitis. The two major sonographic findings are increased pancreatic size and decreased pancreatic echogenicity.[24, 37] The echogenicity marker seems to be more reliable than pancreatic size alternations.[24]

In "normal" children, the pancreatic echodensity is equal to that of the left lobe of the liver. In children, sonography has a positive predictive value of 0.93 and a negative one of 0.78 in acute pancreatitis.[37] Hypoechogenicity was reported in 44% of incidences of acute pancreatitis in children.[20]

The hypodensity of the pancreas in acute pancreatitis was challenged by Swischuk and Hayden,[135] who claimed that, in children, the pancreas is usually sonographically normal, but the pararenal space is hyperechogenic during the inflammation. Overlying gas may present a technical problem that can be overcome by water in the stomach that acts as an acoustic window. Other technical problems can be overcome by intraoperative ultrasonography[141] or CT.

Abdominal Computed Tomography

Contrast-enhanced CT is the imaging method of choice in delineating the pancreas, evaluating the severity of and detecting the complications of acute pancreatitis. In mild pancreatitis, the CT scan demonstrates a normal pancreas in 15% to 30% of patients.[8] In more severe instances, however, nearly always the scan is abnormal. Computed tomographic scan signs include changes in size and texture of the inflamed pancreas, pseudocysts, abscesses, calcifications, duct enlargement, peripancreatic edema, peritoneal exudate, and bowel distention.[8, 13] Dynamic CT pancreatography, in which large doses of intravenous contrast medium are given rapidly and the pancreas is analyzed by thin tomographic cuts, is now used to identify pancreatic perfusion defects that correlate with pancreatic necrosis.[86]

Magnetic Resonance Imaging

Magnetic resonance images identify hydrogen protons and conceivably could detect early pancreatic edema. Experience in children, however, is limited.[133] In adults, MR images of the pancreas did not offer a major advantage over CT scans.[129]

Endoscopic Retrograde Cholangiopancreatography

With a new small endoscopic instrument, ERCP can be performed in infants. In acute pancreatitis, the pediatric indications are evaluation of post-traumatic or postpancreatitis complications, detection of anatomic abnormalities associated with acute pancreatitis, and study of the pancreatic ducts in chronic relapsing pancreatitis or hereditary pancreatitis.[3, 111] In the largest series done, mild pancreatitis was reported after the procedure in 12% of children, but in all it was self-limited.[3] In the most recent report, only 5% of children developed transient pancreatitis owing to the test.[111]

Treatment

Medical Therapy

The treatment of acute pancreatitis is largely supportive, and the intensity of therapy is dictated by the severity of the inflammation. Several specific clinical aims are followed during the treatment, including removal of the initiating offender (i.e., drugs or toxins), reducing the self-perpetuating autodigestive process in the pancreas, treating local and systemic complications, and removal of digestive enzymes or toxins from the circulation or peritoneal cavity.

Although removal of factors that may have precipitated the attack is possible, placing the pancreas at rest is rarely accomplished. Controlled trials have shown that a nasogastric tube does not increase pain relief or shorten hospital stay.[85] Nasogastric suction is indicated in children with ileus or severe vomiting in whom it may afford symptomatic relief. Other measures to "put the pancreas to rest," such as H_2 blockers, atropine, calcitonin, glucagon, somatostatin, and fluorouracil, have not been shown to change the course of the disease, at least in adults.[130] Enzyme inhibitors, such as aprotinin and gabexate, given intravenously or intraperitoneally did not improve the outcome in instances of severe disease.[130] Supportive measures, such as total parenteral nutrition or fresh frozen plasma, also have not proved to be effective. Despite early enthusiasm for peritoneal lavage, subsequent studies were discouraging.[130] However, peritoneal lavage for 7 days decreased the mortality due to pancreatic-abscess formation without affecting the overall mortality.[107] Antibiotic coverage to prevent septic complications using ampicillin did not change the course of acute pancreatitis.[130] A recent study using imipenem was successful in reducing the incidence of pancreatic sepsis in patients with necrotizing pancreatitis.[103]

In practice, children with acute pancreatitis are deprived of oral intake. Nasogastric suction is introduced, and fluid resuscitation is started. Full monitoring of central venous pressure, urinary output, blood gases, and metabolic parameters of serum calcium, glucose, electrolytes, and lipids are performed according to the child's condition.

Analgesic is used, usually meperidine 1 to 2 mg/kg, IM or IV. Appropriate antibiotic is initiated if infection is suspected or proved. Total parenteral nutrition is indicated if an extended period of fasting is anticipated. When clinical improvement occurs, a low-fat elemental diet may be beneficial.[64]

Surgical Treatment

Efforts should be made to treat acute pancreatitis in children medically and to avoid surgery. The traditional indications for surgery include: (1) exploration in the face of an acute abdomen (in children, the most common preoperative diagnosis is acute appendicitis); (2) removal of obstruction in the main pancreatic ducts or common bile duct, which is done preferably on an elective basis; (3) drainage of pancreatic-fluid collections (e.g., cysts and abscesses); and (4) debridement of necrotic tissue.

In the face of limited surgical experience in childhood acute pancreatitis,[136] most information relies on adult experience. Data suggest that removal of impacted stones in severe gallstone-induced pancreatitis is best accomplished by endoscopy with sphincterotomy and not through surgery.[99] With the advance of invasive radiology, infected fluid collections can be drained, but surgical drainage is usually more definitive.[108] The debate of surgical debridement or resection in patients with severe necrotizing pancreatitis has continued during the past century. The debate concerns the type of operation, the timing of surgery, and whether only infected and not sterile necrotic tissue should be debrided. The accepted consensus is that patients with infected necrotic tissue should undergo surgical debridement.[130]

Complications

Pediatricians should be aware of numerous early and late complications. Table 6 summarizes the systemic and organ-specific complications.

The complications of acute pancreatitis can be divided into early and late complications. During the first week of hospitalization, the potential complications are multisystem organ failure involving mainly the pulmonary, cardiovascular, and renal systems. During the first 2 weeks of illness, sterile or infected pancreatic or peripancreatic necrotic tissue can be observed. The two can be distinguished by ultrasound or CT-guided percutaneous aspiration.[41]

The late complications occur after the second week of illness and include pseudocysts and abscess formation.[118] In as many as 15% of patients, an inflammatory mass, such as a pseudocyst, phlegmon, or abscess, develops. The incidence of pancreatic pseudocysts in children is significant.[93] This complication should be suspected whenever symptoms fail to resolve. If hyperamylasemia continues after 4 weeks, surgery probably is needed. In one third of patients, the pseudocyst resolves

Table 6. COMPLICATIONS OF ACUTE PANCREATITIS

Systemic Complications	Organ-specific Complications/Mechanism
Hyperglycemia	Circulatory failure
Hypocalcemia	Fluid sequestration
Hyperlipidemia	Hemorrhage
Hyperkalemia	Kinin activation
Metabolic acidosis	Pericarditis
Disseminated intravascular	Respiratory failure
coagulopathy	Diaphragmatic elevation
	Aspiration
	Pleural effusion
	Surfactant degradation
	Respiratory distress syndrome
	Renal failure
	Acute tubular necrosis
	Hypovolemia
	Vascular thrombosis
	Right-sided hydronephrosis
	Hepatobiliary
	Bile duct obstruction
	Hepatic/portal vein
	Thrombosis
	Hepatorenal syndrome
	Primary liver disease
	Neurologic
	Metabolic disturbances
	Cerebral hypoperfusion
	Analgesics
	Psychosis-demyelination
	Pancreatic
	Necrosis-infected/sterile
	Abscesses
	Pseudocysts
	Hematologic
	Hemolysis
	Sepsis
	Coagulopathy-circulating
	Proteases
	Gastrointestinal
	Stress/ischemic ulcers
	Hemorrhage
	Varices-splenic vein
	Obstruction
	Paralytic ileus

Data from references 6, 9, 10, 17, 20, 24, 30, 31, 34, 37, 48, 49, 62, 76, 105, 130, 131, 135, 139, 141, 149, 150, and 154.

on conservative management. Less frequent complications are jejunal infarction, subcutaneous fat necrosis, pancreatic insufficiency, diabetes millitus, and sudden infant death.[138]

Prognosis

The prognosis is variable because considerable variation exists in the clinical course of acute pancreatitis in children. The clinical picture ranges from mild, transient, self-limited abdominal discomfort to fulminant, rapidly deteriorating discomfort that is complicated by multiorgan failure with a fatal outcome within hours or days. In adults, the mortality rate per attack is estimated to be approximately 9%; however, in patients with severe hemorrhagic pancreatitis, the mortality rate ranges from 15% to 50%. Data regarding mortality in children are scarce. In one report, 13 of 61 (21%) children with acute pancreatitis experienced a fatal outcome.[150]

HEREDITARY PANCREATITIS

Hereditary pancreatitis (HP) is the second most common hereditary disease of the pancreas. It is a form of chronic pancreatitis presenting in childhood but often unrecognized until years later. It represents the second most common cause of chronic or recurrent pancreatitis in childhood, the first being juvenile tropical pancreatitis.

Definition

Hereditary pancreatitis is defined as recurrent inflammation of the pancreas that occurs in families over two or more generations without other known predisposing factors.[88] It was first described by Comfort and Steinberg[21] in 1952, but since then, more then 400 patients were described from more then 95 pedigrees worldwide.[21, 25, 30, 32, 66, 84, 79, 91, 104] The condition is inherited as an autosomal dominant trait with variable (40–80%) penetrance.[91]

Etiology and Pathogenesis

The basic genotypic or phenotypic abnormality has yet to be identified. Because the kindreds presented different clinical pictures and associated conditions, HP may present different entities of hereditary pancreatic diseases.

Several mechanisms were suggested, including: (1) obstructed pancreatic flow with hypertrophy of the sphincter of Oddi and multiple dilatation and constrictions at the pancreatic ducts level[113, 128], although these anatomical alterations may be secondary to the chronic inflammation; (2) inborn error of metabolism (some patients together with asymptomatic family members have generalized or selective aminoaciduria involving cystine, lysine, and arginine)[45, 110]; (3) antioxidant deficiency (lower levels of antioxidants were found in patients with HP, but antioxidant therapy provided relief even in patients with non-HP type of chronic pancreatitis)[15, 92]; and (4) defective production of pancreatic stone protein, which is secreted by the pancreatic acinar cells and functions as a stabilizer of pancreatic juice by preventing calcium precipitation. Decreased levels of stone protein were reported in several chronic calcific lesions of the pancreas and may have a role in HP.[30, 88, 120, 134]

No specific pathologic features were found in the pancreas in patients with HP, and the pancreas resembles other chronic calcific pancreatitis. The pancreas is fibrotic, shrunken with intraductal proteinaceous plugs and occasional calculi. Histologically, extensive fibrosis with loss of the acinar compartment and partial preservation of the islets is observed.

Associated Abnormalities

Several associated conditions were described in patients with HP, including biochemical aberrations, such as hyperlipidemia and especially hypertriglyceridemia,[23] hypercalcemia,[19] and hyperimmunoglobulinemia. On physical examination, developmental anomalies may exist, including nystagmus, strabismus, spina bifida occulta, or mental retardation. The HLA associated to HP is controversial. Increased frequency of HLA B-12, B-13 and BW-50 was described.[5, 8]

Clinical Features

Although the first episode usually occurs between 1 and 13 years of age, the mean age of onset is 10 years.[44, 63] Each episode may last 2 days to 2 weeks, the average being 4 to 8 days. The frequency of the symptoms is variable, occurring almost monthly to once per year. With increased age, the frequency of episodes gradually declines.[125] The attack may be precipitated by a large fatty meal, alcohol, or stress.

The major symptom is abdominal pain, which is severe, prolonged, epigastric, and may radiate to the back. It is alleviated by the knee-chest or fetal position. Often it is associated with nausea and vomiting. The episodes gradually subside, provided there are no complications. Some of the attacks may be very mild or even painless.[110] The physical findings during the attack are typical to acute pancreatitis. Epigastric tenderness and sometimes decreased bowel sounds are observed. Abdominal distension and physical signs of peritoneal irritation are observed less frequently.

Acute episodes of pancreatitis with a positive family history are the mainstay of the diagnosis in HP. All of the known causes of acute pancreatitis should be ruled out. Serum amylase and lipase levels are raised and the amylase creatinine ratio is abnormal.

Plain film radiographs of the abdomen may show a distended sentinal loop, compression of the duodenal sweep, or calcifications; ultrasound can show edema of the pancreas and calcification or a shrunken fibrotic pancreas. Sometimes dilated pancreatic ducts are demonstrated.[127] Computed tomography often is added for better delineation of the pancreas, the ductal system, pancreatic stones, or complications. The presence of large stones within the pancreatic ducts with an "iris" or "bulls-eye" appearance is in keeping with HP. ERCP can delineate more accurately the dilatation or stenosis of the ducts, but occasionally the ductal system appears normal.

Complications are more frequent in patients with HP than in nonhereditary chronic pancreatitis. Calcifications occur in 33% to 50% of patients with HP and are the most frequent complication.[88] Diabetes is reported in between 3% and 30% of patients.[66, 88] It is a late complication in the course of disease.

The major complications of hereditary pancreatitis include pancreatic calcification, diabetes mellitus, pseudocyst, ascites or pleural effusion, portal hypertension, dilatation of the pancreatic ducts, thrombosis of the portal/splenic vein, pancreatic carcinoma, and exocrine pancreatic insufficiency.

Pancreatic exocrine insufficiency manifests itself as steatorrhea. Its incidence is variable, ranging between 5% and 50% in other series.[88] Pseudocyst of the pancreas occurs in 5% to 17% of patients,[66, 88] and carcinoma in 3% to 6% of patients with HP, although a high incidence of 20% was reported in a large survey.[63] It is a late event in the natural history of the disease. Chronic inflammation and pancreatic calcification may present predisposing factors for the development of ductal metaplasia during the course of the disease.

Management

The management resembles any other therapy for acute pancreatitis of any other etiology. Essentially, the treatment is symptomatic and supportive: pain relief; maintenance of fluid, electrolyte, glucose, and calcium homeostasis; and minimization of pancreatic secretion (see section on Acute Pancreatitis). Because pain may present a major problem unalleviated by a strong analgesic, several options can be considered. Somatostatin can reduce pancreatic secretion and help symptomatically.[26, 97] Oral pancreatic enzymes may reduce pain in chronic pancreatitis.[59] Daily antioxidants, such as vitamins C and E or β-carotene, can be helpful.[15, 146] Nutritional management during the acute and chronic stages of the disease is important. Early introduction of parenteral nutrition in the acute phase and gradual introduction of food, carbohydrates as the first step and whole food later, is accepted by most centers. In incidences of steatorrhea and pancreatic insufficiency, pancreatic extracts are added.

Surgical management is reserved for children with intractable pain and complications. Pancreatic abscesses are an indication for surgery, but pseudocyst can be managed conservatively. Surgical drainage is reserved for progressive enlargement of the pseudocyst under ultrasound control. Sphincterotomy, and occasionally removal of pancreatic stones, can be achieved by using ERCP.

In a survey of 42 children with HP, longitudinal pancreaticojejunostomy or resection and drainage procedures were required in 55% of the patients.[94] No surgical mortality was encountered. Postoperative relief of symptoms was obtained in 43% of the patients. The conclusion of the investigators was that longitudinal pancreaticojejunostomy is beneficial for patients with ductal dilatation and associated pseudocysts or pancreatic ascites. Patients without ductal dilatation may eventually lead near-normal lives without surgery.

References

1. Aggett PJ, Cavanagh NPC, Matthew DJ, et al: Shwachman's syndrome: A review of 21 cases. Arch Dis Child 55:331–347, 1980
2. Aggett PJ, Harries JT, Harvey BAM, et al: An inherited defect in neutrophil mobility in Shwachman syndrome. J Pediatr 94:391–394, 1979
3. Allendorph M, Werlin SL, Geenen JE, et al: Endoscopic retrograde cholangiopancreatography in children. J Pediatr 110:206–211, 1987
4. Alonso-Lej F, Rever WB, Pessagno DJ: Congenital choledochal cyst with a report of 2, and an analysis of 94 cases. Int Abstr Surg 108:1–30, 1959
5. Angelini G, Boro P, Merigo F, et al: Morphological and functional finding and HLA antigens of three juvenile brothers with chronic pancreatitis. Digestion 35:4, 1986
6. Arvanitakis C, Cooke AR, Greenberger NJ: Laboratory aids in the diagnosis of pancreatitis. Med Clin North Am 62:107–128, 1978
7. Azzara A, Carulli G, Ceccarelli M, et al: In vivo effectiveness of lithium on impaired neutrophil chemotaxis in Shwachman-Diamond syndrome. Acta Haematol 85:100–102, 1991
8. Balthazar EJ: CT diagnosis and staging of acute pancreatitis. Radiol Clin North Am 27:19–37, 1989
9. Banks PA, Bradley EL, Dreiling DA, et al: Classification of pancreatitis - Cambridge to Marseille. Gastroenterology 89:928–930, 1985
10. Barkin JS, Garrido J: Acute pancreatitis and its complications. Diagnostic and therapeutic strategies. Postgrad Med 79:241–252, 1986
11. Barrios NJ, Kirkpatrick DV: Successful cyclosporin A treatment of aplastic anaemia in Shwachman-Diamond syndrome. Br J Haematol 74:540–541, 1990
12. Bernard JP, Sahel J, Giovannini M, et al: Pancreas divisum is a probable cause of acute pancreatitis: A report of 137 cases. Pancreas 5:248–254, 1990
13. Block S, Maier W, Bittner R, et al: Identification of pancreas necrosis in severe acute pancreatitis: Imaging procedures versus clinical staging. Gut 27:1035–1042, 1986
14. Bodian M, Sheldon W, Lightwood R: Congenital hypoplasia of the exocrine pancreas. Acta Pediatr Scand 53:282–293, 1964
15. Braganza JM, Jeffrey IJM, Foster J, et al: Recalcitrant pancreatitis: Eventual control by antioxidants. Pancreas 2:489–494, 1987
16. Branski D, Groz V, Groz-Kiselshtien H, et al: Shwachman's Diamond syndrome in a child - A case report. Harefuah 105:114–115, 1983

17. Buntain WL, Wood JB, Woolley MM: Pancreatitis in childhood. J Pediatr Surg 13:143–149, 1978
18. Carey LC: Recurrent acute pancreatitis-rarely idiopathic. Can J Surg 33:107–112, 1990
19. Carey MC, Fitzgerald O: Hyperparathyroidism associated with chronic pancreatitis in a family. Gut 9:700–703, 1968
20. Coleman BG, Arger PH, Rosenberg HK, et al: Gray scale sonographic assessment of pancreatitis in children. Radiology 146:145–150, 1983
21. Comfort MW, Steinberg AG: Pedigree of a family with hereditary chronic relapsing pancreatitis. Gastroenterology 21:54–63, 1952
22. Cormier V, Rotig A, Quartino AR, et al: Widespread multitissue deletions of the mitochondrial genome in the pearson marrow-pancreas syndrome. J Pediatr 117:599–602, 1990
23. Cox DW, Breckenridge WC, Little JA: Inheritance of apolipoprotein C-II deficiency with hypertriglyceridemia and pancreatitis. N Engl J Med 299:1421–1424, 1978
24. Cox KL, Ament ME, Sample WF, et al: The ultrasonic and biochemical diagnosis of acute pancreatitis. J Pediatr 96:407–411, 1980
25. Cucchiara S, Staiano A, Minella R, et al: Report of the second kindred in Italy. J Pediatr Gastroenterol Nutr 11:422–424, 1990
26. D'Amico D, Favia G, Biasiato R, et al: The use of somatostatin in acute pancreatitis—Results of a multicenter trial. Hepatogastroenterology 37:92–98, 1990
27. DeLange C, Engelholm L, Cremer M: Pancreas divisum: Congenital anatomical variant or anomaly. Gastroenterology 89:951–958, 1985
28. Demeocq F, Storme B, Schaison G, et al: Anemie refractaire sideroblastique avec vacuolisation des precurseurs medullaires et deficit de la function exocrine du pancreas. Arch Fr Pediatr 40:631–635, 1983
29. Dolan RV, ReMine WH, Dockerty MB: The fate of heterotopic pancreatic tissue. Arch Surg 109:762–765, 1974
30. Durie PR: Pancreatitis. In Walker WA, Durie PR, Hamilton JA, et al (eds): Pediatric Gastrointestinal Disease: Pathophysiology, Diagnosis, Management. Philadelphia, BC Decker, 1991, pp 1209–1236
31. Durie PR, Gaskin KJ, Ogilvie JE, et al: Serial alternations in the forms of immunoreactive pancreatic cationic trypsin in plasma from patients with acute pancreatitis. J Pediatr Gastroenterol Nutr 4:199–207, 1985
32. Elitsur Y, Hunt JA, Chertow BS: Hereditary pancreatitis in the children of West Virginia. Pediatrics 93:528–531, 1994
33. Farbes A, Leung JWC, Cotton PB: Relapsing acute and chronic pancreatitis. Arch Dis Child 59:927–934, 1984
34. Fayne SD, Barkin JS: Acute pancreatitis; update 1986. Mt Sinai J Med 53:396–403, 1986
35. Figarella C, DeCaro A, Deprez P, et al: Un nouveau cas de deficience congenitale en lipase pancreatique avec presence de colipase. Gastro-enterol Clin Biol 3:43–46, 1979
36. Figarella C, DeCaro A, Leupold D, et al: Congenital pancreatic lipase deficiency. J Pediatr 96:412–416, 1980
37. Fleischer AC, Parker P, Kirschner SG, et al: Sonographic findings of pancreatitis in children. Radiology 146:151–155, 1983
38. Gaskin KJ: Hereditary disorders of the pancreas. In Waker AW, Durie PR, Hamilton JR, et al (eds): Pediatric Gastrointestinal Disease: Pathophysiology, Diagnosis, Management. Philadelphia, BC Dekker, 1991, pp 1198–1202
39. Gaskin KJ, Durie PR, Lee L, et al: Colipase and lipase secretion in childhood-onset pancreatic insufficiency. Delineation of patient with steatorrhea secondary to relative colipase deficiency. Gastroenterology 86:1–7, 1984
40. Gershoni-Baruch R, Lerner A, Braun J, et al: Johanson-Blizzard syndrome: Clinical spectrum and further delineation of the syndrome. Am J Med Genet 35:546–551, 1990
41. Gerzof SG, Banks PA, Robbins AH, et al: Early diagnosis of pancreatic infection by computed tomography-guided aspiration. Gastroenterology 93:1315–1320, 1987
42. Ghishan FK, Lee PC, Lebenthal E, et al: Isolated congenital enterokinase deficiency: Recent findings and review of the literature. Gastroenterology 85:727–731, 1983
43. Ghishan FK, Moran JR, Durie PR, et al: Isolated congenital lipase colipase deficiency. Gastroenterology 86:1580–1582, 1984

44. Gross JB, Jones JD: Hereditary pancreatitis: Analysis of experience to May 1969. In Beck IT, Sinclair DG (eds): The Exocrine Pancreas. London, J & A Churchill, 1971, pp 247–272
45. Gross JB, Ulrich JA, Jones JD: Urinary excretion of amino acids in a kindred with hereditary pancreatitis and aminoaciduria. Gastroenterology 47:41–48, 1964
46. Gugulski A, Regula J, Orlowska J, et al: Heterotopic pancreas in the rectum. Endoscopy 26:372, 1994
47. Guillou L, Nordback P, Gerber C, et al: Ductal adenocarinoma arising in a heterotopic pancreas situated in a hiatal hernia. Arch Pathol Lab Med 118:568–571, 1994
48. Gyr KE, Singer MV, Sarles H (eds): Pancreatitis. Concepts and classification. Amsterdam, Excerpta Medica, 1984
49. Haddock G, Coupar G, Youngson GG, et al: Acute pancreatitis in children: A 15 year review. J Pediatr Surg 29:719–722, 1994
50. Hadorn B: The exocrine pancreas. In Anderson CM, Burke V (eds): Pediatric Gastroenterology. Oxford, Blackwell Scientific Publications, 1975, pp 289–327
51. Hadorn B, Tarlow MJ, Lloyd JK, et al: Intestinal enterokinase deficiency. Lancet 1:812–813, 1969
52. Haworth JC, Gourley B, Hadorn B, et al: Malabsorption and growth failure due to intestinal enterokinase deficiency. J Pediatr 78:481–490, 1971
53. Haworth JC, Hadorn B, Gourley B, et al: Intestinal enterokinase deficiency: Occurrence in two sibs and age dependency of clinical expression. Arch Dis Child 50:277–282, 1975
54. Hernanz de la Fuente F, Sandoval Gonzalez F, Fernandez F, et al: Gastric duplication associated with heterotopic pancreas. Circ Pediatr 5:178–181, 1992
55. Hildebrand H, Borgstrom B, Bekassy A, et al: Isolated colipase deficiency in two brothers. Gut 23:243–246, 1982
56. Hill ID, Lebenthal E: Congenital abnormalities of the exocrine pancreas. In Go VLW, Dimango EP, Gardner JD, et al (eds): The Pancreas: Biology, Pathobiology and Disease, ed 2. New York, Raven Press, 1993, pp 1029–1040
57. Howard CP, Go VLW, Infante AJ, et al: Long-term survival in a case functional pancreataic agenesis. J Pediatar 97:786–789, 1980
58. Inceoglu R, Dosluoglu HH, Kullu S, et al: An unusual cause of hydropic gallbladder and biliary colic-heterotopic pancreatic tissue in the cystic duct. Report of a case and review of the literature. Surg Today 23:532–534, 1993
59. Isaksson G, Ihse I: Pain reduction by an oral pancreatic enzyme preparation in chronic pancreatitis. Dig Dis Sci 28:97–102, 1983
60. Johanson A, Blizzard R: A syndrome of congenital aplasia of the alae nasi, deafness, hypothyroidism, dwarfism, absent permanent teeth and malabsorption. J Pediatr 79:982–987, 1971
61. Jones NL, Hofley PM, Durie PR: Pathophysiology of the pancreatic defect in Johanson-Blizzard syndrome: A disorder of acinar development. J Pediatr 125:406–408, 1994
62. Jordan SC, Ament ME: Pancreatitis in children and adolescents. J Pediatr 91:211–216, 1977
63. Kattwinkel J, Lapey A, di Sant'Agnese PA, et al: Hereditary pancreatitis: Three new kindreds and a critical review of the literature. Pediatrics 51:55–69, 1973
64. Keith RG: Effect of a low-fat elemental diet on pancreatic secretion during pancreatits. Surg Gynecol Obstet 151:337–343, 1980
65. Kiernan PD, ReMine SG, Kiernan PC, et al: Annular pancreas: Mayo Clinic experience from 1957 to 1976 with review of the literature. Arch Surg 115:46–50, 1980
66. Konzen KM, Perrault J, Moir C, et al: Long-term follow up of young patients with chronic hereditary or idiopathic pancreatitis. Mayo Clin Proc 68:449–453, 1993
67. Kopelman H: The pancreas, congenital anomalies. In Walker AW, Durie PR, Hamilton JR, et al (eds): Pediatric Gastrointestinal Disease: Pathophysiology, Diagnosis, Management. Philadelphia, BC Decker, 1991, pp 1171–1178
68. Kristjansson K, Hoffman WH, Flannery DB, et al: Johanson-Blizzard syndrome and hypopituitarism. J Pediatr 113:851–853, 1988
69. Lebenthal E: High strength pancreatic exocrine enzyme capsules associated with

colonic stricture in patients with cystic fibrosis: "More is not necessarily better." J Pediatr Gastroenterol Nutr 18:423–425, 1994

70. Lebenthal E, Antonowicz I, Schwachman H: Enterokinase and trypsin activities in pancreatic insufficiency and diseases of the small intestine. Gastroenterology 70:508–512, 1976

71. Lebenthal E, Lee PC: Development of functional response in human exocrine pancreas. Pediatrics 66:556–560, 1980

72. Lebenthal E, Lerner A, Rolston DDK: The pancreas in cystic fibrosis. In VLW Go, EP Dimagno, Gardner JD, et al (eds): The Pancreas: Biology, Pathobiology, and Disease, ed 2. New York, Raven Press, 1933, pp 1041–1081

73. Lebenthal E, Lu RB, Zheng BY, et al: Pancreatic extract lipase activity. JAMA 270:2557–2558, 1993

74. Lebenthal E, Rolston DDK, Holsclaw DS: Enzyme therapy for pancreatic insufficiency: Present status and future needs. Pancreas 9:1–12, 1994

75. Lerner A: Hereditary abnormality of the pancreas. In Lebenthal E (ed): Textbook of Gastroenterology and Nutrition in Infancy. New York, Raven Press, 1989, pp 877–883

76. Lerner A: Acute pancreatitis in children and adolescents. In Lebenthal E (ed): Textbook of Gastroenterology and Nutrition in Infancy, ed 2. New York, Raven Press, 1989, pp 897–906

77. Lerner A, Lebenthal E: The exocrine pancreas In Colon AR, Ziai M (eds): Pediatric Pathophysiology. Boston, Little, Brown, & Co., 1985, pp 242–252

78. Lerner A, Lebenthal E: Hereditary disease of the pancreas. In Go VLW, Dimagno EP, Gardner JD (eds): The Pancreas: Biology, Pathobiology, and Diseases. New York, Raven Press, 1993, pp 1083–1084

79. Lewis MP, Gazet JC: Hereditary calcific pancreatitis in an English family. Br J Surg 80:487–488, 1993

80. Ligumsky M, Granot E, Branski D, et al: Isolated lipase and colipase deficiency in two brothers. Gut 3:416–418, 1990

81. Lilja P, Evander A, Ihse I: Hereditary pancreatitis—A report on two kindreds. Acta Chir Scand 144:35–37, 1978

82. Lillibridge CB, Townes PL: Physiologic deficiency of pancreatic amylase in infancy: A factor in iatrogenic diarrhea. J Pediatr 82:279–289, 1973

83. Lindstrom E, Ihse I: Pancreatic disease caused by pancreas divisium. Eur J Surg 160:385–387, 1994

84. Little JM, Tait N, Richardson A, et al: Chronic pancreatitis beginning in childhood and adolescence. Arch Surg 127:90–92, 1992

85. Loiudice JA, Lang J, Mehta H, et al: Treatment of acute alcoholic pancreatitis: The roles of cimetidine and nasogastric suction. Am J Gastroenterol 79:553–558, 1984

86. London NJM, Leese T, Lavell JM, et al: Rapid-bolus contrast-enhanced dynamic computed tomography in acute pancreatitis: A prospective study. Br J Surg 78:1452–1456, 1991

87. Lowe CV, May DC: Selective pancreatic deficiency: Absent amylase, diminished trypsin and normal lipase. Am J Dis Child 82:459–464, 1951

88. Madrazo-de la Garza JA, Hill ID, Lebenthal E: Hereditary pancreatitis. In Go VLW, Dimagno EP, Gardner JD, et al (eds): The Pancreas: Biology, Pathobiology, and Disease, ed 2. New York, Raven Press, 1993, pp 1095–1101

89. Madrazo-de la Garza A, Lebenthal E: Nutritional considerations in the prognosis and treatment of children with pancreatic disease. In Suskind RM, Lewinter-Suskind L (eds): Textbook of Pediatric Nutrition, ed 2. New York, Raven Press, 1993, pp 363–374

90. Marin du Pan R, Infante F: Quelques etudes biologiques concernant l'intolerance aux farineaux chez l'enfant. Int Z Vitam Ernahrungsforsch (Beih) 1:67–81, 1961

91. Mathew P, Wyllie R, Caulfield M, et al: Chronic pancreatitis in late childhood and adolescence. Clin Pediatr 33:88–94, 1994

92. Mathew P, Wyllie R, Van Lente F, et al: Antioxidant levels in hereditary pancreatitis. Pediatr Res 29:108A, 1991

93. Millar AJW, Rode H, Stunden RJ, et al: Management of pancreatic pseudocysts in children. J Pediatr Surg 23:122–127, 1988

94. Moir CR, Konzen KM, Perrault J: Surgical therapy and long-term follow up of childhood hereditary pancreatitis. J Pediatr Surg 27:282–287, 1992
95. Morris MD, Fisher DA: Trypsinogen deficiency disease. Am J Dis Child 114:203–208, 1967
96. Muller DPR, McCollum JPK, Trompeter RS, et al: Studies on the mechanism of fat absorption in congenital isolated lipase deficiency. [abstract] Gut 16:838, 1975
97. Muller MK, Beglinger C: Effects of somatostatin on the exocrine pancreas. Scand J Gastroenterol 26:129–136, 1991
98. Nagashima K, Yagi H, Kuroume T: A case of Johanson-Blizzard syndrome complicated by diabetes mellitus. Clin Genet 43:98–100, 1993
99. Neoptolemos JP, Carr-Locke DL, London NJ, et al: Controlled trial of urgent endoscopic retrograde cholangiopancreatography and endoscopic sphincterotomy versus conservative treatment for acute pancreatitis due to gallstones. Lancet 2:979–983, 1988
100. Newman BM: Congenital abnormalities of the exocrine pancreas. In Lebenthal E (ed): Textbook of Gastroenterology and Nutrition in Infancy, ed 2. New York, Raven Press, 1989, pp 885–895
101. Pearson HA, Lobel JS, Kocoshis SA, et al: A new syndrome of refractory sideroblastic anemia with vacuolization of marrow precursors and exocrine pancreatic dysfunction. J Pediatr 95:976–984, 1979
102. Pearson S: Aberrant pancreas: Review of the literature and report of 3 cases, one of which produced common and pancreatic duct obstruction. Arch Surg 63:168–184, 1951
103. Pederzoli P, Bassi C, Vesentini S, et al: A randomized multicenter clinical trial of antibiotic prophylaxis of septic complications in acute necrotizing pancreatitis with imipenem. Surg Gynecol Obstet 176:480–483, 1993
104. Perrault J: Hereditary pancreatitis. Gastroenterol Clin North Am 23:743–752, 1994
105. Pieper-Bigelow C, Strocchi A, Levitt MD: Where does serum amylase come from and where does it go? Gastroenterol Clin North Am 19:793–810, 1990
106. Polonovski C, Laplane R, Alison F, et al: Pseudo-deficit en trypsinogene par deficit congenitala en enterokinase: Etude clinique. Arch Fr Pediatr 27:677–688, 1970
107. Ranson JHC, Berman RS: Long peritoneal lavage decreases pancreatic sepsis in acute pancreatitis. Ann Surg 211:708–716, 1990
108. Rattner DW, Legermate DA, Lee MJ, et al: Early surgical debridement of symptomatic pancreatic necrosis is beneficial irrespective of infection. Am J Surg 163:105–109, 1992
109. Rey J, Frezal J, Royer P, et al: L'absence congenital de lipase pancreatique. Arch Fr Pediatr 32:5–12, 1966
110. Riccardi VM, Shih VE, Holmes LB, et al: Hereditary pancreatitis: Nonspecificity of aminoaciduria and diagnosis of occult disease. Arch Intern Med 135:822–825, 1975
111. Richieri JP, Chapoy P, Bertolino JG, et al: Endoscopic retrograde cholangiopancreatography in children and adolescents. Gastroenterol Clin Biol 18:21–25, 1994
112. Richter JM, Schapiro RH, Mulley AG, et al: Association of pancreas divisum and pancreatitis and its treatment by sphincteroplasty of the accessory ampula. Gastroenterology 81:1104–1110, 1981
113. Robechek PJ: Hereditary chronic relapsing pancreatitis: A clue to pancreatitis in general? Am J Surg 113:819–824, 1967
114. Rothbaum RJ, Williams DA, Daugherty CC: Unusual surface distribution of concanavalin A reflects a cytoskeletal defect in neutrophils in Schwachman's syndrome. Lancet 2:800–801, 1982
115. Rotig A, Colonna M, Bonnefont JP, et al: Mitochondrial DNA deletion in Pearson's marrow-pancreas syndrome. Lancet 1:902–903, 1989
116. Ruutu P, Savilahti E, Repo H, et al: Constant defect in neutrophil locomotion but with age decreasing susceptibility to infection in Shwachman's syndrome. Clin Exp Immunol 57:249–255, 1984
117. Sandhu BK, Brueton MJ: Concurrent pancreatic and growth hormone insufficiency in Johanson-Blizzard syndrome. J Pediatr Gastroenterol Nutr 9:535–538, 1989
118. Sanfey H, Aguilar M, Jones RS: Pseudocysts of the pancreas, a review of 97 cases. Am Surg 60:661–668, 1994
119. Sansone G, Masera G, Terzoli S, et al: Congenital refractory anemia with vacuolisation

of bone marrow precursors sideroblastosis and growth failure in a girl with normal endocrine pancreatic function. Haematologica 74:587–590, 1989

120. Sarles H, Camarena J, Bernard JP, et al: Hereditary protein lithiasis and calcium lithiasis: Two different forms of hereditary pancreatitis. Bull Acad Natl Med 177:565–571, 1993

121. Sato T, Oyamada M, Chiba H, et al: Ileal duplication cyst associated with heterotopic pancreas: Report of a case and literature review. Acta Pathol Jpn 43:597–602, 1993

122. Savilahti E, Papola J: Frequent myocardial lesions in Shwachman's syndrome. Eight fatal cases among 16 finnish patients. Acta Pediatr Scand 73:642–651, 1984

123. Sheldon W: Congenital pancreatic lipase deficiency. Arch Dis Child 39:268–271, 1964

124. Schwachman H, Diamond LK, Oski FA, et al: The syndrome of pancreatic insufficiency and bone marrow dysfunction. J Pediatr 65:645–663, 1964

125. Sibert JR: A British family with hereditary pancreatitis. Gut 16:81–88, 1975

126. Skandalakis JE, Gray SW, Rowe JS, et al: Surgical anatomy of the pancreas. Contemp Surg 10:1–31, 1979

127. Spencer JA, Lindsell DR, Isaacs D: Hereditary pancreatitis: Early ultrasound appearances. Pediatr Radiol 20:293–295, 1990

128. Stafford RJ, Grand RJ: Hereditary disease of the exocrine pancreas. Clin Gastroenterol 11:141–170, 1982

129. Stark DD, Moss AA, Goldberg HI, et al: Magnetic resonance and CT of the normal and diseased pancreas: A comparative study. Radiology 150:153–162, 1984

130. Steinberg WM, Tenner S: Acute pancreatitis. N Engl J Med 330:1198–1210, 1984

131. Steinberg WM, Goldstein SS, Davis ND, et al: Diagnostic assays in acute pancreatitis: A study of sensitivity and specificity. Ann Intern Med 102:576–580, 1985

132. Stoddard RA, McCurnin DC, Shultenover SJ, et al: Syndrome of refractory sideroblastic anemia with vacuolization of marrow precursors and exocrine pancreatic dysfunction presenting in the neonate. J Pediatr 99:259–261, 1981

133. Stringer DA: Pediatric gastrointestinal radiology. Toronto, BC Dekker, 1989

134. Suzuki J, Matozaki T, Matsuda K, et al: Analysis of pancreatic stone protein gene of hereditary pancreatitis. Nippon Shokakibyo Gakkai Zasshi 89:633–638, 1992

135. Swischuk LE, Hayden CK Jr: Pararenal space hyperechogenicity in childhood pancreatitis. AJR 145:1085–1086, 1985

136. Synn AY, Mulvihill SJ, Fonkalsrud EW: Surgical management of pancreatitis in childhood. J Pediatr Surg 22:628–632, 1987

137. Szilagyi PG, Cordsetti J, Callahan CM, et al: Pancreatic exocrine aplasia, clinical feature of leprechaunism and abnormal gonadotropin regulation. Pediatr Pathol 7:51–61, 1987

138. Tada T, Wakabayaski T, Kishimota H, et al: Sudden death due to infantile pancreatitis. Acta Pathol Jpn 32:917–923, 1982

139. Tam PKH, Saing H, Irving IM, et al: Acute pancreatitis in children. J Pediatr Surg 20:58–60, 1985

140. Taralow MJ, Hadorn B, Arthurton MW, et al: Intestinal enterokinase deficiency, a newly recognize disorder of protein digdestion. Arch Dis Child 45:651–655, 1970

141. Telander RL, Charboneau JW, Haymond MW: Intraoperative ultrasonography of the pancreas in childhood. J Pediatr Surg 21:262–266, 1986

142. Townes PL: Trypsinogen deficiency disease. J Pediatr 66:275–279, 1965

143. Townes PL, Bryson MF, Miller G: Further observation on trypsinogen deficiency disease: Report of a second case. J Pediatr 71:220–224, 1967

144. Trellis DR, Clouse RE: Johanson-Blizzard syndrome. Progression of pancreatic involvement in adulthood. Dig Dis Sci 36:365–369, 1991

145. Tsai PH, Sahdev I, Herry A, et al: Fatal cyclophosphamide induced congestive heart failure in a 10-year-old boy with Shwachman-Diamond syndrome and severe bone marrow failure treated with allogeneic bone marrow transplantation. Am J Pediatr Hematol Oncol 12:472

146. Uden S, Bilton D, Nathan L, et al: Antioxidant therapy for recurrent pancreatitis: Placebo-controlled trial. Alimentary Pharmacology and Therapy 4:357–371, 1990

147. Ueno S, Ishida H, Hayashi A, et al: Heterotopic pancreas as a rare cause of gastrointestinal hemorrhage in the newborn: Report of a case. Surg Today 23:269–272, 1993

148. Wagner CW, Golladay ES: Pancreas divisum and pancreatitis in children. Am J Surg 54:22–26, 1988
149. Warshaw AL, Lee KH: Serum ribonuclease elevations and pancreatic necrosis in acute pancreatitis. Surgery 86:227–234, 1979
150. Weizman Z, Durie PR: Acute pancreatitis in childhood. J Pediatr 113:24–29, 1988
151. Wilschanski M, van der Hoeven E, Phillips J, et al: Shwachman-Diamond syndrome, presenting as hepatosplenomegaly. J Pediatr Gastroenterol Nutr 19:111–113, 1994
152. Winter WE, Meclaren NK, Riley WJ, et al: Congenital pancreatic hypoplasia: A syndrome of exocrine and endocrine pancreatic insufficiency. J Pediatr 109:465–469, 1986
153. Woods WG, Roloff JS, Lukens GN, et al: The occurrence of leukemia in patients with the Shwachman's syndrome. J Pediatr 99:425–428, 1981
154. Ziegler DW, Long JA, Philippart AI, et al: Pancreatitis in childhood experience with 49 patients. Ann Surg 207:257–261, 1988
155. Zoppi G, Andreotti G, Pajno-Ferrara F, et al: Exocrine pancreas function in premature and full-term neonates. Pediatr Res 6:880–886, 1972

Address reprint requests to

Aaron Lerner, MD
Pediatric Gastroenterology and Nutrition Unit
Department of Pediatrics
Carmel Medical Center
7 Michal Street
Haifa 34362
Israel

PEDIATRIC GASTROENTEROLOGY I   0031–3955/96 $0.00 + .20

CYSTIC FIBROSIS

Gastrointestinal Complications and Gene Therapy*

Linda B. Shalon, MD, and Joel W. Adelson, MD, PhD

BACKGROUND

Cystic fibrosis (CF) is an inherited disease of epithelial cell ion transport that affects multiple organ systems. It is the most common cause of severe, progressive lung disease, and exocrine pancreatic insufficiency in childhood. During the past several years, great progress has been made toward understanding the molecular basis of CF. In 1989, Tsui and colleagues succeeded in cloning the gene responsible for CF and characterized the most frequently occurring mutation in that gene, ΔF508.[108] This gene encodes a large single-chain protein that forms a chloride channel with its associated regulatory regions, named the *cystic fibrosis transmembrane conductance regulator* (CFTR). Combined with physiologic and cell biologic studies, these advances have greatly deepened the understanding of CF and have made further approaches to its clinical management possible.

Pulmonary disease is the main factor limiting longevity in patients with CF. Over the years, advances, mainly in the management of pulmonary disease, have led to an improved prognosis, with a median survival of 29 years in 1993 compared with 16 years in 1970.[27] For individuals with CF born today, median survival has been projected to be 40 years.[15]

---

*The authors dedicate this article to the memory of Hinda R. Kopelman, MD, for her outstanding work on cystic fibrosis and the pancreas.

From the Division of Pediatric Gastroenterology and Nutrition, Department of Pediatrics, Hasbro Children's Hospital, Brown University School of Medicine, Providence, Rhode Island

---

Somatic gene therapy has the potential for definitive treatment for CF pulmonary disease; clinical trials are currently underway at various centers. As longevity improves, gastrointestinal, hepatobiliary, and nutritional considerations are becoming more prominent in the overall care of CF patients. This article provides overviews of the molecular aspects of the pathogenesis of CF, the current status of gene therapy, and a review of the gastrointestinal manifestations and nutritional care of patients with CF.

Incidence

Cystic fibrosis is the most common potentially fatal autosomal recessive childhood disorder among white people. In the United States white population, the reported incidence ranges from 1 in 1900 to 1 in 3700 live births.[143] Worldwide, the incidence in white populations varies considerably on a geographic basis from 1 in 1700 in Northern Ireland to 1 in 7700 in Sweden; certain local populations show a very high incidence, presumably owing to founder effects and inbreeding (i.e., 1 in 377 in Brittany and 1 in 640 in the American Amish).[143] Cystic fibrosis is much less common in nonwhite groups; the incidence in the black population in the United States is estimated at 1 in 17,000.[143] Nevertheless, the disease occurs frequently enough in nonwhite populations that it always should be considered in the differential diagnosis of patients with signs of pancreatic insufficiency, chronic lung disease, or both.

Sweat Test

The detection and diagnosis of CF are relatively straightforward; close to 99% of CF patients having abnormal sweat Cl^- concentrations. Provided the technique is properly carried out, a sweat Cl^- concentration of greater than 60 mEq/L on two separate occasions, in a sample containing at least 100 mg of sweat, confirms the diagnosis of CF. Sweat testing should be performed in a center experienced in the Gibson-Cooke technique, in which a weighed sample of sweat is obtained by pilocarpine iontophoresis and Cl^- concentration is determined chemically.[33] Sweat-test results may be false-positive (elevated) in malnutrition and false-negative (normal range) in the presence of hypoalbuminemia and edema.[86] Normal newborns may have elevated sweat Cl^- levels in the first 2 days of life; newborns in general may have insufficient sweat for sampling. Diagnosis by genotype analysis is useful in these circumstances.

Newborn Screening

In almost all newborns with CF, pancreatic insufficiency (exocrine pancreatic failure resulting in maldigestion) is associated with elevated levels of serum trypsinogen, presumably owing to ductal obstruction or subclinical pancreatitis. Detection of elevated levels of serum trypsino-gen on dried filter paper blood specimens using an immunoreactive trypsinogen (IRT) assay is the basis for mass neonatal CF screening programs. Neonates with CF and pancreatic sufficiency (i.e., sufficient residual exocrine pancreatic function to permit adequate nutrient diges-tion) also can be recognized by this method.[53] By adding genotypic analysis of a duplicate blood sample for neonates with high IRT levels, the rate of false-positive results can be reduced, and the initial use of the far more costly genotypic analysis as a screening tool thereby avoided.[127] Routine neonatal screening for CF has not been widely recommended thus far; although short-term morbidity may be reduced by early diagno-sis, long-term benefits have not been demonstrated to date.[38]

MOLECULAR AND CELLULAR ASPECTS

The Basic Gene Defect

Cystic fibrosis is caused by mutations in the *CFTR* gene, located on the long arm of chromosome 7 at position 7q31, which encodes a cyclic AMP-regulated chloride channel protein of 1480 amino acids.[108] The most common mutation is referred to as ΔF508, indicating a 3 nucleotide base-pair deletion that results in a missing phenylalanine at position 508 in the amino acid sequence. Numerous other mutations exist; of over 350 mutations characterized so far, about half are due to amino acid substitutions, and the remainder includes frame shift, nonsense, and mRNA-splicing mutations. ΔF508 is by far the most common mutation, occurring in approximately 70% of the North American CF genes stud-ied.[85] In certain populations, mutations other than ΔF508 are more com-mon; among Ashkenazi Jews, for example, only 22% of the CF genes carried ΔF508, whereas the nonsense mutation W1282X occurred with a frequency of 60%.[133]

Genotype Analysis

Cystic fibrosis genotyping is highly useful in several clinical set-tings. Gene carriers among relatives of probands with CF can be readily identified and the future risk of having affected children assessed. Prena-tal diagnosis of CF can be accomplished by analysis of fetal tissue obtained by chorionic villus sampling or aminocentesis. A definitive diagnosis also can be obtained in newborns with meconium ileus who may have insufficient sweat to test at this age. Commercial laboratories routinely offer analysis of a panel of the 20 to 30 most common CF mutations, which together account for approximately 89% of alleles associated with the classic CF phenotype in North American popula-tions.[32] Detection by this panel is less frequent in populations with less common alleles, such as Africans, Asians, African-Americans, and

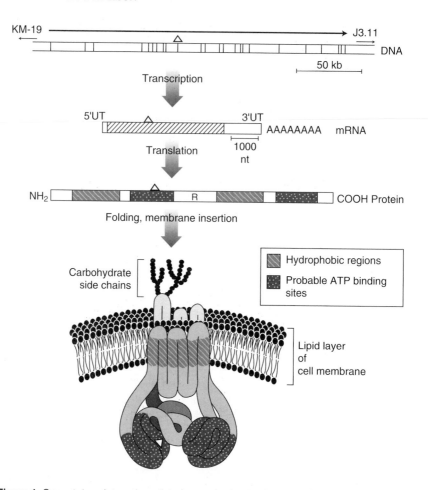

Figure 1. Gene, transcript, and predicted structure for the CFTR protein. The gene contains 27 exons and is flanked by the genetic markers KM-19 and J3.11. The mRNA is 6129 bp long, including 5' and 3' untranslated (UT) regions. The protein includes two hydrophobic transmembrane domains, two nucleotide-binding sites, and a highly charged R (regulatory) domain. The diagram of the folding of the protein is hypothetical. The triangle ($\triangle$) shows the location of the 3-bp deletion in exon 10 that generates ΔF508, the most common mutation in CF patients. (*Reprinted with permission from* Collins FS: Cystic fibrosis: Molecular biology and therapeutic implications. Science 256:775, Copyright 1992, American Association for the Advancement of Science.)

Hispanics.[143] Additional methods for the detection of rare mutations are available through research centers.

CFTR Protein

CFTR is a membrane-associated glycoprotein that functions as a cyclic AMP-regulated chloride channel. CFTR is a member of a general family of proteins called the *traffic ATPases* or *ABC* (A̲TP-b̲inding c̲assette) transporters (Figs. 1 and 2).[143] CFTR is located on the apical membrane of many types of epithelial cells.[108] Immunocytochemical studies have localized CFTR to the apical region of epithelial cell types known to be affected by CF, including pancreatic, intestinal crypt, salivary, sweat, airway, vas deferens, and biliary duct. CFTR has also been localized to kidney tubules and the basolateral membrane of sweat duct epithelium. CFTR has been found intracellularly also, on specific vesicular membranes within airway epithelial cells, possibly functioning in parallel with proton pumps to acidify these vesicles.[5]

The Chloride Channel Defect

The general mechanisms that underlie CFTR dysfunction are illustrated in Figure 3. The ΔF508 mutation results in defective processing of CFTR protein leading to failure of CFTR to traffic to the correct cellular location. The ultimate result of all mutations found to date that interfere with CFTR function is the same: failure of Cl⁻ transport.[142]

General Principles

Movement of water across all cell membranes is directly dependent on ion transport; water follows the transported ions. Failure to transport

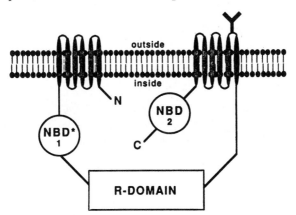

Figure 2. The predicted structure of the CFTR, adapted from the model proposed by Riordan et al. Two groups of six transmembrane-spanning domains are shown traversing the plasma membrane lipid bilayer with the inside and outside of the cell marked. The majority of the protein is intracellular. Structural domains are labeled: N, amino terminus; C, carboxy terminus; NBD1, first nucleotide-binding fold; NBD2, second nucleotide-binding fold; R-domain, regulatory domain; Y, extracellular carbohydrate moiety. The asterisk identifies the NBD containing the ΔF508 mutation. Features that placed CFTR in the traffic ATPase/ABC transporter family include sequence similarity in the two NBDs, the prediction of two membrane-spanning domains, and overall configuration. (*From* Marino CR, Gorelick FS: Scientific advances in cystic fibrosis. Gastroenterology 103: 684, 1992; *as adapted from* Riordan JR, Rommens JM, Kerem B, et al: Identification of the cystic fibrosis gene: Cloning and characterization of complementary DNA. Science 245:1066, 1989; with permission.)

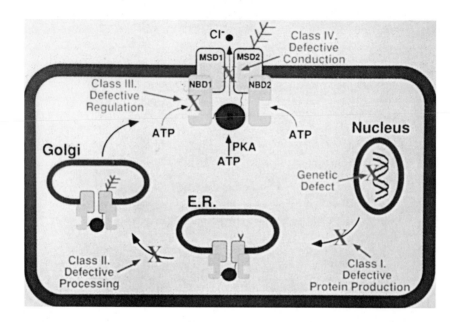

Figure 3. The biosynthesis and function of CFTR in an epithelial cell and of mechanisms of dysfunction associated with CF mutations. The ΔF508 mutation is a class II mutation; defective protein processing results in failure of CFTR to traffic to the correct cellular location. (*Adapted from* Welsh MJ, Smith AE: Molecular mechanisms of CFTR chloride channel dysfunction in cystic fibrosis. Cell 73:1251, Copyright 1993, Cell Press, with permission.)

Cl⁻ in CF, therefore, ultimately results in insufficient secretion of fluid with consequent inadequate hydration of various macromolecules. Thus, alterations occur in the physical and chemical properties of secretions in affected organs; macromolecules tend to gel or precipite, inspissating within the small secretory ducts of these organs. Poor clearance of these secretions predisposes the ducts to distention and obstruction (Fig. 4).[77]

Defective Cl⁻ transport may also result in altered glycoprotein synthesis through mechanisms that are as yet unclear; decreased sialylation and increased fucosylation and sulfation of various glycoproteins have been reported.[143] Defective Cl⁻ transport results in impaired intracellular organelle acidification, thereby altering glycoprotein processing.[5] Some researchers have suggested that the excessively sulfated glycoproteins in CF airway epithelia may lead to increased adherence by *Pseudomonas aeruginosa,* possibly explaining the increased colonization by this organism found in CF patients.[113]

The Sweat Gland

In the normal sweat gland, Cl⁻ transport by epithelial cells of the secretory coil is accomplished by two channels—CFTR and a second, distinct calcium-activated Cl⁻ channel—which together produce an isotonic fluid (Fig. 5).

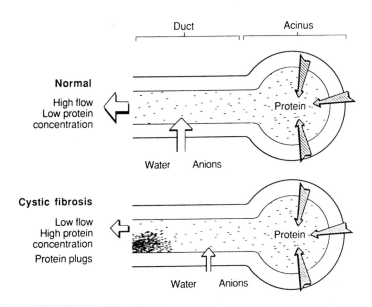

Figure 4. Pancreatic pathophysiology in CF. When ductal water flow is reduced owing to decreased anion secretion, the protein concentration in the duct rises. High concentrations of protein favor microprecipitation and plugging of duct lumina. [*From* Forstner G, Durie PR: Cystic fibrosis. *In* Walker WA, Durie PR, Hamilton JR, et al (eds): Pediatric Gastrointestinal Disease, vol 2, ed 1. Philadelphia, BC Decker Inc, 1991, p 1180; with permission.]

As the isotonic sweat flows distally, epithelial cells lining the duct lumen absorb Na^+ and Cl^-, producing hypotonic sweat. Both the initial secretion of Cl^- by secretory coil epithelial cells and the later resorption of Cl^- by ductular epithial cells are dependent on CFTR, which is localized on the apical membrane of epithelial cells.[8] Failure to open these Cl^- channels in CF ultimately results in the production of hypertonic sweat with a high residual Cl^- and Na^+ concentration. General mechanisms of epithelial cell Cl^- secretion are similar in the sweat gland secretory coil, airway, epididymis, and vas deferens; anion accumulation processes occur at the basolateral membrane and CFTR channels transport intracellular Cl^- at the apical membrane (see Fig. 5).[143]

The Pancreas

The exocrine pancreas normally produces an alkaline fluid containing high levels of HCO_3^- and pancreatic enzymes, which are secreted by pancreatic ductal and acinar cells, respectively. Pancreatic fluid neutralizes gastric acid and establishes an optimal pH for pancreatic enzyme activity. In normal pancreatic ducts, apical CFTR transports Cl^- into the pancreatic duct lumen (Fig. 6). Cl^-/HCO_3^- exchangers, also located on the apical surface, subsequently reabsorb lumenal Cl^- in exchange for intracellular HCO_3^-.[90] HCO_3^- exchange is directly depen-

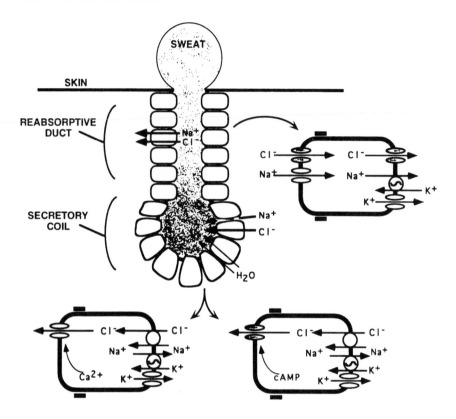

Figure 5. Sweat production and electrolyte transport by the sweat gland. Reabsorptive duct and secretory coil are indicated. Insets show cellular mechanisms of electrolyte transport by duct and coil epithelial cells. Note that cAMP-dependent and Ca^{2+}-dependent Cl^- secretion seem to occur in two different types of cells in the secretory coil. The CFTR Cl^- channel that is defective in CF is indicated by shading; all other channels, transporters, and pumps are indicated by open symbols. Transport processes in the airway and vas deferens are similar to those in the secretory coil. [*Adapted from* Welsh MJ, Tsui L-C, Boat TF, et al: Cystic fibrosis. *In* Scriver CR, Beaudet AL, Sly WS, et al (eds): Metabolic and Molecular Bases of Inherited Disease. New York, McGraw-Hill, 1995, p 3829; with permission of McGraw-Hill, Inc.]

dent on the presence of lumenal Cl^-. CFTR dysfunction leads to lumenal Cl^- levels insufficient for HCO_3^- exchange and, consequently, insufficient secretion of pancreatic fluid. Failure to provide sufficient quantities of pancreatic fluid results in plugging and obstruction of the pancreatic ducts, leading to ultimate destruction of the organ. Failure to alkalinize pancreatic fluid impairs gastric acid neutralization, further interfering with pancreatic digestive enzyme function in the intestinal lumen. Intestinal crypt and biliary duct epithelial cells exhibit similar Cl^- transport mechanisms, including HCO_3^- and Cl^- exchange, suggesting that similar pathophysiologic mechanisms occur in these tissues in CF (Fig. 7).[14, 90]

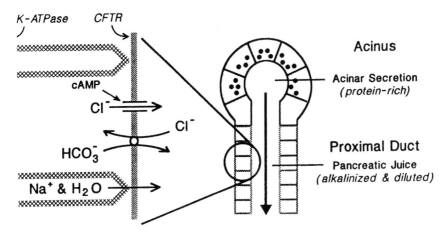

Figure 6. How CFTR may function during pancreatic secretion. As pancreatic juice flows through the duct, the protein-rich acinar secretions are diluted and alkalinized by the duct epithelial cells. CFTR, localized to the apical domain of these cells, exists near the site of the cAMP-regulated chloride channel, which has been implicated in the control of bicarbonate secretion. If CFTR is required for normal regulation of this channel, then failure of the channel to open properly in patients with CF could lead to a decrease in bicarbonate secretion resulting in impaired fluid secretion. Thus, a defect in CFTR function in the duct cell may promote the formation of protein plugs and thereby contribute to the ductal obstruction and progressive pancreatic insufficiency that occur in CF. (*Adapted from* Marino CR, Matovcik LM, Gorelick FS, et al: Localization of the cystic fibrosis transmembrane conductance regulator in pancreas. J Clin Invest 88:716, Copyright 1991; with permission of the American Society for Clinical Investigation.)

Phenotype-Genotype Correlations

In the CF population at large, approximately 85% of patients are considered to have pancreatic insufficiency (PI) on the basis of the presence of steatorrhea, defined as excessive losses of fat in the stool. The remainder have pancreatic sufficiency (PS), with sufficient exocrine pancreatic function to allow nutrient digestion without the need for exogenously administered pancreatic enzyme supplements; however, PI eventually develops in approximately 10% to 20% of these patients.[139] As a group, CF patients with PS are less likely to have meconium ileus or distal intestinal obstruction syndrome develop, and they maintain better nutritional status.[52] They are also more likely to be diagnosed at an older age, have relatively lower sweat chloride levels, maintain better pulmonary function, and have lower colonization rates with *Pseudomonas aeruginosa* than patients with PI.[131] Consequently, these patients have a better overall prognosis.

It has long been suspected that the degree of pancreatic dysfunction in patients with CF may correlate with certain CF genotypes. Despite the wide variations in pancreatic dysfunction that are observed in the general CF population, siblings with the disease often exhibit striking similarities, suggesting the importance of specific genetic factors.[20] Muta-

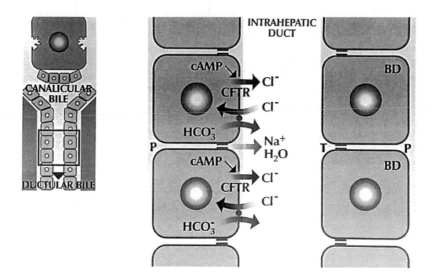

Figure 7. Changes in canalicular bile during passage through bile ductules. BD, bile duct cells; CFTR, cystic fibrosis transmembrane regulator; P, paracellular route; T, tight junction. (*From* Colombo C, Battezzati PM, Dodda M: Hepatobiliary disease in cystic fibrosis. Semin Liver Dis 14:262, 1994; with permission of Thieme Medical Publishers, Inc.)

tional analysis has confirmed that the degree of pancreatic insufficiency is indeed primarily determined by the specific nature of the CF mutation.[59] Various mutant alleles are associated with either PS or PI; fortunately, the PS allele seems to have a dominant effect over the PI allele. Patients who are found to have two alleles of the severe type should thus be followed expectantly for the development of PI. ΔF508 is associated with PI; other genotype-phenotype associations may be found in Table 1.[79]

To date, the genotypic correlations with other gastrointestinal manifestations of CF are not as convincing as for pancreatic disease. One study showed a lower incidence of meconium ileus in patients with the mild G551D mutation.[60] In adult patients with CF who had liver disease, an increased frequency of homozygous ΔF508 status has been found in one study; in contrast, a second study of children and young adults with CF found no correlation between genotype and the development of liver disease.[30, 37]

Thus far, reports of genotype correlations with pulmonary status have also been inconsistent. Whereas most studies have shown no correlation, one study did show an association of homozygous ΔF508 genotype with the early development of airway obstruction in neonates screened for CF; one study showed a relatively lower frequency of the ΔF508 mutation in older adult patients with CF; and a study of Dutch patients demonstrated a correlation between the A455E mutation and mild pulmonary disease.[40, 47a, 88]

Table 1. CLASSIFICATION OF CF GENE MUTATIONS AS SEVERE OR MILD WITH RESPECT TO PANCREATIC FUNCTION

| | Associated Pancreatic Phenotype Type of Mutation | | | | |
	Missense	Single Amino Acid Deletion	Nonsense	Splice Site	Frameshift
Insufficiency	I148T G480C G551D R560T N1303K	ΔF508 ΔI507	Q493X G542X R553X W1282X	621 + 1G→T 1717 − 1G→A	556delA 3656delC
Sufficiency	R117H R334W R347P A455E P574H				

Adapted from Kristidis P, Bozon D, Corey M, et al: Genetic determination of exocrine pancreatic function in cystic fibrosis. Am J Hum Genet 50:1178, 1992 and Cutting GR: Genotype-phenotype relationships in cystic fibrosis: Current progress and future avenues of research. New Insights into Cystic Fibrosis 2:1, 1994; with permission.

GASTROINTESTINAL MANIFESTATIONS OF CYSTIC FIBROSIS

Pancreas

Digestive Function

The primary clinical manifestations of pancreatic involvement in cystic fibrosis are due to incomplete fat and protein digestion. Pancreatic lipase, in conjunction with the cofactor pancreatic colipase, normally accounts for hydrolysis of the major proportion of dietary triglycerides. Exocrine pancreatic insufficiency in CF does not appear to result in overt steatorrhea until the secretion of lipase falls by about 98%, which commonly occurs in CF due to destruction of the pancreas.[51]

Histopathology

In contrast with the lungs, which are essentially unaffected by CF in utero, pancreatic involvement begins in utero with the arrest of acinar development.[65] Infants and children with CF almost always have evidence of an abnormal pancreas at autopsy, which, in its mildest form, may be manifested simply by an abnormal ratio of acinar to connective tissue. The earliest lesion seems to consist of dilated intralobular ductules filled with secretory material occluding the lumen. A mild degree of acinar atrophy and interstitial fibrosis may be evident at birth. During the first year of life in patients with PI, progressive ductular obstruction leads to acinar disruption and atrophy, possibly exacerbated by damage caused by the release of proteolytic enzymes. By the time these patients are 1 year of age, advanced acinar destruction has occurred with replacement by fibrous tissue and fat. Eventually ductules and acini disappear completely, with replacement of both pancreatic lobules and islets; the gland appears grossly shrunken. Late destructive changes to the pancreas may also include cyst formation and calcification.[101, 102]

Pancreatitis

Pancreatitis has been considered to be a complication of CF that exclusively occurs in patients with PS. Residual acinar tissue has been presumed to be required for the generation of an active inflammatory response. In one clinical population of patients with CF who had PS, pancreatitis developed in 15%.[4] Contrary to previous impressions, in the 1990 national registry of patients with CF, only 8% of the 64 CF patients with pancreatitis had PS, whereas the remaining 92% had PI; only 1 of 10 patients fewer than 10 years of age with pancreatitis had PS.[41] Hence, the diagnosis of pancreatitis should be considered in all CF patients with a suggestive clinical presentation, including abdominal pain, vomiting, and elevated serum amylase and lipase levels. Young children with CF, as well as older children and adults, may develop pancreatitis.[123] Because pancreatitis may be the presenting feature of CF in some patients, the diagnosis of CF should at least be considered in all patients who develop acute or recurrent pancreatitis, in whom the disease is otherwise unexplained.[4]

Diabetes

The incidence of diabetes mellitus (DM) in CF patients has been estimated to be 40- to 200-fold higher than in the general pediatric and young adult population.[80] Frank DM develops in approximately 1% of children, and in as many as 13% of adults with CF; subtler problems with glucose intolerance occur in approximately 50% of patients with CF.[80, 94] The development of DM invariably is associated with histopathologic abnormalities of the pancreas and is generally restricted to patients with CF who have PI. Early in CF-associated pancreatic disease, islets of Langerhans are preserved among the fibrous strands; with advancing disease, the total number of islet cells and the relative proportion of β cells decrease.[121, 122, 125] Diabetes mellitus in patients with CF is relatively mild in most cases, infrequently resulting in ketosis. The increasing incidence of DM with advancing age in patients with CF suggests that the prevalence rises as the size of the adult CF population increases. The frequency of serious secondary complications due to diabetic microangiopathy in patients with CF is also increasing, indicating that careful control of glucose in patients with CF may prove to be important to avoid the sequelae of DM.[35] Other endocrine abnormalities demonstrated in CF patients with PI include diminished secretion by alpha and pancreatic polypeptide-secreting cells, as measured by peak glucagon and pancreatic polypeptide secretion in response to hypoglycemia; the clinical significance of these abnormalities has not been established to date.[94]

Detection of Malabsorption

Fat malabsorption is generally defined as stool fat losses greater than 15% of the dietary intake in infants fewer than 6 months of age, and greater than 7% thereafter.[44] Steatorrhea is the first indication of CF in many patients with PI; however, grossly visible fat or oil in the stools often is not evident. Furthermore, the stools are rarely either watery or explosive and may even manifest as constipation, leading parents to describe the stool pattern as normal.

Stool Smear or 'Spot Stool Fat.' Pancreatic lipase hydrolyzes dietary triglycerides (neutral fat) to fatty acids (split fats) and glycerol. In patients with PI, an excessive number of neutral fat droplets may be rapidly and easily detected microscopically using water or alcohol in combination with Sudan II or oil red O. This serves as a basic screening tool only; quantification of fecal fat losses with a 72-hour fecal fat study is necessary for patients with an abnormal stool smear or patients suspected of having PI. False-negative results may occur in patients with low dietary fat intake at the time of testing.

Seventy-two–hour Fecal Fat Study. The 3- (or 5-) day stool collection with determination of fecal fat losses provides a reliable, quantitative estimation of fat absorption when performed properly. For accuracy, 3 days prior to and during the test, the dietary fat intake should be greater than 100 g/d in adults and at least 3 g/kg/d in infants.[75] The coefficient of fat absorption is calculated from estimation of the amount of fat ingested in the diet and direct assay of the amount excreted in the stool: coefficient of absorption = [(gm fat ingested − gm fat excreted) ÷ gm fat ingested] × 100. Generally, absorption should be greater than 85% of the dietary fat intake in infants fewer than 6 months of age and 93% thereafter, unless the dietary fat intake is excessive.[75] The mean dietary fat absorption in CF patients with PI who are not receiving enzyme replacement is approximately 60% (range, 10%–80%).[48] When performed properly, this test is the gold standard for the diagnosis of fat malabsorption. In patients with PI, this test is very useful for following the response to pancreatic enzyme replacement therapy. Because the commonly used van de Kamer laboratory method of fecal fat extraction does not detect medium-chain triglycerides (MCT), patients receiving formulas or supplements with MCT require an alternate method of fecal fat extraction, which may not be readily available, an easier alternative is placement on a long-chain triglyceride-containing diet during the testing period.[67, 137]

Assessment of Pancreatic Function

Stool Chymotrypsin Activity. An improved method for the qualitative estimation of exocrine pancreatic function that measures chymotrypsin activity in stool samples has been introduced.[72] The stool sample is collected, homogenized, and centrifuged in a specially designed test tube.[56] This is useful as a screening test for PI; the sensitivity has been reported as 80%, and specificity as 84%.[114]

Orally Administered Enzyme Substrates. BT-PABA (Bentiromide) and fluorescein dilaurate (Pancreolauryl) are orally administered substrates that are hydrolyzed by the pancreatic enzymes chymotrypsin and cholesterol ester hydrolase, respectively. Once hydolyzed, an absorbable product can be measured in either blood or urine.[56, 114] Although these tests are complicated to perform, they are more sensitive and specific than is the stool chymotrypsin assay.

Direct Pancreatic Stimulation Testing. Although the indirect tests described earlier are noninvasive, none offer the quantitative information and sensitivity available from direct pancreatic stimulation testing or reliably detect the subtler degrees of diminution of pancreatic function in CF patients prior to the overt development of PI.[58] Direct pancreatic stimulation with intravenously administered pancreatic secretagogues stimulates the pancreas to secrete fluid, HCO_3^-, and digestive enzymes at maximal capacity, thereby allowing identification of subtle defects in secretory capacity. Although the exact methodology used for direct pancreatic stimulation testing varies, usually two gastrointestinal hormones are simultaneously administered by continuous intravenous infusion; secretin stimulates water and HCO_3^- secretion by pancreatic ductular and centroacinar cells, and cholecystokinin stimulates the release of digestive enzymes from acinar cells.[56] Rates of pancreatic secretion of water, HCO_3^-, total protein, and specific digestive enzymes can then be determined from data derived from the collected duodenal fluid.

Patients with CF who have apparent pancreatic sufficiency at the clinical level have proved to exhibit a wide range of exocrine function when subjected to pancreatic stimulation testing, with lipase and colipase secretion ranging from normal to as low as 1% to 2% of normal.[51] Those patients with PS who eventually develop PI have been found to have greatly reduced outputs of enzyme, fluid, and electrolytes on pancreatic stimulation testing when compared with those who continue to have pancreatic sufficiency.[22] Thus, direct pancreatic stimulation testing may identify those PS patients who are at eventual risk of pancreatic failure.

Direct pancreatic stimulation testing has provided invaluable information regarding the pathophysiology of the pancreatic secretory defect in CF. Kopelman and colleagues demonstrated that pancreatic fluid from CF patients with PS or PI exhibited a high concentration of digestive enzyme protein and a low fluid volume; as fluid secretion dropped, protein output also fell, suggesting that the defect in fluid secretion resulted in reduced digestive enzyme secretion.[77] The hyperconcentrated protein secretions most likely lead to ductal obstruction and pancreatic damage, resulting in impairment of digestive enzyme secretion.[77] Gaskin and co-workers found that mean HCO_3^- secretion was defective in CF patients at all levels of pancreatic enzyme secretion.[50] Subsequently, Kopelman and colleagues found that Cl^- output, as well as HCO_3^- and fluid secretion, was decreased in patients with CF, independent of the residual extent of pancreatic enzyme secretion.[76] Thus, the basic pancreatic abnormality in CF is the anion secretion defect, which directly results in low pancreatic fluid secretion, and eventually results in ductal obstruction with loss of pancreatic enzyme secretion.[76] These results confirmed and extended earlier work by Johansen and colleagues.[68]

Gastrointestinal Tract

Patients with CF who have PI are predisposed to partial or complete obstruction of the lumen of the gastrointestinal tract, manifesting as meconium ileus at birth or distal intestinal obstruction syndrome (DIOS) later, often in adolescence. Presumably, the viscid, adherent lumenal contents lead to intestinal distention and obstruction. The viscid intestinal contents most likely result from the impaired digestion of lumenal proteins due to insufficient secretion of pancreatic enzymes, and the inadequate hydration of luminal macromolecules due to defective pancreatic, intestinal, and biliary fluid secretion. Characteristic histopathologic abnormalities of the gastrointestinal tract may be found in the small bowel, rectum, and appendix; these include bulging mucin-filled goblet cells, dilated mucin-filled intestinal crypts, and eosinophilic casts; the villous and microvillous structures remaining normal.[2, 101] These findings on intestinal resection may serve to raise the suspicion of CF in previously undiagnosed patients.

Meconium Ileus

Meconium ileus may be the earliest clinical manifestation of CF, occurring in 10% to 20% of patients.[36] Polyhydramnios may be found by antenatal fetal ultrasonographic examination, because bowel obstruction caused by meconium ileus may occur in utero; in most cases, however, bowel obstruction does not manifest until birth or the immediate postnatal period. Obstruction of the terminal ileum results in the failure to pass meconium, with progressive abdominal distention and bilious vomiting. Abdominal examination may reveal generalized distention with palpable stool-filled loops of bowel in the right lower quadrant; digital rectal examination may demonstrate a tight rectum and stimulate the passage of small amounts of sticky meconium or a dry mucus plug. Meconium plugs or delayed passage of meconium in the newborn may be early indicators of CF and probably represent a milder form of meconium disease in these patients.

Typical radiographic findings in meconium ileus include distended loops of small bowel associated with bubbles of gas and stool, described as a ground-glass appearance (i.e., Neuhauser's sign), with no air in the distal unused colon. The bubbles are due to gas trapped within viscous stool. Obstruction may be reflected by development of air-fluid levels (Fig. 8) and perforation may be indicated by extralumenal air; the earlier occurrence of perforation in utero may be exhibited by intra-abdominal calcifications. A barium enema usually reveals an unused, collapsed microcolon and may delineate the obstructing meconium mass in the distal ileum (see Fig. 8). In uncomplicated meconium ileus, intestinal obstruction may at times be relieved by administering iso-osmolar contrast enemas, under fluoroscopic control. The potential development of fluid and electrolyte imbalances may be avoided by the use of nonionic water-soluble agents [Hypaque (Winthrop, New York, NY), or Gastrografin (Squibb, Princeton, NJ)], diluted to isotonicity. Risks of this treatment include fluid and electrolyte shifts, intestinal perforation, and enterocolitis. If the patient's condition remains stable, repeated therapeutic enemas may be attempted over several days.

Surgical intervention is necessary if enemas fail to relieve the obstruction; an enterotomy with intestinal irrigation may enable removal of the meconium plug in some cases, but more extensive ileal resection may be required. The intralumenal mass of inspissated meconium may act as a fulcrum for volvulus of the bowel, leading to bowel necrosis, perforation, and peritonitis. Meconium peritonitis may lead further to ascites, adhesions, intra-abdominal calcifications, and meconium pseudocyst formation. In utero, ileal atresia may develop, presumably owing to vascular compromise. The reported incidence of CF is 30% in patients with meconium peritonitis and 20% in patients with intestinal atresias,

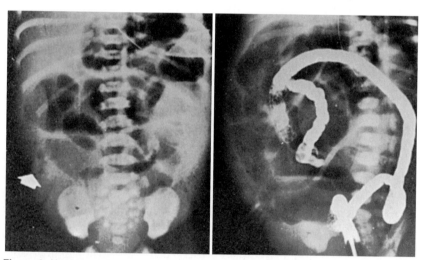

Figure 8. Newborn with intestinal obstruction. Abdomen film *(left)* shows distended bowel loops with "bubbly" pattern of inspissated meconium in terminal ileum *(arrow)*. Barium enema *(right)* shows a microcolon from disuse secondary to intrauterine obstruction. (*From* Boat TF, Welsch MJ, Beaudet AL: Cystic fibrosis. *In* Scriver CR, Beaudet AL, Sly WS, et al (eds): The Metabolic Basis of Inherited Disease, ed 6. New York, McGraw-Hill, 1989, p 2655; with permission.)

indicating that individuals with these conditions should undergo evaluation for CF.[97]

Meconium ileus occurs almost exclusively in association with PI and occurs more frequently in CF patients in families in which the first sibling with CF initially presented with meconium ileus.[58] In rare CF patients with meconium ileus and PS, pancreatic stimulation testing has revealed subtler degrees of impairment of pancreatic enzyme secretion, further lending support to the idea that pancreatic dysfunction is essential for the development of meconium ileus.[81] The prognosis for CF patients with meconium ileus is more than 96% survival in the first year of life; beyond 1 year, survival is the same as for the overall CF population.[31]

Distal Intestinal Obstruction Syndrome

Cystic fibrosis patients, primarily adolescents and adults, may suffer from recurrent episodes of partial obstruction due to DIOS. This condition occurs in approximately 15% of patients with CF and may occasionally be the presenting feature of CF.[105] DIOS is almost always associated with PI, although there are occasional reports of DIOS in CF patients with PS. The pathogenic mechanisms that contribute to the development of DIOS are thought to be similar to those in meconium ileus.

DIOS typically manifests as recurrent episodes of crampy or colicky abdominal pain, often in the right lower quadrant. A palpable fecal mass may be found in the right ileac fossa due to fecal impaction, which occurs first in the ileocecal region and then spreads distally. Frank obstructive symptoms may develop, frequently following years of persistent intermittent abdominal pain in the epigastrium or right lower quadrant. It is relatively unusual for patients with DIOS to develop full-blown episodes of complete intestinal obstruction with bilious vomiting, abdominal distention, and tenderness. Some patients are pain-free between episodes; others may complain of unremitting discomfort with associated weight loss. Abdominal radiographs in DIOS characteristically show bubbly-appearing fecal material in the distal small bowel and proximal colon. Air fluid levels may be present with a variable degree of small bowel dilatation. A barium enema may outline a fecal mass; if the appearance is difficult to distinguish from an appendical abscess or cecal neoplasm, ultrasound or computed tomography scan may be helpful.

Other gastrointestinal conditions may be confused with DIOS. Appendicitis is particularly difficult to distinguish, as demonstrated by the reported delay in the diagnosis of appendicitis in CF patients.[120] Intussusception occurs in 1% of CF patients; presumably the inspissated stool forms the lead point for the intussusceptum.[62] The classic symptoms of intussusception may not be present; patients may describe only mild crampy abdominal pain, and the stools are often heme-negative. Crohn's disease, ovarian pathology, hepatobiliary conditions, and pancreatitis should also be considered. Volvulus occurs very rarely as a complication of DIOS and is a surgical emergency.

Uncomplicated DIOS usually responds to medical management. Oral administration of a balanced electrolyte lavage solution (GoLytely; Colyte), which contains the nonabsorbable iso-osmolar agent polyethylene glycol, is considered safe and effective and has generally replaced other treatments used in the past.[13] Adults may be able to drink the large volume (5–6 L) required to relieve impaction, but children may require nasogastric tube placement for administration of 20 to 40 mL/ kg body weight per hour (maximum 1 L/h). The appearance of a clear rectal effluent does not exclude the possibility of incomplete evacuation; a repeat physical examination or abdominal radiograph are necessary. If further therapy is required, water-soluble contrast enemas containing the detergent Tween 80 (Hypaque, Gastrografin) may be diluted to iso-osmolar concentration and administered under fluoroscopic guidance to both confirm the diagnosis and provide additional treatment. If the patient remains clinically stable, enemas can be repeated over several days. Medical therapy is contraindicated if complete bowel obstruction or peritoneal irritation is evident, whereupon decompression with a nasogastric tube and urgent surgical consultation are required.

DIOS is a recurrent condition that requires prevention of onset. Once the acute episode has resolved, the adequacy of pancreatic enzyme therapy should be re-evaluated and appropriately adjusted. In addition, a high fiber diet and laxatives, including mineral oil and psyllium, may be helpful. For patients with persistent symptoms, efforts to prevent recurrence of episodes may include the administration of the prokinetic agent cisapride (Propulsid), stimulant laxatives, or, in refractory cases, the routine oral intake of N-acetylcysteine or Gastrografin.[74] Hypomagnesemia has been described as a complication of chronic N-acetylcysteine treatment.[55]

Rectal Prolapse

Rectal prolapse occurs in almost 20% of the CF population. In approximately half of this group, it is a presenting sign of CF. The onset usually occurs during the first few years of life, often during toilet training, and spontaneous resolution generally occurs by the age of 5 years. The degree of prolapse varies from the mucosal layer alone to all layers of the anorectum. The tendency to prolapse often improves dramatically with the initiation of pancreatic enzyme replacement, suggesting an etiologic role for the passage of large bulky stools; indeed, in a series of CF patients with PS, rectal prolapse was found in only 4%.[52] When rectal prolapse occurs in already-supplemented patients, the condition is often refractory. Further possible precipitating factors include diarrhea, constipation, malnutrition, and forceful coughing. Parents and patients should be taught to manually reduce the prolapse to avoid the onset of edema in the prolapsed segment. Surgical intervention is rarely warranted unless the episodes are painful, very frequent, difficult to reduce, or accompanied by incontinence.

Constipation

The symptoms of constipation in patients with CF are typical of those in the normal population, including crampy abdominal pain, difficulty passing stools, and infrequent evacuation. A stool mass located in the sigmoid colon and extending proximally may be noted by examination or abdominal radiograph. In contrast, in DIOS, the mass initially forms in the ileocecal region and extends distally.[26] Acute episodes may require enemas followed by intestinal lavage with a balanced electrolyte solution. In patients with CF, constipation is often associated with inadequate doses of pancreatic enzyme replacement rather than with excessive dosages. Additional options for therapy are the same as for the general population, including a high-fiber diet, various laxatives, and enemas.

Gastroesophageal Reflux Disease

Infants, children, and adults with CF are prone to gastroesophageal reflux (GER) disease. pH-probe studies have demonstrated abnormal levels of GER in infants and in malnourished patients with CF.[28, 116] The incidence of regurgitation (21%) and heartburn (27%) were also higher in children and adults with CF compared with their healthy siblings (0% and 4%, respectively).[116] The predominant mechanism in CF has been reported to be an increased number of inappropriate transient relaxations of the lower esophageal sphincter, rather than tonically low lower esophageal sphincter pressure.[25] Patients with advanced respiratory disease are especially prone to develop GER; coughing, wheezing, and physiotherapy tend to increase intra-abdominal versus thoracic pressure gradients, and certain medications used to treat bronchospasm may reduce lower esophageal sphincter pressure.[45] Patients with CF who have severe pulmonary disease have a high frequency of esophagitis demonstrated by endoscopy.[39] Gastroesophageal reflux disease, especially if severe or prolonged, may contribute to weight loss and may lead to the development of esophagitis, esophageal stricture, and Barrett's esophagus. Esophageal stricture and Barrett's esophagus may require surgical intervention. Aggressive and timely medical management should be a priority to improve patient comfort and nutritional status and to avoid the sequelae of GER disease and the need for surgery.

Gastrointestinal Malignancy

Anecdotal reports of gastrointestinal tract cancers and leukemia in patients with CF have suggested the possibility of an increased risk of cancer. A recent retrospective cohort study of more than 25,000 patients with CF found that the overall risk of cancer was similar to that of the general population; however, cancers specific to the digestive tract occurred more frequently in patients with CF, including cancers of the esophagus, stomach, small intestine, colon, rectum, liver, biliary tract, and pancreas.[96] Thus, gastrointestinal tract cancer should be actively considered in CF patients with otherwise unexplained gastrointestinal symptoms.

HEPATOBILIARY DISEASE

The hepatobiliary conditions associated with CF become increasingly apparent with advancing age. Liver disease in infancy and childhood is often asymptomatic, but serious complications arising from advanced disease, including cirrhosis with portal hypertension, occur more frequently in the adolescent and adult population. An increased prevalence of the severe complications of liver disease may be expected to accompany the increasing number of older patients with CF.

Liver Disease

Incidence

The reported incidence of CF-associated liver disease is variable (Table 2). The most reliable reports of the incidence of liver disease are found retrospectively in autopsy studies of patients with CF; an age-related increase in both the prevalence and severity of CF-associated liver disease has been clearly shown.[138] Clinical studies report a much lower incidence overall due to the lack of reliable noninvasive tests. Two large clinical series that included children and adults have been reported recently.[41, 118] Overt liver disease, manifested by hepatomegaly or splenomegaly, was found in 4.4% of 1100 patients with CF overall, with a peak incidence of 8.7% in adolescence.[118] A fall in prevalence was found after 20 years of age; possible reasons include the increased incidence of malnutrition-induced hepatomegaly in adolescence or ear-

Table 2. LIVER AND BILIARY TRACT DISORDERS

Location	Complication	Incidence
Liver	Steatosis	20–66%
	Focal biliary cirrhosis	10–72%
	Multilobular biliary cirrhosis	<1–24%
	Portal hypertension	<5–28%
Gallbladder	Nonvisualized gallbladder	12–40%
	Microgallbladder	30%
	Distended gallbladder	3–20%
	Atretic cystic duct	16%
	Cholelithiasis	0–33%
Common bile duct	Distal stenosis	10–33%
	Sclerosing cholangitis	1%
	Cholangiocarcinoma	Rare

From Gaskin K: The liver and biliary tract in cystic fibrosis: *In* Suchy FJ (ed): Liver Disease in Children. St. Louis, Mosby, 1994, p 707; with permission.

lier mortality associated with advanced liver disease in adolescence.[118] Data from the National Cystic Fibrosis Foundation Registry in the United States revealed the presence of cirrhosis, indicated by esophageal varices or splenomegaly, in 1.4% of 16,000 patients with CF overall, with a peak frequency of 2.7% in patients aged 16 to 20 years.[41] In a smaller series of 233 CF patients, which took into account the presence of abnormal liver biochemistry and overt liver disease, the incidence of liver disease was found to be 24.5% in patients more than 15 years of age.[95] Cystic fibrosis–associated liver disease has been found in patients who have PS, although it is more commonly associated with PI.[49] Cystic fibrosis–associated liver disease also may be a presenting feature in some patients with minimal lung involvement.

The exact mechanism of the pathogenesis of CF-associated liver disease is unclear to date. CFTR has been localized to biliary ductal epithelium, suggesting that the ubiquitous chloride channel dysfunction present in patients with CF may result in deficient biliary electrolyte and fluid secretion.[14] Even in the absence of overt clinical liver disease, biliary ductal epithelial cell abnormalities have been demonstrated by electron microscopy in patients with CF.[83] Thus, the specific hepatic conditions associated with CF, focal biliary cirrhosis, and multilobular biliary cirrhosis, possibly result from the intrahepatic biliary ductal epithelial cell transport defect.[17]

Specific Hepatic Disorders

Fatty Liver

Fatty liver—hepatic steatosis—may occur either as an isolated condition in patients with CF or in conjunction with the other CF-associated liver diseases. When fatty liver occurs alone, the liver is usually found to be enlarged, and a smooth soft edge is apparent. The condition is usually benign, but severe fatty infiltration can lead to massive hepatomegaly, especially in severely malnourished patients.[66] Resolution of the steatosis may occur with enzyme replacement and dietary therapy. In an infant with CF, resolution of massive steatosis occurred after supplementation with carnitine.[132]

Focal Biliary Cirrhosis

This condition is pathognomonic for CF. Eosinophilic material is found to occlude small bile ducts, and obstructive changes are found proximal to these, including small ductular dilatation, bile duct proliferation, portal tract fibrosis, and cholangiolitis (Fig. 9).[100] Sparing of the hepatocytes and parenchymal architecture is characteristic of focal biliary cirrhosis (FBC); the focal lesions are limited to the bile ducts. Thus, most patients with FBC are asymptomatic, and the only clinical sign is a firm, enlarged or tender liver.

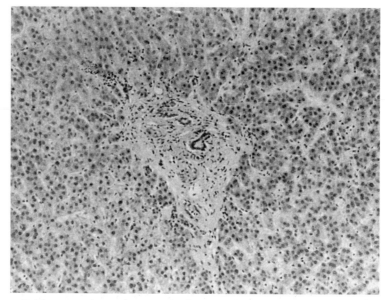

Figure 9. Biopsy specimen of a patient with cystic fibrosis demonstrates changes typical of focal biliary cirrhosis. (*From* Balistreri WF, Schubert WK: Liver disease in infancy and childhood: *In* Schiff L, Schiff ER (eds): Diseases of the Liver, vol 2, ed 7. Philadelphia, JB Lippincott, 1993, p 1119; with permission.)

The explanation for why only a minority of patients develop FBC remains unknown. In patients with liver disease, there is a relatively higher frequency of the CF genes associated with pancreatic insufficiency, and there is a decreased incidence of the "mild" or missense types of mutations.[37] An increased incidence of cirrhosis in patients with CF who have a history of meconium ileus or DIOS also has been reported, suggesting that biliary and intestinal epithelial cell dysfunction may be associated.[91] Other CF-associated abnormalities, such as lithogenic bile, malnutrition, or bile duct strictures, may further contribute to the development of FBC.[16, 54]

Multilobular Biliary Cirrhosis

In some patients, the fibrous lesions of FBC progress further, eventually coalescing to form the multilobular pattern characteristic of multilobular biliary cirrhosis (MBC). Whereas patients with FBC are usually asymptomatic, patients with MBC may develop portal hypertension, variceal bleeding, and, rarely, liver failure. Findings on liver biopsy include large irregular nodules, regenerative microscopic nodules, bile duct proliferation, and extensive fibrosis.[109] The uneven pattern of lobular fibrosis, in which fibrous tissue surrounds some hepatic lobules and spares others, is characteristic of MBC and explains the infrequent development of liver failure, despite the prevalence of portal hypertension.

Patients with MBC usually present with hepatomegaly. The liver edge may be firm and nodular. Splenomegaly due to portal hypertension is often the first indication of advanced liver disease, with variceal bleeding developing later. The hepatic transaminases may be either normal or minimally elevated; gamma glutamyltranspeptidase (GGT) may be the first to rise. In patients with CF, increasing levels of GGT correlate with the presence of MBC.[112] Hyperbilirubinemia is uncommon. Further signs of impaired hepatic function, such as coagulopathy, ascites, and encephalopathy, are not seen until very late in the disease. The major morbidity and mortality in patients with CF-associated liver disease is due to the complications of portal hypertension, especially variceal hemorrhage.

Neonatal Cholestasis

Hepatobiliary involvement in neonates with CF ranges from hepatomegaly or mild cholestatic jaundice to severe cholestasis with acholic stools. Clinically apparent liver disease in infancy, as indicated by hepatomegaly or cholestasis, was found in more than 35% of patients in one CF clinic.[112] Histologic evidence of FBC was found in 10% of CF infants fewer than 3 months of age at autopsy, and cholestasis was found in 38%.[100] The histopathologic abnormalities found in neonates with CF and cholestasis are variable and include the lesions associated with neonatal cholestasis in the general population, such as giant cell hepatitis, paucity of interlobular bile ducts, and correctable biliary atresia, as well as specific CF-associated lesions, such as FBC and distal common duct stricture.[47, 71, 110, 115] Biliary obstruction in neonates with CF is usually due to inspissation of biliary secretions and generally resolves by 3 to 4 months of age; however, biliary atresia should certainly be excluded in patients with acholic stools. Neonatal cholestasis may be the presenting feature of CF; thus, patients with neonatal cholestasis should undergo sweat testing unless another diagnosis is evident.

Evaluation of Liver Disease

Although conventional liver enzyme biochemistries are frequently found to be abnormal in many patients with CF who undergo screening for hepatobiliary involvement, these abnormal values do not correlate well with liver histology, nor does the finding of normal values exclude advanced liver disease. The synthetic functions of the liver usually are preserved until late in the disease; these can be determined by testing prothrombin and partial thromboplastin times and the serum albumin level, if vitamin K and protein intake requirements have been met.

Ultrasonography is the most widely used screening test for hepatobiliary involvement in CF. Abdominal ultrasound may show an echogenic pattern in the hepatic parenchyma suggestive of either steatosis or cirrhosis, or may reveal varices and spontaneous vascular shunts indicating portal hypertension; Doppler studies may demonstrate portal flow reversal due to advanced portal hypertension. Hepatobiliary scintigraphy is useful for evaluation of hepatobiliary function as well as for determination of ductular patency and anatomy of the biliary tract. An impression of biliary tree obstruction obtained by scintigraphy should be confirmed with cholangiography, which offers the most definitive demonstration of anatomy. The utility of percutaneous liver biopsy is limited by the possibility of sampling error due to the patchy distribution of lesions of FBC and MBC; however, it may be helpful in providing prognostic information if the degree of scarring is evident and in enabling differentiation of FBC or MBC from other hepatic conditions.

Management of Liver Disease

Cholestasis

In cholestatic conditions, serum levels of potentially hepatotoxic bile acids increase owing to impaired hepatic secretion. Hepatotoxicity is directly related to bile acid hydrophobicity. Ursodeoxycholic acid (URSO), which is a bile acid found in very low concentrations in humans, is thought to be capable of exerting an hepatoprotective effect when administered to patients with cholestasis by its relatively increased hydrophilicity. URSO has been reported to improve the biochemical parameters indicative of hepatocyte injury and pruritus in patients with a variety of cholestatic liver diseases; however, the biochemical profiles often return to pretreatment levels when URSO is discontinued.[136] URSO may protect the liver by replacing endogenous hepatotoxic bile acids in the circulating bile acid pool, enhancing clearance of toxic bile acids by stimulating bile flow, and inhibiting intestinal absorption of toxic bile acids. URSO may also have cytoprotective and immunomodulatory effects in the liver.[12, 136] URSO administration to patients with CF-associated liver disease, who were on prior taurine supplementation to enhance fat absorption, was shown to result in dose-dependent improvement in liver biochemistry profiles.[18] Optimal improvement was achieved with URSO doses of at least 20 mg/kg/d, which is greater than the dose required in most other liver diseases, perhaps because of impaired absorption in CF.[18] Patients with severe steatorrhea who are placed on high-dose URSO supplements should have their steatorrhea monitored closely, because URSO may interfere with lipid solubilization.[10] Further studies are needed to assess whether URSO administration consistently improves other parameters of liver injury, such as histologic abnormalities, and whether long-term benefits of therapy, such as slower progression of portal hypertension, can be achieved.

Portal Hypertension

Prophylactic treatment of variceal bleeding prior to the first episode of bleeding is not currently recommended for patients with CF. The use of propranolol in prevention of bleeding is contraindicated in patients with CF-associated lung diasease due to the risk of inducing bronchospasm. Sclerotherapy or variceal bonding should be considered after the onset of the first episode of bleeding; it is effective and well-tolerated in CF patients. In the general population, endoscopic variceal ligation has been shown to be equally effective in treating varices and has been associated with fewer complications compared with variceal sclerotherapy.[42, 130] Portosystemic shunting is also an option when sclerotherapy or variceal ligation fail to control bleeding in patients with mild to moderate lung disease. The relatively less invasive transjugular intrahepatic portosystemic shunt placement may be advantageous for patients with severe lung disease.

Hepatic Failure

Patients with CF who have intractable bleeding or signs of progressive hepatic insufficiency, such as coagulopathy, hypoalbuminemia, or ascites, may be candidates for liver transplantation. The severity of the patient's respiratory disease and the presence of malnutrition, diabetes, or infection are factors determining the patient's suitability for transplantation. Survival of patients with CF after liver transplantation has thus far been comparable with other liver transplant recipients, but experience is limited.[23] Some patients require both liver and lung transplantation.

Biliary Tract Disease

Nonvisualization of the Gallbladder and Microgallbladder

The most common biliary tract condition found in patients with CF is the "nonvisualized" or microgallbladder, a condition that is defined radiologically as either the inability to identify a gallbladder or the finding of a gallbladder measuring less than 1.5 cm in length and 0.5 cm in breadth.[49] Patients initially found to have nonvisualized gallbladders often later develop microgallbladders; both occur independently of liver disease. The atrophic gallbladder is usually filled with thick, grayish, translucent bile. The gallbladder wall and cystic duct exhibit small mucus-filled epithelial cysts; the cystic duct may also be atretic or functionally stenotic, due to marked mucosal hyperplasia.[102] Presumably, the gallbladder atrophies as a result of obstruction of the cystic duct by thick mucus. The patients are usually asymptomatic and do not require further evaluation.

Cholelithiasis

The incidence of cholestasis increases with advancing age. Patients with CF who have PI seem to be predisposed to the development of cholesterol gallstones, whereas gallstones are rare in those patients with PS.[112] The large fecal bile acid losses found in patients with CF are thought to play a role in cholesterol gallstone formation; these losses are associated with a diminished bile acid pool, predisposing to the formation of lithogenic bile.[111, 140] Because normal bile acid absorption has been found in patients with CF who have PS, the existence of a primary intestinal mucosal bile acid transport defect in CF is considered doubtful.[141] However, support for an etiologic role for malabsorption in the development of CF-associated cholelithiasis was suggested by the observation that raising the pancreatic enzyme replacement dosage in patients with steatorrhea resulted in doubling of the bile acid pool, reduced fecal bile acid losses, and decreased steatorrhea.[140]

Patients with CF who become symptomatic from cholelithiasis present in typical fashion, with intermittent right upper quadrant pain, nausea, vomiting, jaundice, and dietary fat intolerance; fever may be indicative of cholecystitis. Ultrasonography usually identifies gallstones. Owing to reports of distal common bile duct stricture in at least two CF patients with cholelithiasis, it may be beneficial to assess common bile duct patency and anatomy prior to surgery with scintigraphy; cholangiography may be used when further evaluation is warranted.[49] Cholecystectomy should be considered in patients with CF who have symptomatic gallstones and mild to moderate respiratory disease. Laparoscopic cholecystectomy usually reduces postoperative recovery time and may be especially preferable to open abdominal surgery in patients with respiratory compromise from CF lung disease. Therapy with biliary stone dissolution agents, such as URSO, may be considered as an alternative, but the recurrence rate is high.

Distal Common Duct Stricture

The most common abnormality of the bile duct in patients with CF is distal common duct stricture, although sclerosing cholangitis may be more common than previously recognized.[54, 98] Stricture in the region of the intrapancreatic bile duct segment may be caused by external compression resulting from fibrosis of the head of the pancreas or by intramural fibrosis.[49] In one report, distal common duct stricture was demonstrated in 96% of patients with CF who had clinical or biochemical evidence of liver disease, but these results have been contradictal by later studies that showed a much lower incidence of this anomaly.[54, 95, 98]

The presence of recurrent colicky right upper quadrant abdominal pain, especially in the absence of gallstones, should raise suspicion of common duct stenosis. Hepatomegaly and right upper quadrant tenderness are often apparent on physical examination. The majority of patients are anicteric.[54] Among patients with common duct stricture, some had been previously diagnosed with DIOS, suggesting the possibility that the symptoms of common duct stricture had been confused earlier with those due to DIOS. Persistent steatorrhea also may be noted despite high dosages of enzyme replacement.[49] Common bile duct dilatation or gallbladder distention on ultrasonography may suggest the presence of a distal common duct stricture; however, a normal study does not exclude it. Although hepatobiliary scintigraphy may be used as a screening tool to assess biliary tree function and anatomy, a definitive diagnosis of distal common duct stricture requires cholangiography; endoscopic retrograde cholangiopancreatography may be the procedure of choice. Surgery may be necessary in patients who develop recurrent pain or biliary tree obstruction but should be restricted to patients with mild to moderate respiratory disease. A cholecystojejunostomy may be done if the gallbladder is functioning, whereas a choledochojejunostomy may be required with a nonvisualized or microgallbladder.[49]

NUTRITION

Patients with CF are at very high risk for malnutrition. Substantial energy losses due to steatorrhea, increased energy requirements, and poor intake may converge, placing these patients in a precarious nutritional state. It is very important to recognize that impaired growth and malnutrition in CF are not inherent to the disease and can frequently be overcome or postponed by aggressive nutritional intervention.[106] Nutrition evaluation and support should begin at the time of diagnosis. When treatment plans are individualized according to the specific risk of malnutrition in each patient, aggressive nutritional therapy can be expected to achieve near normal nutritional status and age-appropriate growth in most patients.

Energy Intake

In past years, the energy intake of patients with CF may have been adversely affected by widely held misconceptions about the role of dietary fat. To avoid steatorrhea, recommendations were for diets low in long-chain fats and high in less concentrated sources of calories, such as carbohydrates, as well as less palatable sources of calories, such as medium-chain triglycerides (MCT). It is now clear that liberal fat intake, accompanied by proportionate increases in pancreatic enzyme replacement, is associated with increased survival and growth in patients with CF.[21] Although patients with CF who are on non-restricted diets tend to exhibit age-appropriate caloric intakes that are sufficient for the general population, they generally do not consume sufficient calories to compensate for the multiple CF-associated increases in energy requirements.[7] Severe anorexia may result from many factors, including pulmonary infection, liver disease, gastroesophageal reflux with painful esophagitis leading to dysphagia, and abdominal discomfort due to DIOS or constipation. A multidisciplinary approach is needed to identify and control the multiple factors that lead to diminished caloric intake.

Energy Losses

Contributions to energy loss in patients with CF may include such diverse causes as inadequate pancreatic digestive enzyme supplementation, a history of intestinal resection resulting in decreased absorptive surface, reduced permeability of viscid intestinal mucus leading to decreased nutrient absorption, impaired carbohydrate utilization due to CF-associated diabetes, and vomiting associated with gastroesophageal reflux, among many others. Steatorrhea is exacerbated by bile acid losses, which may result from precipitation of bile salts in the abnormally low pH of the duodenum, binding to unabsorbed protein and fat, distal ileal resection, and liver disease. Patients with CF who continue to have high caloric losses in the stool despite adequate enzyme replacement need to increase their daily intake to compensate.

Energy Utilization

Energy balance in patients with CF may be further disrupted by an increased resting energy expenditure (REE); increases as high as 180% of normal have been demonstrated in malnourished patients with CF who have moderate to severe pulmonary disease.[109] Resting energy expenditure was shown to be only slightly higher than predicted in patients with CF who have normal nutritional status and good lung function.[46] Thus, deteriorating lung function is a major factor contributing to increased REE, particularly at FEV_1 values below 75% of those predicted.[135] The presence of superimposed pulmonary infection further increases the energy requirements of patients with CF who have moderate to severe respiratory disease.[129] Refeeding undernourished patients with CF also has been shown to increase REE.[134]

Nutrient Deficits

Macronutrients

Stool fat losses in patients with CF who have PI average 40% (range 10–80%) in the absence of pancreatic enzyme administration; 40% to 60% of patients normalize on enzyme replacement therapy.[49] Unfortunately, 5% to 10% of patients maintain fat losses higher than 25% during enzyme replacement, perhaps owing to insufficient alkalinization of the small intestine or other factors that are not yet understood.[48] Essential fatty acid (EFA) deficiency may occur as a result of steatorrhea and marginal fat intake; characteristic signs are thrombocytopenia, skin desquamation, poor wound healing, increased infections, and growth retardation.[61] Although full-blown clinical EFA deficiency is rare in patients with CF after infancy, the biochemical abnormalities associated with EFA are relatively common, such as decreased plasma levels of linoleic acid.[63] The lipid profile often normalizes when caloric supplementation is sufficient to support weight gain, most likely by preventing the utilization of EFA as an energy source.[103]

In the absence of enzyme replacement, total dietary protein losses, reflected by stool nitrogen content, average 30% (range 10–50%).[48] This generally decreases to approximately 18% when sufficient digestive enzymes are given.[82] The greatest risk for protein deficiency occurs in infancy, because protein requirements are highest then. Compared with cow's milk formula, human milk is lower in protein; soy protein has a lower biologic value than cow's milk protein. Clinical signs of protein deficiency, with hypoproteinemia, edema, and growth failure have been found prior to enzyme replacement in infants who are breast fed or on soy formula. For infants with PI, enzyme replacement is recommended with any type of milk. The risk for protein-energy malnutrition increases again in early adolescence, as evidenced by decreased weight gain, growth, and pubertal development that may become apparent in this age group.[93]

Large-scale carbohydrate malabsorption is not characteristic of patients with CF, owing to the presence of α-amylases in saliva and glucoamylase in the intestinal brush border that act to hydrolyze dietary glucose polymers and starch.

Vitamins

Patients with CF are at risk for deficiency of the fat-soluble vitamins A, D, E, and K, particularly at the time of diagnosis. In infants with CF identified by newborn screening, biochemical evidence of vitamin A deficiency was present in 21%, vitamin D in 35%, and vitamin E in 38% of infants by age 3 months; whereas none were deficient in vitamin K, most likely owing to the administration of this vitamin at the time of delivery.[126] Standard vitamin supplementation served to normalize vitamin A and D levels, but serum vitamin E levels remained low in 10% of infants. Hence, serum fat-soluble vitamin levels should be closely monitored until normalization is achieved. It is not uncommon for older children with CF to develop biochemical evidence of fat-soluble vitamin deficiency; clinically apparent signs of vitamin deficiency are infrequent but do occur. The risk is further increased in patients with bile acid losses due to ileal resection following meconium ileus or cholestatic liver disease. Antibiotic usage may lead to decreased vitamin K production by intestinal flora. Vitamin B_{12} is the only water-soluble vitamin that is poorly absorbed in CF patients with PI, but pancreatic enzyme replacement usually normalizes absorption; supplementation is generally necessary only in patients with ileal resection.[107]

Minerals and Trace Metals

Patients with CF are prone to hyponatremic dehydration during periods of exercise and heat stress due to the high losses of sodium in sweat. Breast-fed infants should be supplemented with sodium chloride, particularly during the summer months, with 2 to 4 mEq/kg body weight per day (1/4 tsp = 1437.5 mg NaCl ~ 24 mEq/d).[107] No overt abnormalities in the absorption or metabolism of minerals or trace metals have been described in CF, although the occurrence of iron deficiency is common.[3] As in all patients with severe malnutrition, nutritional rehabilitation may be associated with hypokalemia, hypomagnesemia, and hypophosphatemia.

Nutrition Support in Cystic Fibrosis

Assessment

The Cystic Fibrosis Foundation guidelines recommend that children with CF be seen routinely every 3 to 4 months, and infants weekly or biweekly, until normal weight gain is established.[106] At each visit, anthropometric measurements should be taken, including weight, height, midarm circumference, triceps skinfold thickness, and, in children under 2 years of age, head circumference and length. Assessment of energy balance is necessary at the time of diagnosis and as part of the yearly evaluation; more frequent evaluations are required in children who are not gaining weight or height normally for age. Energy balance is evaluated by determining energy intake, coefficient of fat absorption, and energy expenditure. In well-nourished CF patients, the caloric intakes suggested by the Manual of Recommended Dietary Allowances provide adequate energy requirements.[19] In patients who are growing poorly, an accurate estimation of energy requirements can be derived from calculation of the basal metabolic rate followed by adjustments for activity level, pulmonary function, and degree of fat malabsorption, as detailed in the Cystic Fibrosis Consortium consensus on nutrition.[106] Biochemical indices of nutritional status should be evaluated at the time of diagnosis and yearly thereafter, including a complete blood count, serum or plasma retinol, α-tocopherol, albumin, and electrolytes. Further evaluation is required on an individual basis.

Pancreatic Enzyme Replacement Therapy

The enzymes in most preparations are derived from desiccated extracts of porcine pancreas. Enzyme content varies among preparations, including lipase, which is the most important factor determining the efficacy of enzyme replacement therapy. pH-sensitive enteric-coating of the enzymes is used to minimize oral ulceration by preventing enzyme release in the mouth; however, infants may not swallow the enteric-coated microspheres unless they are mixed with solids. Infants with PI require pancreatic enzyme supplements with any type of milk, including protein hydrolysate and breast milk; supplements should be administered with each feed. Similarly, children require enzyme replacement with each meal or snack. Guidelines for enzyme supplementation are available, but therapy should be individualized. Initial enzyme dosages appropriate for infants are 1000 to 2000 U lipase in pH-sensitive microspheres per 120 mL of formula.[106] Initial dosing in children and adults is 500 U lipase/kg/meal using enteric-coated microcapsule products;

the dosage should be increased in a stepwise fashion.[6] A requirement greater than 2000 U lipase/kg/meal is considered a poor response to therapy and should be further investigated.[6] Fibrosing colonopathy has been found in CF patients taking very high-dose enzyme replacement (> 6000 lipase U/kg/meal); colonic strictures occur in the advanced stage of this condition.[6, 92] Enzyme dosages above 2000 U lipase/kg/meal should be avoided to prevent the development of this condition; at any rate, the maximal clinical response for treatment of steatorrhea, usually occurs below this dosage. Enzyme dosage should not presumptively be increased above the recommended range without first specifically documenting improvement via a 3-day fecal fat collection.[6]

Despite adequate digestive enzyme supplementation, some patients continue to have severe stool losses of both fat and protein. This may be in part due to the low intestinal pH, which results from reduced pancreatic HCO_3^- secretion in CF. This prevents dissolution of the coating on the enzyme preparation, inhibits exogenous pancreatic enzyme activity, and promotes bile acid precipitation. Therapeutic options for improving fat absorption in these patients include gastric acid suppression therapy with antacids, H_2 blocking agents, omeprazole (Prilosec), or taurine supplementation.[11, 124] Other medical approaches include the addition of pancreatic powder preparations at the beginning of the meal for early onset of action, or perhaps choosing an alternate enzyme preparation, because the dissolution profiles of the various enteric-coated microspheres and microtablets may vary.[6]

Nutrition Therapy

General dietary recommendations should include a high calorie diet with liberal fat intake, vitamin/mineral supplementation (Table 3), and, in patients with PI, pancreatic enzyme supplements. The addition of behavioral group treatment programs has resulted in sustained improvements in caloric intake in patients with CF.[128] Anticipatory guidance is especially important during periods of rapid growth, as in infancy and adolescence. The importance of the role of one-on-one, continuous nutritional evaluation and counseling over the years cannot be overemphasized.

In mildly undernourished patients, high calorie oral supplementation should be initiated. Infants who are growing slowly may benefit from continued intake of infant formula, with introduction of the less nutritionally complete cow's milk delayed to 24 months of age.[107] Patients with intestinal resection or cholestatic liver disease may require formulas or caloric supplements that contain a portion of fat as MCT. The failure to reverse moderate to severe degrees of malnutrition by noninvasive interventions, such as oral supplements, necessitates direct enteral feeding. Over the short term, nasogastric tube-feeding is useful; over the long term, either gastrostomy or jejunostomy tube feedings are effective. Usually overnight enteral feeding by continuous drip is used in combination with a regular diet during the daytime. Although gas-

Table 3. DAILY VITAMIN SUPPLEMENTATION FOR CYSTIC FIBROSIS PATIENTS

Vitamin	Dosage
Vitamins A and D*	
Infants and children ≤2 years	1 mL Poly-Vi-Sol (Mead Johnson Nutritionals, Evansville, IN) or a similar preparation
Children 2–8 years	1 standard multivitamin tablet containing vitamin D 400 IU and vitamin A 5000 IU
Children >8 years, adolescents, and adults	1–2 standard multivitamin tablets
Vitamin E†	
0–6 months	25 IU
6–12 months	50 IU
1–4 years	100 IU
4–10 years	100–200 IU
>10 years	200–400 IU
Vitamin K	
0–12 months	2.5 mg/wk, or 2.5 mg twice weekly if on antibiotics
>1 year	5.0 mg twice weekly if on antibiotics or if cholestatic liver disease is present

*Water-miscible vitamin A preparations are available (Aquasol A, Rover Pharmaceuticals, Fort Washington, PA) for patients with inadequate serum vitamin A concentrations on a standard multivitamin preparation.

†Vitamin E is given as Aquasol E (Rover Pharmaceuticals, Fort Washington, PA) or Liqui-E (Twin Labs, Ronkonkoma, NY) for the first year or two of age. After that, capsules of α-tocopherol or d-α-tocopherol acetate may be used. Excessive doses of vitamin E (>1000/d) may exacerbate vitamin K-induced coagulopathy.

Adapted from Ramsey BW, Farrell PM, Pencharz P, and the Consensus Committee: Nutritional assessment and management in cystic fibrosis. Am J Clin Nutr 55:108, 1992; with permission.

trostomy tube placement has been found to increase the frequency of gastroesophageal reflux in malnourished patients, no increase was found in the total time esophageal pH was below 4 or in the frequency of clinical symptoms.[117] Adjunctive medications, including an acid secretory blocker such as omeprazole, and a prokinetic agent such as cisapride, may reduce the number or severity of reflux episodes. Total parenteral nutrition is usually reserved for acute short-term gastrointestinal conditions, but may be helpful in otherwise intractable malnutrition.

There are substantial gains to be achieved by optimizing the nutritional status in patients with CF. It has been long recognized that the degree of malnutrition correlates with the severity of pulmonary disease and patient survival rates.[78] It is also clear that respiratory and nutritional status influence each other; as one deteriorates, so does the other. In malnourished patients with CF, aggressive long-term nutritional intervention has been shown to achieve improvements in patient well-being, catch-up growth, slower deterioration of pulmonary function, decreased incidence of pulmonary infection as well as improved exercise capacity, and respiratory muscle strength.[9, 84, 119] It seems highly possible that improvements in pulmonary status, achieved through a sustained reversal of malnutrition, may ultimately improve longevity, because the severity of the pulmonary disease is the major determinant of long-term survival.

SOMATIC GENE THERAPY

In patients with autosomal recessive genetic diseases, such as CF, introduction of a normal copy of the involved gene into the homozygous recessive mutant host cell should enable the host cell to function normally. Certain features specific to CF have suggested that somatic gene therapy might be feasible in this disease. In normal postnatal airways, CFTR expression occurs at very low levels and in only a few cells, suggesting the possibility that gene therapy would be beneficial in CF, even if CFTR expression were only achieved at very low levels in a small percentage of cells.[94] Indeed, an in vitro study demonstrated restoration of normal chloride transport function in a sheet of CF airway epithelial cells, after gene transfer corrected only 6% to 10% of cells.[70]

In patients with most of the other diseases for which gene therapy protocols are considered, cells are removed from the organ, genetically modified, and then reinfused into the organ, in an ex vivo approach. Due to the lack of accessibility of the branching airways in patients with CF, gene transfer instead requires the use of vectors which encode the normal CFTR gene, which can be safely delivered in vivo into the airways, and selectively infect the appropriate cell population.[69]

There are two general approaches to gene therapy using vectors. In the integrative approach, vectors are used that directly integrate into the host cell genome by insertion of normal DNA.[43] If a normal gene were successfully integrated into the host genome, it would potentially function indefinitely. The principal vectors used are retroviruses and adeno-associated viruses. The nonintegrative approach uses vectors that function as extrachromosomal DNA in the host cell nucleus and that do not require chromosomal integration for transcription.[43] The current nonintegrative methods for gene therapy include administration of liposomes, various molecular conjugates, and adenovirus.[69] Gene expression resulting from this approach is transient, typically lasting from days to weeks. Clinical trials of gene therapy in CF patients are currently using nonintegrative vectors; liposomes are being used in the United Kingdom and adenovirus in the United States.[69, 99]

Liposomes

The development of cationically charged liposomes has enabled the use of DNA-liposome complexes for liposome-mediated gene transfer.[69] To accomplish this, CFTR DNA is first cloned into a plasmid vector. The negatively charged plasmid DNA binds to cationic liposomes forming a complex that is then incorporated into the host cell, mainly through endocytosis.[69] Cationic liposomes have been used in CFTR-deficient transgenic mice to deliver normal CFTR genes to the airways by nebulization and have restored chloride transport function in most of the animals.[89] In clinical trials in the United Kingdom, patients with CF are undergoing liposome-mediated gene transfer into the epithelium of the nasal cavity.[1] The advantages of the cationic liposome approach include low toxicity, avoidance of risks associated with viral vectors, and ability to transfect nondividing cells rendering them functional. The main disadvantage is that repetitive dosing is required.[99]

Adenoviruses

Adenoviruses are double-stranded DNA viruses that infect the respiratory and gastrointestinal tracts of humans and other primates. The major potential advantages of using adenoviral vectors in patients with CF is their specific tropism for respiratory epithelia and their ability to infect nondividing cells.[69] In constructing the vector, a portion of the viral gene sequence is replaced by the CF gene, thereby forming a hybrid sequence that is packaged into the infective virus particle. This enables viral attachment to the host cell–surface receptors, followed by cell entry via receptor-mediated endocytosis and subsequent avoidance of lysosomal degradation.[69] Adenoviral vectors encoding normal human CFTR gene have achieved transgene expression following in vivo delivery to the nasal epithelium of rhesus monkeys and humans, and to the airways of cotton rats, baboons, and humans.[24, 146, 147] Adenovirus vectors also have been used to achieve CFTR gene expression in rat biliary duct epithelium in vivo and in human biliary duct epithelium ex vivo, suggesting the possibility of using endoscopic retrograde cholangiopancreatography (ERCP) to deliver the CFTR gene for the treatment of CF-associated hepatobiliary disease.[57, 145] The eventual feasibility of gene therapy for treatment of exocrine pancreatic insufficiency was suggested by the recent demonstration of adenovirus-mediated transfer of human pancreatic lipase–complementary DNA into sheep gallbladder, using in vitro and ex vivo approaches.[87]

The potential for adverse effects is currently under study. In some animal models, adenovirus vector administration has produced inflammatory reactions, including acute mixed cellular responses, antibody-mediated immune processes, or late lymphocyte predominant responses.[69, 99] After receiving adenoviral vector delivery to the lungs, a lung infiltrate in the region of vector administration developed in one patient with CF, with a transient episode of fever, hypotension, and reduced lung function.[24] Theoretic risks include overexpression of CFTR, ectopic expression of CFTR by nonepithelial cell function, viral replication, and expression of viral proteins. Human studies designed to determine in vivo safety and efficacy of adenovirus-mediated gene transfer to nasal or airway epithelium are in progress at six centers to date.[144] One controlled study of 12 patients with CF showed that adenoviral-vector–mediated transfer of the CF gene did not correct functional defects in nasal epithelium, and local inflammation limited the dose of adenovirus that could be administered to improve efficacy.[73a] The feasibility of somatic gene therapy will become evident in the very near future.

SUMMARY

Cystic fibrosis is an autosomal recessive disorder of epithelial cell chloride transport that affects multiple organs. The gastrointestinal manifestations of CF are diverse, with potential dysfunction of the pancreas, intestine, liver, and biliary tree. Not only pancreatic disease but also pulmonary and gastrointestinal involvement may contribute to compromised nutritional status. Aggressive nutritional intervention can achieve normal growth in most patients and may improve pulmonary function. Improved longevity in patients with CF is most likely due to the positive impact of comprehensive, multidisciplinary management on pulmonary and nutritional status. Clinical trials are underway at multiple centers to explore the use of somatic gene therapy as a potentially definitive treatment for pulmonary disease.

References

1. Alton EWFW, Middleton PG, Caplen NJ, et al: Non-invasive liposome-mediated gene delivery can correct the ion transport defect in the cystic fibrosis mutant mice. Nat Genet 5:135, 1993
2. Andersen D: Pathology of cystic fibrosis. Ann N Y Acad Sci 93:500, 1962
3. Ater JL, Herbst JJ, Landaw SA, et al: Relative anemia and iron deficiency in cystic fibrosis. Pediatrics 71:810, 1983
4. Atlas AB, Orenstein SR, Orenstein DM: Pancreatitis in young children with cystic fibrosis. J Pediatr 120:756, 1992
5. Barasch J, Kiss B, Prince A, et al: Defective acidification of intracellular organelles in cystic fibrosis. Nature 352:70, 1991
6. Beall RJ: Summary outline from consensus conference on fibrosing colonopathy: National Cystic Fibrosis Foundation, official communication to directors of cystic fibrosis centers, April 1995
7. Bell L, Linton WL, Corey ML, et al: Nutrient intakes of adolescents with cystic fibrosis. J Can Diet Assoc 42:1, 1981
8. Bell CL, Reddy MM, Quinton PM: Reversed anion selectivity in cultured cystic fibrosis sweat duct cells. Am J Physiol 262:C32, 1992
9. Boland MP, Stoski DS, MacDonald, et al: Chronic jejunostomy feeding with a non-elemental formula in undernourished patients with cystic fibrosis. Lancet 1:232, 1986
10. Carey MC, Montet J-C, Phillips MC, et al: Thermodynamic and molecular basis for dissimilar cholesterol-solubilizing capacities by micellar solutions of bile salts. Biochemistry 20:3634, 1981
11. Carroccio A, Pardo F, Montalto G, et al: Use of famotidine in severe exocrine pancreatic insufficiency with persistent maldigestion on enzymatic replacement therapy. Dig Dis Sci 9:1441, 1992
12. Cirillo NW, Zwas FR: Ursodeoxycholic acid in the treatment of chronic liver disease. Am J Gastroenterol 89:1447, 1994
13. Cleghorn GJ, Forstner GG, Stringer DA, et al: Treatment of distal intestinal obstruction syndrome in cystic fibrosis with a balanced intestinal lavage solution. Lancet i:8, 1986
14. Cohn JA, Strong TV, Picciotto MR, et al: Localization of the cystic fibrosis transmembrane conductance regulator in human bile duct epithelial cells. Gastroenterology 105:1857, 1993
15. Collins FS: Cystic fibrosis: Molecular biology and therapeutic implication. Science 256:774, 1992
16. Colombo C, Apostolo MG, Ferrari M, et al: Analysis of risk factors for the development of liver disease in CF. J Pediatr 124:393, 1994
17. Colombo C, Battezzati PM, Podda M: Hepatobiliary disease in cystic fibrosis. Sem Liver Dis 14:3, 1994
18. Colombo C, Crosignani A, Assaisso M, et al: Ursodeoxycholic acid therapy in cystic fibrosis-associated liver disease: A dose-response study. Hepatology 16:924, 1992
19. Committee on Dietary Allowances: Recommended Dietary Allowances (ed 9): National Academy of Sciences, Washington, DC, 1980

20. Corey M, Durie P, Moore D, et al: Familial concordance of pancreatic function in cystic fibrosis. J Pediatr 115:274, 1989
21. Corey M, McLaughlin FJ, Williams M, et al: A comparison of survival, growth, and pulmonary function in patients with cystic fibrosis in Boston and Toronto. J Clin Epidemiol 41:583, 1988
22. Couper RTL, Corey M, Moore DJ, et al: Decline of exocrine pancreatic function in cystic fibrosis patients with pancreatic sufficiency. Pediatr Res 32:179, 1992
23. Cox KL: The role of liver transplantation in cystic fibrosis patients. Pediatr Pulmonol Suppl 5:78, 1990
24. Crystal RG, et al: Nat Genet 8:42, 1994
25. Cucchiara S, Santamaria F, Andreotti MR, et al: Mechanisms of gastroesophageal reflux in cystic fibrosis. Arch Dis Child 66:617, 1991
26. Cystic Fibrosis Foundation: Patient Registry 1993 Annual Data Report, Bethesda, Maryland, September, 1994
27. Cystic Fibrosis Foundation: Concepts in Care Consensus Conference: Gastrointestinal problems in CF II:1, 1991
28. Dab I, Malfroot A: Gastroesophageal reflux: A primary defect in cystic fibrosis? Scand J Gastroenterol 23 (Suppl 143):125, 1988
29. Daniels L, Davidson GP, Cooper, DM: Assessment of nutrient intake of patients with cystic fibrosis compared with healthy children. Hum Nutr Appl Nutr 41A:157, 1987
30. De Arce M, O'Brien S, Hegarty J, et al: Deletion of delta F508 and clinical expression of cystic fibrosis-related liver disease. Clin Genet 42:271, 1992
31. Del Pinn CA, Czyrko C, Ziegler MM, et al: Management of survival of meconium ileus: A 30-year review. Ann Surg 215:179, 1992
32. DeMarchi JM, Beaudet AL, Caskey CT, et al: Experience of an academic reference laboratory using automation for analysis of cystic fibrosis mutations. Arch Pathol Lab Med 118:26, 1994
33. Denning CR, Huang NN, Cusay LR, et al: Cooperative study comparing three methods of performing sweat tests to diagnose cystic fibrosis. Pediatrics 66:752, 1980
34. Deren JJ, Arora B, Toskes PP, et al: Malabsorption of crystalline vitamin B_{12} in cystic fibrosis. N Engl J Med 288:949, 1973
35. Dodge JA, Morrison G: Diabetes mellitus in cystic fibrosis: A review. JR Soc Med 85(Suppl 19):25, 1992
36. Donnison AB, Shwachman H, Gross RE: A review of 164 children with meconium ileus seen at the Children's Hospital Medical Center, Boston. Pediatrics 37:833, 1966
37. Duthie A, Doherty DG, Williams C, et al: Genotype analysis for F508, G551D and R553X mutations in children and young adults with cystic fibrosis with and without chronic liver disease. Hepatology 15:660, 1992
38. Farrell PM, Mischler EH: Newborn screening for cystic fibrosis. Adv Pediatr 39:35, 1992
39. Feigelson J, Girault F, Pecau Y: Gastro-esophageal reflux and esophagitis in cystic fibrosis. Acta Paediatr Scand 76:989, 1987
40. Ferec, Verlinque C, Guillermit H, et al: Genotype analysis of adult cystic fibrosis patients. Hum Mol Genet 2:1557, 1993
41. FitzSimmons SC: The changing epidemiology of cystic fibrosis. J Pediatr 122:1, 1993
42. Fix VL, Carr-Locke DL, Connors PJ, et al: Endoscopic ligation of esophageal varices in children. Pediatr Gastroenterol Nutr 20:202, 1995
43. Flotte TR: Prospects for virus-based gene therapy for cystic fibrosis. J Bioenerg Biomembr 25:37, 1993
44. Fomon SJ, Ziegler ER, Thomas LN, et al: Excretion of fat by normal full-term infants fed various milks and formulas. Am J Clin Nutr 23:1299, 1970
45. Foster AC, Voyles JB, Murray BL, et al: Twenty-four hour pH monitoring in children with cystic fibrosis: Association of chest physical therapy to gastroesophageal reflux. Pediatr Res 17:188A, 1983
46. Fried MD, Durie PR, Tsui L-C, et al: The cystic fibrosis gene and resting energy expenditure. J Pediatr 119:913, 1991
47. Furuya KN, Roberts EA, Canny GJ, et al: Neonatal hepatitis syndrome with paucity of interlobular bile ducts in cystic fibrosis. J Pediatr Gastroenterol Nutr 12:127, 1991

47a. Gan King-Han, Veeze HJ, Van den Ouweland Ans MW, et al: A cystic fibrosis mutation associated with mild lung disease. N Engl J Med 333:95, 1995
48. Gaskin KJ: Cystic fibrosis: Nutritional problems and their management. Sem Pediatr Gastroenterol Nutr 4:9, 1993
49. Gaskin KJ: The liver and biliary tract in cystic fibrosis. In Suchy FJ (ed): Liver Disease in Children. St. Louis, Mosby, 1994, p 705
50. Gaskin KJ, Durie PR, Corey M, et al: Evidence for a primary defect of pancreatic HCO_3^- secretion in cystic fibrosis. Pediatr Res 16:554, 1982
51. Gaskin KJ, Durie PR, Lee L, et al: Colipase and lipase secretion in childhood-onset pancreatic insufficiency: Delineation of patients with steatorrhea secondary to relative colipase deficiency. Gastroenterology 86:1, 1984
52. Gaskin KJ, Gurwitz D, Durie PR, et al: Improved respiratory prognosis in patients with cystic fibrosis with normal fat absorption. J Pediatr 100:857, 1982
53. Gaskin KJ, Waters D, Dorney S, et al: Assessment of pancreatic function in screened infants with cystic fibrosis. Pediatr Pulmonol Suppl 7:69, 1991
54. Gaskin KJ, Waters D, Howman-Giles R, et al: Liver disease and common-bile-duct stenosis in cystic fibrosis. N Engl J Med 318:340, 1988
55. Godson C, Ryan MP, Brady HR, et al: Acute hypomagnesaemia complicating the treatment of meconium ileus equivalent in cystic fibrosis. Scand J Gastroenterol Suppl 143:14, 1988
56. Goldberg DM, Durie PR: Biochemical tests in the diagnosis of chronic pancreatitis and in the evaluation of pancreatic insufficiency. Clin Biochem 26:253, 1993
57. Grubman SA, Fang SL, Mulberg AE, et al: CFTR gene complementation in intrahepatic biliary epithelial cell lines derived from CF patients. Pediatr Pulmonol 18(Suppl 10):228(175A), 1994
58. Hadorn B, Zoppi G, Shmerling D, et al: Quantitative assessment of exocrine pancreatic function in infants and children. J Pediatr 73:39, 1968
59. Hamosh A, Corey M: Correlation between genotype and phenotype in patients with cystic fibrosis. N Engl J Med 329:1308, 1993
60. Hamosh A, King TM, Rosenstein BJ, et al: Cystic fibrosis patients bearing both the common missense mutation Gly→Asp at codon 551 and the delta F508 mutation are clinically indistinguishable from delta F508 homozygotes, except decreased risk of meconium ileus. Am J Hum Genet 51:245, 1992
61. Hansen AE, Wiese HF, Boelsche AN, et al: Role of linoleic acid in infant nutrition. Pediatrics 331:171, 1963
62. Holsclaw DS, Rocmans C, Shwachman H: Intussusception in patients with cystic fibrosis. Pediatrics 48:51, 1971
63. Hubbard VS, Dunn GD, di Santi' Agnese PA: Abnormal fatty acid composition of plasma lipids in cystic fibrosis. Lancet ii:1302, 1977
64. Hyde SC, Gill DR, Higgins CF, et al: Correction of the ion transport defect in cystic fibrosis transgenic mice by gene therapy. Nature 362:250, 1993
65. Imrie J, Fagan D, Sturgess J: Quantitative evaluation of the development of the exocrine pancreas in CF and control infants. Am J Pathol 95:697, 1979
66. Isenberg JN: Cystic fibrosis: Its influence on the liver, biliary tree, and bile salt metabolism. Sem Liver Dis 2:312, 1982
67. Jeejeebhoy KN, Ahmed S, Kozak G: Determination of fecal fats containing both medium and long chain triglycerides and fatty acids. Clin Biochem 3:157, 1970
68. Johansen PG, Anderson CM, Hadorn B: Cystic fibrosis of the pancreas: A generalized disturbance of water and electrolyte movement in exocrine tissue. Lancet 1:455, 1968
69. Johnson LG: Gene therapy for cystic fibrosis. Chest 107:77S, 1995
70. Johnson LG, Olsen JC, Sarkadi B, et al: Efficiency of gene transfer for restoration of normal airway epithelial function in cystic fibrosis. Nat Genet 2:21, 1992
71. Jones MC, Sakai H, Rogerson AG: Intravenous cholangiography in children with fibrocystic disease of the pancreas: A pilot study. J Pediatr 53:172, 1958
72. Kaspar P, Moeller G, Wahlefeld AW, et al: A new photometric method for the determination of chymotrypsin in stool. Fresenius Z Anal Chem 311:391, 1982
73. Kerem E, Cory M, Kerem B, et al: Clinical and genetic comparisons of patients with cystic fibrosis, with or without meconium ileus. J Pediatr 114:767, 1989
73a. Knowles MR, Hohneker KW, Zhou Zhaoging, et al: A controlled study of adenoviral-

vector-mediated gene transfer in the nasal epithelium of patients with cystic fibrosis. N Engl J Med 333:823, 1995

74. Koletko S, Corey M, Ellis L, et al: Effects of cisapride in patients with cystic fibrosis and distal intestinal obstruction syndrome. J Pediatr 117:815, 1990

75. Kopelman H: Pancreatic function testing. In Wyllie R, Hyams JS (eds): Pediatric Gastrointestinal Disease. Philadelphia, WB Saunders, 1993, p 854

76. Kopelman H, Corey M, Gaskin K, et al: Impaired chloride secretion, as well as bicarbonate secretion, underlies the fluid secretory defect in the cystic fibrosis pancreas. Gastroenterology 95:349, 1988

77. Kopelman H, Durie P, Gaskin K, et al: Pancreatic fluid secretion and protein hyper-concentration in cystic fibrosis. N Engl J Med 312:329, 1985

78. Kraemer P, Rudeberg A, Hadorn B, et al: Relative underweight in cystic fibrosis and its prognostic value. Acta Paediatr Scand 67:33, 1978

79. Kristidis P, Bozon D, Corey M, et al: Genetic determination of exocrine pancreatic function in cystic fibrosis. Am J Hum Genet 50:1178, 1992

80. Krueger LJ, Lerner A, Katz SM, et al: Cystic fibrosis and diabetes mellitus: Interactive or idiopathic. J Pediatr Gastroenterol Nutr 13:209, 1991

81. Lands L, Ainman P, Wise M, et al: Pancreatic function testing or meconium ileus in cystic fibrosis: Two case reports. J Pediatr Gastroenterol Nutr 7:276, 1988

82. Lapey A, Kattwinkel J, Di Sant' Agnese PA, et al: Steatorrhea and azotorrhea and their relation to growth and nutrition in adolescents and young adults with cystic fibrosis. J Pediatr 84:328, 1974

83. Lendblad AL, Hultcrantz R, Strandvik B: Bile duct destruction and collagen deposition: A prominent ultrastructural feature of the liver in cystic fibrosis. Hepatology 16:372, 1991

84. Levy L, Durie P, Pencharz PB, et al: Effects of long-term nutritional rehabilitation on body composition and clinical status in malnourished children and adolescents with cystic fibrosis. J Pediatr 107:225, 1985

85. Lucotte G, Loirat F: A more detailed map of the cystic fibrosis mutation delta F508 frequencies in Europe. Hum Biol 65:503, 1993

86. MacLean W, Tripp R: Cystic fibrosis with edema and falsely negative sweat test. J Pediatr 83:85, 1973

87. Maeda H, Danel C, Crystal RG: Adenovirus-mediated transfer of human lipase complementary DNA to the gallbladder. Gastroenterology 106:1638, 1994

88. Mahon RT, Wagener JS, Abman SH, et al: Relationship of genotype to early pulmonary function in infants with cystic fibrosis identified through neonatal screening. J Pediatr 122:550, 1993

89. Marino CR, Gorelick FS: Scientific advances in cystic fibrosis. Gastroenterology 103:681, 1992

90. Marino CR, Matovcik LM, Gorelick FS: Localization of the cystic fibrosis transmembrane conductance regulator in pancreas. J Clin Invest 88:712, 1991

91. Maurage C, Lenerts C, Weber AM, et al: Meconium ileus and its equivalent as a risk factor for the development of cirrhosis: An autopsy study in cystic fibrosis. J Pediatr Gastroenterol Nutr 9:17, 1989

92. Milla CE, Wielinski CL, Warwick WJ: High-strength pancreatic enzymes. Lancet 343:599, 1994

93. Mitchell-Heggs P, Mearns M, Battern JC: Cystic fibrosis in adolescents and adults. Q J Med 45:479, 1976

94. Moran A, Diem P, Klein D, et al: Pancreatic endocrine function in cystic fibrosis. J Pediatr 118:715, 1991

95. Nagel RA, Javaid A, Meire HB, et al: Liver disease and bile duct abnormalities in adults with cystic fibrosis. Lancet ii:1422, 1989

96. Neglia JP, Fitzsimmons SC, Maisonneuve P, et al: The risk of cancer among patients with cystic fibrosis. N Engl J Med 332:494, 1995

97. Noblett H: Meconium ileus. In Ravithc M, Welch K, Benson C, et al (eds): Pediatric Surgery. Chicago, Year Book Medical Publishers, 1979, p 943

98. O'Brien S, Keogan M, Casey M, et al: Biliary complications of cystic fibrosis. Gut 33:387–391, 1992

99. O'Neal WK, Beaudet AL: Somatic gene therapy for cystic fibrosis. Hum Mol Genet 3:1497, 1994
100. Oppenheimer EH, Esterly JF: Hepatic changes in young infants with cystic fibrosis: Possible relation to focal biliary cirrhosis. J Pediatr 86:683, 1975
101. Oppenheimer EH, Esterly JF: Pathology of cystic fibrosis, review of the literature and comparison with 146 autopsied cases. In Perspectives in Pediatric Pathology, vol 2. Chicago, Year Book Publishers 1975, p 2451
102. Park RW, Grand RJ: Gastrointestinal manifestations of cystic fibrosis: A Review. Gastroenterology 81:1143, 1981
103. Parsons HG, O'Loughlin EV, Forbes D, et al: Supplemental calories improve essential fatty acid deficiency in cystic fibrosis patients. Pediatr Res 24:353, 1988
104. Pencharz P, Hill R, Archibald E, et al: Energy needs and nutritional rehabilitation in undernourished adolescents and adults with cystic fibrosis. J Pediatr Gastroenterol Nutr 3 (Suppl 1):147, 1984
105. Quinlan M, Way N, Joske R: Adult cystic fibrosis presenting with meconium ileus equivalent and diagnosed by selenomethionine scanning of the pancreas. Aust Ann Med 16:84, 1967
106. Ramsey BW, Farrell PM, Pencharz P, and the Consensus Committee: Nutritional assessment and management in cystic fibrosis. Am J Clin Nutr 55:108, 1992
107. Ramsey BW, Farrell PM, Pencharz P, and the Consensus Committee: Nutritional assessment and management in cystic fibrosis. Consensus Conferences Volume I, Section V, April 1990, p 1
108. Riordan JR, Rommens JM, Kerem B, et al: Identification of the cystic fibrosis gene: Cloning and characterization of complementary DNA. Science 245:1066, 1989
109. Roberts WC: The hepatic cirrhosis of cystic fibrosis of the pancreas. Am J Med 32:324, 1962
110. Rosenstein BJ, Oppenheimer EH: Prolonged obstructive jaundice and giant cell hepatitis in an infant with cystic fibrosis. J Pediatr 91:102, 1977
111. Roy CC, Weber AM, Morin CL, et al: Abnormal biliary lipid composition in cystic fibrosis: Effect of pancreatic enzymes. N Engl J Med 297:1301, 1977
112. Roy CC, Weber AM, Morin CL, et al: Hepatobiliary disease in cystic fibrosis: A survey of current issues and concepts. J Pediatr Gastroenterol Nutr 1:469, 1982
113. Saiman L, Cacalano G, Gruenert D, et al: Comparison of adherence of Pseudomonas aeruginosa to respiratory epithelial cells from cystic fibrosis patients and healthy subjects. Infect Immun 60:2808, 1992
114. Schmidt E, Schmidt FW: Advances in the enzyme diagnosis of pancreatic diseases. Clin Biochem 23:383, 1990
115. Schwarz HP, Kraemer R, Thurnheer U, et al: Liver involvement in cystic fibrosis. Helv Paediatr Acta 33:351, 1978
116. Scott RB, O'Loughlin EV, Gall DG: Gastroesophageal reflux in patients with cystic fibrosis. J Pediatr 106:223, 1985
118. Scott-Jupp R, Lama M, Tanner MS: Prevalence of liver disease in cystic fibrosis. Arch Dis Child 66:698, 1991
119. Shepherd RW, Holt TL, Thomas BJ, et al: Nutritional rehabilitation in cystic fibrosis. Controlled studies of effects on nutritional growth retardation, body protein turnover, and course of pulmonary disease. J Pediatr 109:788, 1986
120. Shields MD, Levison H, Reisman JJ, et al: Appendicitis in CF. Arch Dis Child 65:307, 1991
121. Shwachman H: Cystic fibrosis. Curr Probl Pediatr 8:1, 1978
122. Shwachman H, Kowalski M, Khaw KT: Cystic fibrosis: A new outlook, 70 patients above 25 years of age. Medicine 56:24, 1977
123. Shwachman H, Lebenthal E, Khaw K: Recurrent acute pancreatitis in patients with cystic fibrosis with normal pancreatic enzymes. Pediatrics 55:86, 1975
124. Smith LJ, Laaille F, Lepage G, et al: Taurine decreases fecal fatty acid and sterol excretion in cystic fibrosis. Am J Dis Child 145:1401, 1991
125. Soejima K, Landing BH: Pancreatic islets in older patients with cystic fibrosis with and without diabetes mellitus: Morphometric and immunocytologic studies. Pediatr Pathol 6:25, 1986

126. Sokol RJ, Reardon MC, Accurso FJ, et al: Fat-soluble vitamin status during the first year of life in infants with cystic fibrosis identified by screening of newborns. Am J Clin Nutr 50:1064, 1989
127. Spence WC, Paulus-Thomas J, Orenstein DM, et al: Neonatal screening for cystic fibrosis: Addition of molecular diagnostics to increase specificity. Biochem Med Metab Biol 49:200, 1993
128. Stark LJ, Knapp LG, Bowen AM, et al: Increasing calorie consumption in children with cystic fibrosis: Replication with 2-year follow-up. J Appl Behav Anal 26:435, 1993
129. Steinkamp G, Drommer A, von der Hardt H: Resting energy expenditure before and after treatment for *Pseudomonas aeruginosa* infection in patients with cystic fibrosis. Am J Clin Nutr 57:685, 1993
130. Stiegmann GV, Goff JS, Michaletz-Onody PA, et al: Endoscopic sclerotherapy as compared with endoscopic ligation for bleeding esophageal varices. N Engl J Med 326:1527, 1992
131. The Cystic Fibrosis Genotype-Phenotype Consortium: Correlation between genotype and phenotype in patients with cystic fibrosis. N Engl J Med 329:1308, 1993
132. Treem WR, Stanley CA: Massive hepatomegaly, steatosis and secondary plasma carnitine deficiency in an infant with CF. Pediatrics 83:993, 1989
133. Tsui L-C: The spectrum of cystic fibrosis mutations. Trend Genet 8:392, 1992
134. Vaisman N, Clarke R, Pencharz PB: Nutritional rehabilitation increases resting energy expenditure without affecting protein turnover in patients with cystic fibrosis. J Pediatr Gastroenterol Nutr 13:380, 1991
135. Vaisman N, Pencharz PB, Corey M, et al: Energy expenditure of patients with cystic fibrosis. J Pediatr 111:496, 1987
136. Van de Meeberg PC, van Erpecum KJ, van Berge-Henegouwen GP: Therapy with ursodeoxycholic acid in cholestatic liver disease. Scand J Gastroenterol 200(Suppl 28):15, 1993
137. Van de Kamer JK, ten Bokkel Huinink H, Weyers HA: Rapid method for the determination of fat in feces. J Biol Chem 177:347, 1949
138. Vawter GF, Shwachman H: Cystic fibrosis in adults: An autopsy study. Pathol Ann 14:357, 1979
139. Waters DL, Dorney SFA, Gaskin KJ, et al: Pancreatic function in infants identified as having cystic fibrosis in a neonatal screening program. N Engl J Med 322:303, 1990
140. Watkins JB, Tercyak AM, Szczepanik P, et al: Bile salt kinetics in cystic fibrosis: Influence of pancreatic enzyme replacement. Gastroenterology 73:1023, 1977
141. Weber AM, Roy CC, Chartrand L, et al: Relationship between bile acid malabsorption and pancreatic insufficiency in cystic fibrosis. Gut 17:295, 1976
142. Welsh MJ, Smith AE: Molecular mechanisms of CFTR chloride channel dysfunction in cystic fibrosis. Cell 73:1251, 1993
143. Welsh MJ, Tsui L-C, Boat TF, et al: Cystic fibrosis. *In* Scriver CR, Beaudet AL, Sly WS, et al (eds): Metabolic Basis of Inherited Disease, ed 7. New York, McGraw-Hill, 1995, p 3799
144. Wilson JM: Prospects for human gene therapy. Highlights: Eighth annual North American cystic fibrosis conference. Orlando, October 20, 1994, p 20
145. Yang Y, Raper SE, Cohn JA, et al: An approach for treating the hepatobiliary disease of cystic fibrosis by somatic gene transfer. Proc Natl Acad Sci U S A 90:4601, 1993
146. Zabner J, Couture LA, Gregory RJ, et al: Adenovirus-mediated gene transfer transiently corrects the chloride transport defect in nasal epithelia of patients with cystic fibrosis. Cell 75:207, 1993
147. Zabner J, Petersen DM, Puga AP, et al: Safety and efficacy of repetitive adenovirus-mediated transfer of CFTR cDNA to airway epithelia of primates and cotton rats. Nat Genet 6:75, 1994

Address reprint requests to

Linda B. Shalon, MD
Pediatric Gastroenterology and Nutrition
Hasbro Children's Hospital
593 Eddy Street (MPS 126)
Providence, RI 02903

0031–3955/96 $0.00 + .20

GASTROESOPHAGEAL REFLUX
Diagnostic and Therapeutic Approaches

A. Craig Hillemeier, MD

The term *gastroesophageal reflux* (GER) is merely descriptive and refers to the presence of gastric contents in the esophagus proximal to the stomach. Reflux of gastric contents is a physiologic occurrence that takes place more often during infancy and decreases with advancing age. Although virtually all infants have some degree of GER, the severity of symptoms ranges widely from an occasional burp to persistent emesis. The evaluation of most of these infants usually reveals no definable anatomic, metabolic, infectious, or neurologic cause for GER. The clinical importance of these symptoms of spitting up or vomiting early in life is derived from their potential association with other related medical conditions, such as failure to thrive or respiratory symptoms.

The past two decades have seen a virtual explosion in the number of diagnostic tests that are available to analyze and quantitate GER in infants. The clinical challenge of determining the medical conditions that are casually associated with obvious symptoms of GER and what diagnostic tests are appropriate to define this relationship is substantial. To determine which infants may be suffering from pathologic conditions associated with subtle signs of GER is even more challenging. This determination is essential to avoid subjecting many healthy infants to costly and potentially invasive testing.

PHYSIOLOGY OF UPPER GASTROINTESTINAL TRACT MOTILITY

The muscular layers of the upper gastrointestinal tract distal to the mid-esophagus are composed of smooth muscle and are not, therefore,

From the Division of Pediatric Gastroenterology, University of Michigan, Ann Arbor, Michigan under voluntary control. The esophagus functions as a muscular tube. Peristaltic waves of contraction are responsible for the forces that transport an ingested food bolus through the body of the esophagus and ultimately past a relaxed lower esophageal sphincter into the stomach. The external circular muscle layer is primarily responsible for the generation of force identified as a *peristaltic wave* and the maintenance of lower esophageal sphincter tone.

The lower esophageal sphincter at the distal end of the esophagus has attracted the greatest amount of interest in attempts to explain why infants seem to have a greater tendency to GER than do older children or adults. The lower esophageal sphincter is an area of thickened circular muscle that is tonically contracted at rest. The relaxation that occurs at the end of an esophageal peristaltic sequence is integrated by a network of neurons that are coordinated to ensure that relaxation occurs at the appropriate time. This tonically contracted zone is relatively independent of neurotransmitters in the generation of tone at rest in the basal state[10]; however, neural input is important in the production of the inhibitory neurotransmitters that are responsible for relaxation of the lower esophageal sphincter. These neurotransmitter agents are non-cholinergic, non-adrenergic, and current investigation suggests vasoactive intestinal peptide and nitric oxide as likely candidates.

This tonically contracted muscle, known as the *lower esophageal sphincter,* has long been theorized to be abnormal in people who have symptoms of GER. Although initial manometric studies suggested a decreased basal tone in the lower esophageal sphincter of infants who have significant GER,[19] animal models[28] and human studies have suggested that, in newborns, the muscle of the lower esophageal sphincter is not weaker than in the adult. Some evidence suggests, however, that the lower esophageal sphincter is at a mechanical disadvantage in generating its basal pressure because of anatomic pressure diameter relationships.[30] Another possible explanation for pathologic reflux that has received increasing support is that inappropriate relaxation of the lower esophageal sphincter[12] is responsible for many instances of GER. This inappropriate relaxation of the lower esophageal sphincter may be related to abnormal functioning of the central nervous system or developmentally exaggerated enteric reflexes. These abnormal enteric reflexes could be either proximal (i.e., esophageal) or distal (i.e., gastric) in origin. An example of an abnormal proximal enteric reflex is the initiation of a swallow that is not picked up in the body of the esophagus but does result in lower esophageal sphincter relaxation.[52] Distal enteric reflexes could be initiated by abnormal gastric motor function, causing distention that results in retrograde peristalsis and lower esophageal sphincter relaxation (i.e., the "vomiting reflex").[31] Recent evidence from animal models suggests that newborn gastric muscles may function differently than adult gastric musculature.[28] These differences may give risk to more retrograde peristalsis in the newborn.

Speculation as to the pathogenesis of GER has very practical implications. The understanding that most infants with GER have normal lower esophageal sphincter tone explains why the use of agents such as bethanechol, which primarily increases lower esophageal sphincter pressure, is not very successful in treating this disorder. Gastric prokinetic agents, such as cisapride, which increase gastric emptying rates, may be effective by allowing ingested food less time to undergo reflux in the stomach during inappropriate relaxation. They also may modify gastric motor activity in such a way as to allow less retrograde peristalsis. However, the inability to understand the most effective means to control inappropriate relaxation of the lower esophageal sphincter is likely the reason that pharmacologic therapy of this disorder is only modestly effective at best.

CLINICAL PRESENTATIONS

Although many older children with GER complain of symptoms, such as heartburn, that are quite similar to those of adults, infants often present with a different spectrum of clinical manifestations. As noted previously, all infants have some degree of reflux in the newborn period, and spitting or vomiting during the first year of life is common. It must be remembered that infants who suffer from significant regurgitation or vomiting might be responding to disease process outside the gastrointestinal tract. It is, therefore, important to perform a careful history and physical to ensure that no easy definable anatomic, metabolic, infectious, or neurologic cause for GER is present.

Anatomic disorders, such as pyloric stenosis, often have a typical history of projectile nonbilious vomiting following eating. Bilious emesis usually indicates more distal obstructions, such as congenital webs, atresias, or malrotations. Children with metabolic diseases or central nervous system tumors may present with emesis during infancy. Because most infants have some degree of GER, one should not automatically assume a cause-and-effect relationship between the symptoms of GER and other health-related conditions, such as growth problems, respiratory disease, apnea, or behavioral problems. Unfortunately, clinical determination of the relationship between these conditions and GER is often difficult, and their relationship must be approached with a degree of skepticism.

The vast majority of infants with GER who are symptomatic of spitting up during the first year of life resolve their overt symptoms between the ages of 9 and 24 months. Because most infants with symptoms of GER are thriving and healthy, they require no diagnostic or therapeutic maneuvers other than a careful history and physical examination, with appropriate reassurance to the parents if anxiety is present. Infants and older children who have significant neurologic deficits or psychomotor retardation often have significant GER and may suffer from serious sequela secondary to GER.[59] Recurrent pneumonia or blood loss from erosive esophagitis in these children is not uncommon. Often, the symptoms of GER in children with significant neurologic impairments are associated with anatomic problems, such as large hiatal hernias, and they are more likely to require aggressive or definitive therapy, such as surgical fundoplication, to reduce their likelihood of esophagitis with bleeding, aspiration pneumonia, or both.

Another group of children likely to present with symptoms of GER are older school-aged children and adolescents who have significant amounts of heartburn. These children often have worsening symptoms associated with exercise, stress, obesity, or body braces. These children seem to represent a spectrum of disease observed in adults and may suffer from recurrent symptoms after discontinuation of medical therapy.

Relationship Between GER and Respiratory Symptoms

The cause-and-effect relationship between GER and respiratory symptoms in children is often difficult to determine. The anatomic proximity of the trachea to the esophagus and the precise coordination that is required between the epiglottis, which protects the trachea from esophageal contents, and esophageal peristalsis, have been the basis for the frequent assumption that aspiration of esophageal contents leads to respiratory tract pathology. Although it has been demonstrated in some patients with recurrent respiratory symptoms that GER occurs into the proximal esophagus,[44] experience suggests that prevention of GER does not necessarily result in resolution of respiratory tract disease.

Many case reports of upper respiratory tract disorders are being associated with GER in children.[8,56] It is thought that aspiration of esophageal contents causes inflammation and edema resulting in stridor or that neural reflexes cause laryngospasm. If evaluation of the upper airway suggests a chronic inflammatory component, it is prudent to consider GER as a possible cause. In this population, the use of an acid profusion test to reproduce the symptoms may be of benefit.

The possible role of GER in apnea and bradycardia has been of great interest because of the life-threatening nature of these disorders. Some animal studies suggest that installation of foreign substances in the hypopharynx or esophagus may be associated with apnea.[72] Unfortunately, instances in which these events are clearly associated in a cause-and-effect relationship are uncommon. Although studies sometimes show that infants with a history of apnea have greater-than-normal amounts of GER, the correlation of apneic episodes with GER usually does not exist.[35, 54]

The association between asthma, bronchitis, or pneumonia with GER is often equally difficult to document. Although case reports have attempted to demonstrate the presence of GER in these disorders,[9, 18, 65] it is often unclear whether GER is an etiologic agent or secondary to increased respiratory effort or coughing. An example is cystic fibrosis, in which a large percentage of the patient population has GER, although the precise pathophysiology is unclear.[13] The presence of pneumonia in inpatients who have neurologic impairment and psychomotor retardation is well established, and aspiration of esophageal contents during swallowing or episodes of reflux must be considered strongly in this patient population. The use of macrophages may be helpful in detecting which children have respiratory symptoms on the basis of aspiration of gastric contents.[36, 42]

Miscellaneous Clinical Conditions Associated with GER

Abnormal behavioral and posturing with the tilting of the head to one side and bizarre contortions of the trunk have been noted in many children who have symptoms of reflux. These symptoms are often referred to as *Sandifer's syndrome*.[38] The use of pH probes may be helpful in determining which children are having abnormal behavioral problems because of GER. GER is occasionally associated with a variety of head and neck complaints that occur in children, such as recurrent otalgia[22] and dental erosions in older children.[1, 64]

DIAGNOSIS AND EVALUATION OF GER

Because the term *GER* refers to a symptom complex without a specific etiology, any process, intestinal or extraintestinal, that disrupts gastrointestinal motility may result in GER. Many of the diagnostic tests available to assess GER merely quantitate the presence of GER and do not give any information as to the etiology of this disorder.

Barium Swallow

Specific anatomic intestinal abnormalities that may give rise to symptoms of GER include pyloric stenosis; gastric outlet obstruction from a variety of conditions; malrotation; or even more distal intestinal obstruction, such as intestinal webs, stenosis, or atresia. Many of these intestinal tract anomalies can be readily picked up by a contrast study of the upper gastrointestinal tract. This study should be readily performed if history and physical examination suggest an anatomic obstruction in the intestinal tract is likely. GER symptoms can be the initial manifestation of more diffuse disorders of gastrointestinal motility that involve enteric neural or muscular function (i.e., postinfectious motility disorders or intestinal pseudo-obstruction) that may be indicated by diffuse dilation of the intestinal tract.

Roentgenologic contrast studies of the upper gastrointestinal tract were one of the first techniques used to study idiopathic GER in infants. Although early studies suggested that most infants with GER had hiatal hernias demonstrable by barium swallow, further experience has shown that this is not true. Some infants and children, especially those with profound central nervous system impairments have large hiatal hernias that may be linked to their symptoms of GER. Although many radiologists believe that they can quantitate the degree of GER on a barium swallow or an upper gastrointestinal tract study, most clinicians do not find these tests particularly helpful. The ability to accurately reproduce quantitative GER on this study requires a supervising pediatric radiologist who has a large amount of experience and interest in performing the study.[40] However, infants with severe symptoms of GER must have a contrast study of the upper gastrointestinal tract to rule out the presence of a large hiatal hernia; esophageal stricture; or other intestinal obstructions, such as a typical pyloric stenosis, duodenal web, gastric web, or the anatomic cause for recurrent vomiting. To rule out these abnormalities, the contrast study should proceed at least to the ligament of Treitz.

The barium swallow is a sensitive way of detecting reflux but has a very low specificity rate because many infants who have little or no clinical symptoms of reflux experience reflux of some barium into the esophagus. The barium swallow is not helpful also in terms of evaluating rates of gastric emptying, because barium is physiologically inert and does not activate any of the normal duodenal receptor mechanisms that tend to modulate gastric emptying function.

pH Probe

The use of thin, flexible probes that are able to detect pH in the distal esophagus has created an inexpensive way to accurately detect the amount of acid reflux in the distal esophagus. pH probes are restricted by their ability to detect only episodes that cause a change in the esophageal pH. They are unable to determine the volume of reflux material into the distal esophagus, but they are able to detect the frequency of episodes of reflux, the time it takes for an episode of acid reflux to be cleared, and, over a given period of time, the frequency of episodes of acid reflux in the distal esophagus. This has allowed standardized norms to be published, which permits one to know how often reflux occurs in a particular age group.[69] A 24-hour pH probe study can obtain fairly reproducible information on the amount of reflux that is occurring in an infant. There have been attempts to reproduce the validity of the 24-hour pH probe by reducing the amount of time to 12 hours or even to 4 hours. In many instances, however, it may be important to monitor the sleeping and nonsleeping period because infants who have significant reflux during the sleep phase may have altered esophageal clearance of reflux gastric contents.[63]

The recent availability of a more portable recording apparatus allows children to be monitored for GER in a more physiologic setting with normal dietary intake. Many pH probes can now be performed on children as outpatients with the ambulatory device being read by an automated system at a later point.[24, 45] One problem of pH probe monitoring is that they are often unable to detect acid reflux during the postprandial period because many ingested foodstuffs buffer the gastric acidity for varying periods of time and thereby alter the ability of the pH probe to detect reflux episodes. Some researchers have suggested the use of relatively low-buffering food during at least one feeding during pH probe study allows more accurate determination of GER during the postprandial period.[24]

Although pH probes have proven effective at quantitating the phenomenon, they have offered little information about the pathogenesis of GER during infancy. A diagnostic test such as the pH probe may, therefore, be valuable in associating a specific time-related clinical problem with GER or evaluating specific pharmacologic or surgical therapy for problems with GER. However, because the overt symptoms of GER are obvious and do not need to be quantitated by a pH probe in general practice, it is important not to overuse this test because it adds very little to the diagnostic evaluation of the typical child with GER. The indiscriminate use of a pH probe to associate GER with a wide variety of clinical disorders (i.e., colic or feeding problems) is usually fruitless.

Endoscopy and Esophageal Biopsy

The increased use of small fiberoptic endoscopes in recent years has resulted in many infants and children with symptoms of GER undergoing an endoscopic procedure. This technique allows direct visualization of the esophageal mucosa and biopsy to determine the severity of reflux esophagitis.

Basal cell hyperplasia of esophageal mucosa epithelium resulting in an increased length of the stroma pili has long been established as the histologic criteria for reflux esophagitis in the adult population.[33] Often, however, this is not observed in the distal esophagus of the infant who has reflux esophagitis. Although inflammatory cells, such as lymphocytes and polymorphic nuclear cells, have been seen in reflux esophagitis, these cells can be observed under normal conditions, and eosinophilic infiltrates have been found to be far more specific indicators of reflux esophagitis in infants.[74] One or more of epithelial eosinophils are considered sufficient to establish the presence of GER in an infant. Although these intraepithelial eosinophils are a sensitive indicator for esophagitis secondary to GER in infants, there has been little if any correlation of this finding with the course of idiopathic GER during infancy. Therefore, whether the presence of eosinophils on esophageal biopsy of an infant mandates more aggressive therapy remains to be shown. Esophageal strictures in normal infants with symptoms of GER are uncommon but have been reported.[60]

The increasing number of biopsies performed in pediatric-age patients has resulted in increased findings of Barrett's esophagus or gastric metaplasia of the normal stratified squamous epithelium in the esophagus. This conversion of the squamous epithelium of the esophagus into columnar epithelium with glandular elements was initially thought to be a congenital anomaly[58] but now seems to be more commonly observed in children with severe, long-standing GER.[25] Some evidence suggests that prevention of reflux by surgical means or aggressive medical therapy may result in the reversion of the Barrett's esophagus.[26] Some researchers have claimed that Barrett's esophagus can be seen in many children with endoscopically documented esophagitis[16] and that children with Barrett's esophagus often have associated esophageal strictures. It is hoped that, in the near future, studies will address the concerns about the malignant potential of the dysplasia that is often noted in these ectopic areas of intestinal glandial epithelium seen in the esophagus of patients who have GER.[11]

Manometric

Initially, there was great hope that the measurement of changing pressure profiles in the upper gastrointestinal tract and changes in basal lower esophageal sphincter tone would be of great value in evaluating GER during infancy. Manometric studies are difficult to perform in the unsedated infant, however, and have proven to be of little clinical use for patients and remain primarily a research tool. Manometry has been more helpful than any other modality in understanding more about the pathophysiology of GER in infants. Although initial reports suggested that many infants with GER had decreased lower esophageal sphincter pressure,[19] later studies have suggested basal or tonic lower esophageal sphincter pressure in the majority of infants who have GER is within the normal range. Although a subset of patients have markedly reduced basal lower esophageal sphincter pressure, some infants actually have increased lower esophageal sphincter pressure.[6, 27, 43, 70]

One reason that it may be difficult to compare lower esophageal sphincter pressure in infants who have GER is that manometric catheters produce different amounts of stretch in the lower esophageal sphincter in infants of different size and age. This may result in varying deformation of the lower esophageal sphincter by the manometric catheter, and it may change the pressure that is measured in this region.[30] The understanding that decreased lower esophageal sphincter is unlikely to account for most reflux that is observed during infancy has caused other possibilities, such as increased gastric pressure overcoming the basal lower esophageal sphincter tone and transient relaxation of the lower esophageal sphincter, to be considered as other possible etiologies. Careful studies of large populations of adults have shown that inappropriate relaxation of the lower esophageal sphincter may be the primary etiologic agent for most GER. There have been indications that similar events occur during infancy.[71] These episodes of relaxation of the lower esophageal sphincter seem to occur during the day and night in children and may be fundamental to understanding GER during infancy and children.[12] The pathogenesis of inappropriate relaxation during infancy remains essentially unexplored.

Changes in the body of the esophagus associated with GER have been well documented in adult patients. A decreased amplitude of peristalsis and a loss of peristaltic activity with some simultaneous, and perhaps even reversed, peristalsis often have been shown in infants or children who have severe GER. This loss of peristaltic activity in the distal esophagus may be responsible for delayed clearance of acid that is observed during reflux episodes of children who have severe esophagitis.[63] Some investigators have suggested that aggressive medical or surgical treatment of the reflux esophagitis resolves these abnormalities and results in a return to normal peristaltic activity in the esophagus.[12] The exception to this is in infants who have neurologic impairment or severe psychomotor retardation, in whom the esophageal abnormalities are likely neural in origin and do not improve with aggressive medical or surgical treatment of the GER.

Scintigraphy

The ingestion of radionuclide-labeled formula allows the performance of a nuclear medicine scan known as *gastroesophageal scintiscan*. After ingestion of the formula or meal, the infant or child is placed under a gamma counter. If anterior/posterior, and lateral views are obtained, then it is possible to calculate how much radionuclide empties from the stomach over a given period of time and for how often reflux occurs into the esophagus. This test has the advantages of being noninvasive, low in radiation, and widely available. In practice, however, the value of this test in documenting and quantitating GER is small. The studies are difficult to reproduce, and frequent images, perhaps as frequent as every 30 to 60 seconds, are necessary to accurately quantitate the amount of reflux that occurs into the distal esophagus.[48] It also has the disadvantage of being performed over a relatively short period of time in a rather nonphysiologic setting. In theory, the esophageal scintiscan has an advantage over the traditional pH probes because it can detect postprandial reflux when an esophageal pH probe may not be able to detect reflux because the gastric contents are buffered by ingested food. The esophageal scintiscan also has the advantage of being able to detect a volume of reflux without observing the fact that the reflux has occurred. Investigators have shown, however, that gastroesophageal scintiscan does not correlate closely with pH probes,[67] and the gastroesophageal scintiscan has not proven to be a practical test to quantitate GER. This test has not become widely used because it is not as sensitive as an upper gastrointestinal study in ruling out anatomic obstruction and does not provide the precise quantitation of GER that a pH probe does.

The gastroesophageal scintiscan does allow the detection of rates of gastric emptying that may be helpful in the evaluation of children who have GER. This may be particularly valuable in those children who are undergoing surgical fundoplication and suggest whether or not they need to have a procedure to facilitate gastric emptying simultaneously with the fundoplication.[21] Although the vast majority of infants with GER have gastric emptying rates that fall into the normal range, many infants with severe GER have shown delayed gastric emptying.[29] At this time, many pediatric surgeons prefer to obtain a gastric emptying study prior to performing a fundoplication to determine which patients would benefit from a surgical procedure to facilitate gastric emptying, such as pyloroplasty or gastric antroplasty.

Some researchers have also suggested that the gastroesophageal scintiscan may be useful in detecting pulmonary aspiration of radionuclide. Although some investigators have claimed that it has sufficient sensitivity to be clinically useful,[41] most attempts to document the aspiration of this radionuclide have not been uniformly successful, most likely because of technical limitation of the technique.[53]

THERAPY

The traditional therapy of placing a child in an infant seat to reduce the amount of GER has not been shown to be effective either by clinical observation or by pH probe studies that have quantitated the amount of GER that occurs in various positions. Some evidence indicates that placing the infant in a head-elevated prone position resulted in both fewer and briefer episodes of reflux[47] but that the decreases in reflux time are small, and the possible increased risk of sudden infant death syndrome for children in this position has led to less enthusiasm for its use.

Many infants often can be treated effectively with small or more frequent feedings. This feeding program likely reduces the volume of ingested food in the stomach that is available for reflux at any one time. Continuous infusions, either by nasal, gastric, or even postduodenal tubes, have been shown to be successful in getting adequate weight gain and may allow surgical intervention to be avoided in infants in whom the risk is unacceptably high.[20] Some investigators have suggested that if the infant does not show catch-up growth during the first week of nasogastric feedings, he or she is unlikely to benefit from longer periods of therapy.

Thickened Feedings

Thickening the child's food (e.g., rice cereal in formula) to reduce the clinical symptoms of children with GER has long been an accepted practice. This assumption has been tested with pH probe data, and thickened feedings (e.g., apple juice thickened with rice cereal) were found to have no effect on reflux time unless the child was in a head-elevated prone position after the feeding.[2] However, although infants with GER who are given thickened feedings might not have significantly reduced reflux time as measured by a pH probe, other criteria, such as episodes of emesis, time spent crying, and time spent awake, may be reduced. In addition, their effects may often result in the therapeutic success of thickened feedings.[50] Some researchers also have suggested that thickened feedings in some infants may result in an increased number of coughing episodes.[51]

Surgical Correction

It is clear that if one has unacceptable symptoms associated with GER, a fundoplication that increases the barrier in the region of the lower esophageal sphincter and, therefore, prevents reflux of gastric contents into the esophagus is an effective means of controlling the symptoms. These surgical procedures are not without complication, however, and the benefits must be weighed carefully. The value of fundoplication has caused this procedure to become one of the more common surgical procedures in many pediatric surgical centers. Long-term follow-up varies greatly, however, and efficacy rates may range from 60% to 90%.[17, 46] The Nissen fundoplication that involves a 360-degree wrap of the fundus around the distal 3.5 cm of the esophagus is a common procedure. Although some studies have shown good follow-up in the 5 years following the procedure, many researchers claim that there is a large percentage of breakdown within a relatively short period of time.[66] In addition, some investigators have suggested that an anterior gastric fundoplication may be equally therapeutic.[5]

By far, the most common patient to have a fundoplication in the pediatric age group is one who has psychomotor retardation. Many studies have suggested that the incidence of small intestinal obstruction, secondary to the adhesions, from the surgery ranges from 5% to 10%[6, 27, 43, 70] compared with 1% for other causes of laparotomy. Complication of small intestinal obstruction is particularly unfortunate in the patient who has been made unable to vomit. In one series of patients with obstruction secondary to adhesions following fundoplication, fewer than 20% were able to vomit. This patient population has a significant neurologic impairment and may not be able to bring rapid attention to problems with intestinal obstruction.[7] It is, therefore, important that patients who have had a fundoplication be rapidly evaluated for signs of intestinal obstruction if clinical signs arise.[39]

The frequent use of gastrostomy feeding tubes in the pediatric age group has led to the observation that, often, a child who previously had no mild or moderate symptoms of GER may have considerable problems with GER after placement of a gastrostomy tube. Many children, especially those who have neurologic impairments and who are not symptomatic for a reflux prior to gastrostomy tube placement, are symptomatic after the procedure.[44] Performance of a pH probe prior to placement of a gastrostomy tube may indicate some children who are likely to have this problem. If a pH probe reveals significant GER prior to the placement of a gastrostomy tube, it may be prudent to perform a fundoplication at the time of the gastrostomy.

Many pediatric surgeons have suggested that children should be carefully evaluated for gastric emptying problems prior to the performance of a fundoplication.[21] The use of pyloroplasty or gastric antraplasty together with the fundoplication may prevent problems with gastric bloating and vomiting after the fundoplication. The gastric dumping syndrome has been reported after a fundoplication or fundoplication with gastrostomy and should be looked for and treated medically when observed.[55]

Pharmacologic Therapy

The widespread nature of GER in infants has generated considerable interest in developing a specific pharmacologic therapy for this disorder; however, the observation that many episodes of GER are transitory in nature and caused by inappropriate relaxation of the lower esophageal sphincter explains the inability of many therapeutic agents to alleviate symptoms of GER. The use of antacids or H_2 antagonists certainly can reduce the amount of gastric acid produced in the stomach and may have an effect on peptic esophagitis.[14] The rationale for the indiscriminate treatment of reflux of the esophagitis in infants fewer than 2 years of age has received little justification in medical literature, however. In older patients who are likely to have chronic reflux, symptoms often return when the acid inhibition therapy is terminated.

Bethanechol, a muscarinic agonist, has been shown to increase basal lower esophageal sphincter pressure in many patients; however, researchers have had difficulty in showing whether it has any effect in reducing GER.[49] It has a high frequency of undesirable side effects, such as cramping and diarrhea.[37] The relative lack of success using bethanechol may be due to the fact that most infants with GER do not have reduced basal lower esophageal sphincter pressure.

Metoclopramide and a related agent, domperidone, mildly increase resting lower esophageal sphincter pressure and somewhat increase gastric emptying under many conditions. Domperidone has marginal benefits at best[23] and is not widely used to treat GER during infancy. Metoclopramide has been used much more widely; however, few studies have demonstrated its effectiveness in widespread use for treatment of GER during infancy. It has a high range of side effects, the occurrence rate of which ranges from 11% to 34%. Although drowsiness and restlessness are the most common side effects, the most troublesome is an extrapyramidal reaction that seems to occur with increased frequency in children. This is an acute dystonic type of extrapyramidal reaction that manifests neck pain, rigidity, trismus, and oculogyric crisis.[57] Although occasional studies have shown metoclopramide to be somewhat effective in treating GER in the pediatric age group, many researchers have argued that it is either ineffective or that high doses, which may increase the incidence of its side effects, are necessary to cause these therapeutic results.[32, 49]

Cisapride is a relatively new agent in the United States used to treat GER.[3] The mechanism of action is thought to work primarily by enhancement of release of neurotransmitters, which seems to stimulate smooth muscle contraction throughout the intestinal tract. Most of the side effects observed with cisapride are related to the gastrointestinal tract. Clinical trials suggest that it may have some benefit in treating GER in the pediatric age group,[14, 61, 68] although results are not dramatically impressive.

References

1. Aine L, Baer M, et al: Dental erosions caused by gastroesophageal reflux disease in children. ASDC J Dent Child 60:210–214, 1993
2. Bailey DJ, Andres JM, et al: Lack of efficacy of thickened feeding as treatment for gastroesophageal reflux. J Pediatr 110:187–189, 1987
3. Barone JA, Jessen LM, et al: Cisapride: A gastrointestinal prokinetic drug. Ann Pharmacother 28:488–500, 1994
4. Bauman NM, Sandler AD, et al: Reflex laryngospasm induced by stimulation of distal esophageal afferents. Laryngoscope 104:209–214, 1994
5. Bliss D, Hirschl R, et al: Efficacy of anterior gastric fundoplication in the treatment of gastroesophageal reflux in infants and children. J Pediatr Surg 29:1071–1074, 1994
6. Boix-Ochoa J, Canals J: Maturation of the lower esophagus. J Pediatr Surg 11:749–754, 1976
7. Borgstein ES, Heij HA, et al: Risks and benefits of antireflux operations in neurologically impaired children. Eur J Pediatr 153:248–251, 1994
8. Burton DM, Pransky SM, et al: Pediatric airway manifestations of gastroesophageal reflux. Ann Otol Rhinol Laryngol 101:742–749, 1992
9. Chen PH, Chang MH, et al: Gastroesophageal reflux in children with chronic recurrent bronchopulmonary infection. J Pediatr Gastroenterol Nutr 13:16–22, 1991
10. Christensen J, Freeman BW, et al: Some physiological characteristics of the esophagogastric junction in the opossum. Gastroenterology 64:1119–1125, 1973
11. Cooper JE, Spits L, et al: Barrett's esophagus in children: A histologic and histochemical study of 11 cases. J Pediatr Surg 22:103–108, 1987
12. Cucchiara S, Bortolotti M, et al: Fasting and postprandial mechanisms of gastroesophageal reflux in children with gastroesophageal reflux disease. Dig Dis Sci 1:86–92, 1993
13. Cucchiara S, Santamaria F, et al: Mechanisms of gastroesophageal reflux in cystic fibrosis. Arch Dis Child 66:617–622, 1991
14. Cucchiara S, Staiano A, et al: Antacids and cimetidine treatment for gastroesophageal reflux and peptic oesophagitis. Arch Dis Child 59:842–847, 1984
15. Cucchiara S, Staiano A, et al: Cisapride for gastroesophageal reflux and peptic oesophagitis. Arch Dis Child 62:454–457, 1987
16. Dahms B, Rothstein FC: Barrett's esophagus in children: A consequence of chronic gastroesophageal reflux. Gastroenterology 86:318–323, 1984
17. Dedinsky GK, Vane DW, et al: Complications and reoperation after Nissen fundoplication in childhood. Am J Surg 153:177–183, 1987
18. Eid NS, Shepherd RW, et al: Persistent wheezing and gastroesophageal reflux in infants. Pediatr Pulmonol 18:39–44, 1994
19. Euler AR, Ament M: Value of esophageal manometric studies in the gastroesophageal reflux of infancy. Pediatrics 59:58–62, 1977
20. Ferry GD, Selby M, et al: Clinical response to short-term nasogastric feeding in infants with gastroesophageal reflux and growth failure. J Pediatr Gastroenterol Nutr 2:57–61, 1983

21. Fonkalsrud EW, Ament ME, et al: Gastric antroplasty for the treatment of delayed gastric emptying and gastroesophageal reflux in children. Am J Surg 164:327–331, 1992
22. Gibson WS Jr, Cochran W: Otalgia in infants and children–A manifestation of gastroesophageal reflux. Int J Pediatr Otorhinolaryngol 28:213–218, 1994
23. Grill BB, Hillemeier AC, et al: Effects of domperidone therapy on symptoms and upper gastrointestinal motility in infants with gastroesophageal reflux. J Pediatr 106:311–316, 1985
24. Haase GM, Meagher DP, et al: A unique teletransmission system for extended four channel esophageal pH monitoring in infants and children. J Pediatr Surg 22:68–74, 1987
25. Hassall E: Barrett's esophagus: Congenital or acquired? Am J Gastro 88:819–824, 1993
26. Hassall E, Weinstein WM: Partial regression of childhood Barrett's esophagus after fundoplication. Am J Gastroenterol 87:1506–1512, 1992
27. Herbst J, Book L, et al: The lower esophageal sphincter in gastroesophageal reflux in children. J Clin Gastroenterol 1:119–122, 1979
28. Hillemeier AC, Bitar KN, et al: Developmental characteristics of the kitten antrum. Gastroenterology 101:339–343, 1991
29. Hillemeier AC, Lange R, et al: Delayed gastric emptying in infants with gastroesophageal reflux. J Pediatr 98:190–193, 1981
30. Hillemeier AC, McCallum R, Biancani P: Developmental characteristics of the lower esophageal sphincter in the kitten. Gastroenterology 89:760–766, 1985
31. Holloway RH, Berger K, McCallum RW: Gastric distention: A mechanism for postprandial gastroesophageal reflux. Gastroenterology 89:779–784, 1985
32. Hyams JS, Zamett LO, Walters JK: Effect of metoclopramide on prolonged intraesophageal pH testing in infants with gastroesophageal reflux. J Pediatr Gastroenterol Nutr 5:716–720, 1986
33. Ismail-Beigi F, Horton CE, et al: Histologic consequences of gastroesophageal reflux in man. Gastroenterology 58:163–174, 1970
34. Jolley SG, Tunell WP, et al: Lower esophageal pressure changes with tube gastrostomy: A causative factor of gastroesophageal reflux in children? J Pediatr Surg 21:624–627,1986
35. Kahn A, Rebuffat E, et al: Lack of temporal relation between acid reflux in the proximal oesophagus and cardiorespiratory events in sleeping infants. Eur J Pediatr 151:208–212, 1992
36. Kurlandsky L, Vaandrager V, et al: Lipoid pneumonia in association with gastroesophageal reflux. Pediatr Pulmonol 13:184–188, 1992
37. Levi P, Marmo F, et al: Bethanechol versus antacids in the treatment of gastroesophageal reflux. Helvetica Paediatric Acta 40:349–359, 1985
38. Mandel H, Tirosh E, et al: Sandifer syndrome reconsidered. Acta Paediatr Scand 78:797–799, 1989
39. Martinez DA, Ginn-Pease ME, et al: Sequelae of antireflux surgery in profoundly disabled children. J Pediatr Surg 27:271–273, 1992
40. McCauley RG, Darling DB, et al: Gastroesophageal reflux in infants and children. A useful classification and reliable physiologic technique for its demonstration. AJR Am J Roentgenol 130:47–50, 1978
41. McVeagh P, Howman GR, et al: Pulmonary aspiration studied by radionuclide milk scanning and barium swallow roentgenography. Am J Dis Child 141:917–921, 1987
42. Moran JR, Block SM, et al: Lipid-laden alveolar macrophage and lactose assay as markers of aspiration in neonates with lung disease. J Pediatr 112:643–645, 1988
43. Moroz S, Espinoza J, et al: Lower esophageal sphincter function in children with/without gastroesophageal reflux. Gastroenterology 89:760–766, 1976
44. Narcy P: Gastropharyngeal reflux in infants and children. A pharyngeal pH monitoring study. Arch Otolaryngol Head Neck Surg 118:1028–1030, 1992
45. Newman LJ, Berezin S, et al: A new ambulatory system for extended esophageal pH monitoring. J Pediatr Gastroenterol Nutr 4:707–710, 1985
46. Opie JC, Chaye H, et al: Fundoplication and pediatric esophageal manometry: Actuarial analysis over 7 years. J Pediatr Surg 22:935–938, 1987

47. Orenstein SR, Whitington PE: Positioning for prevention of infant gastroesophageal reflux. J Pediatr 103:534–537, 1983
48. Orenstein SR, Klein HA, et al: Scintigraphy versus pH probe for quantification of pediatric gastroesophageal reflux: A study using concurrent multiplexed data and acid feedings. J Nucl Med 34:1228–1234, 1993
49. Orenstein SR, Lofton SW, et al: Bethanechol for pediatric gastroesophageal reflux: A prospective, blind, controlled study. J Pediatr Gastroenterol Nutr 5:549–555, 1986
50. Orenstein SR, Magill LH, et al: Thickening of infant feedings for therapy of GER. J Pediatr 110:181–186, 1987
51. Orenstein SR, Shalaby TM, et al: Thickened feedings as a cause of increased coughing when used as therapy for gastroesophageal reflux in infants. J Pediatr 121:913–915, 1992
52. Paterson WG, Rattan S, et al: Pathophysiology of inappropriate lower esophageal relaxation. Gastroenterology 88:1533, 1985
53. Paton JY, Cosgriff PS, et al: The analytical sensitivity of Tc-99m radionuclide milk scanning in the detection of gastroesophageal reflux. Pediatr Radiol 15:381–383, 1985
54. Paton JY, Nanayakkara CS, et al: Observations of gastroesophageal reflux, central apnoea and heart rate in infants. Eur J Pediatr 149:608–612, 1990
55. Pittschieler K: Dumping syndrome after combined pyloroplasty and fundoplication. Eur J Pediatr 150:410–412, 1991
56. Putnam PE, Orenstein SR: Hoarseness in a child with gastroesophageal reflux. Acta Paediatr 81:635–636, 1992
57. Putnam PE, Orenstein SR, et al: Tardive dyskinesia associated with use of metoclopramide in a child. J Pediatr 121 6:983–985, 1992
58. Rector LE, Connerley ML: Aberrant mucosa in the esophagus in infants and children. Arch Pathol Lab Med 31:285–294, 1941
59. Reyes AL, Cash AJ, et al: Gastroesophageal reflux in children with cerebral palsy. Child Care Health Dev 19:109–118, 1993
60. Rode H, Millar AJ, et al: Reflux strictures of the esophagus in children. J Pediatr Surg 27:462–465, 1992
61. Saye An, Forget PP, et al: Effect of Cisapride on gastroesophageal reflux in children with chronic bronchopulmonary disease: A double-blind cross over pH monitoring study. Pediatr Pulmonol 3:8–12, 1987
62. Smith CD, Othersen HB, et al: Nissen fundoplication in children with profound neurologic disability. High risks and unmet goals. Ann Surg 215:654–658, 1992
63. Sondheimer JM, Hoddes E: Gastroesophageal reflux with drifting onset in infants: A phenomenon unique to sleep. J Pediatr 15:418–425, 1992
64. Taylor G, Taylor S, et al: Dental erosion associated with asymptomatic gastroesophageal reflux. ASDC J Dent Child 59:182–185, 1992
65. Tucci F, Resti M, et al: Gastroesophageal reflux and bronchial asthma: Prevalence and effect of cisapride therapy. J Pediatr Gastro Nutr 17:265–270, 1993
66. Turnage RH, Oldham KT, et al: Late results of fundoplication for gastroesophageal reflux in infants and children. Surgery 105:457–464, 1995
67. Vandenplas Y, Derde MP, et al: Evaluation of reflux episodes during simultaneous esophageal pH monitoring and gastroesophageal reflux scintigraphy in children. J Pediatr Gastroenterol Nutr 14:256–260, 1992
68. Vandenplas Y, deRoy C, et al: Cisapride decreases prolonged episodes of reflux in infants. J Pediatr Gastroenterol Nutr, 1991
69. Vandenplas Y, Goyvaerts H, et al: Gastroesophageal reflux, as measured by 24-hour pH monitoring, in 509 healthy infants screened for risk of sudden infant death syndrome. Pediatrics 88:834–840, 1991
70. Vanderhoof JA, Rapoport PJ, et al: Manometric diagnosis of lower esophageal sphincter incompetence in infants: Use of a small, single-lumen perfused catheter. Pediatrics 62:805–808, 1978
71. Werlin S, Dodds W, et al: Mechanisms of gastroesophageal reflux in children. J Pediatr 97:244–248, 1980
72. Wetmore RF: Effects of acid on the larynx of the maturing rabbit and their possible significance to the sudden infant death syndrome. Laryngoscope 103:1242–1254, 1993

73. Wilkins BM, Spitz L: Adhesion obstruction following Nissen fundoplication in children. Br J Surg 74:777–779, 1987
74. Winter HS, Madara JL, et al: A new diagnostic criterion for reflux esophagitis. Gastroenterology 83:818–823, 1982

Address reprint requests to

A. Craig Hillemeier, MD
1500 East Medical Center Drive
F6854 C, S. Mott
Ann Arbor, MI 48109–0200

PEDIATRIC GASTROENTEROLOGY I 0031–3955/96 $0.00 + .20

HELICOBACTER PYLORI AND PEPTIC DISEASE IN THE PEDIATRIC PATIENT

Yoram Bujanover, MD, Shimon Reif, MD, and Jacob Yahav, MD

Peptic disease in the adult population has been estimated to affect as many as 10% of people in the United States. In children, peptic ulcer is uncommon but the exact incidence is unknown. The literature quotes numbers such as four to six new ulcer cases per year or 1 in 2500 pediatric hospital admissions in large pediatric centers. These numbers include primary and secondary ulcers. Since the primary method of diagnosis was changed from radiography to endoscopy, the diagnosis of peptic disease in children has become more accurate, and the histopathology more definite. Endoscopy also has demonstrated what was shown first in adults: the linkage between *Helicobacter pylori* and peptic disease in children.

BACTERIOLOGY

Nearly a decade ago, the pathogenesis of peptic disease expressed as gastritis, gastric ulcer duodenitis, and duodenal ulcer was attributed to an imbalance between acid secretion and mucosal defense mechanisms. In 1983, Marshall and Warren introduced a new pathogenic factor, a microorganism called *H pylori*.[16] This organism was originally named *Campylobacter pyloridis* because of its structural similarity to the *Campylobacter* species. Later it was named *C pylori*.

From the Pediatric Gastrointestinal Unit, Dana Children's Hospital, Sourasky-Tel Aviv Medical Center, Tel Aviv (YB, SR); and the Pediatric Gastroenterology Unit, Sheba Hospital, Tel Hashomer (JY), Israel

Only in 1989, after defining its distinct functional and enzymatic properties, C pylori acquired its recognition as a new genus and was named H pylori.[51] In retrospect, Helicobacter-like organisms were observed in animal mucosa in the 1800s, and in humans in the early part of the 20th century.[26, 27] However, the interest in the bacteria was resurrected by Marshall and Warren, who isolated for the first time the bacteria that was nestled in the interface between the gastric epithelial cell surface and the overlying mucosa.

Helicobacter pylori is a spiral-shaped, gram-negative rod measuring 0.5×3.0 μm with 4 to 6 sheathed flagella. In prolonged culture or exposure to oxygen, bacteria can appear in coccoidal forms. An afibrial pilus-like structure has also been described.[50]

Studies of the organism, biotyping, genome, and plasmid profile diversity revealed the existence of approximately 40 epidemiologically unrelated strains of H pylori.

One of the typical features of this organism is its possession of a high molecular weight 600,000 urease enzyme that enables it to catalyze urea into ammonium and bicarbonate.[37] The alkaline microenvironment produced by this action protects the organism from gastric acid. H pylori is an obligatory microaerophilic. The optimal O_2 concentration is 2% to 8%. In addition, CO_2 is important for primary isolation. The basal media should be supplemented with whole blood or serum and urea.[94]

The organism derives its energy from the metabolism of organic acids and amino acids. It cannot use carbohydrates for this purpose.[94] The binding of H pylori to the stomach is mediated by cell-bound and soluble hemagglutinins and its surface proteins and lipopolysaccharides.[36]

PATHOGENESIS

Helicobacter pylori infection almost always is associated with inflammation. The mechanisms by which the bacteria produces the different pathologic conditions in the stomach or duodenum are not completely elucidated. Several factors contribute to the virulence of H pylori in the unfriendly environment of the stomach. Due to its flagella, the organism has active motility that allows it to penetrate the mucus layer of the gastric mucosa.[33] Urease, which hydrolyzes urea into ammonia and water, produces an alkaline environment that defends the organism from gastric acidity. A protein inhibitor of gastric acid secretion possessed by the bacteria has a similar role.[106] Catalase protects the bacteria against reactive oxygen radicals produced by neutrophils.[63]

Bacterial adhesins and receptors that are mainly localized in gastric mucous cells also are important virulence factors.[39]

Goodwin proposed the "leaking roof" hypothesis to explain the contribution of H pylori to the gastroduodenal injury. The submucosal tissue is protected by the mucin gel and epithelial cells (the "roof") from the gastric acid ("rain").[49] Injury to the protective elements causes a "leak," namely back diffusion of H^+ ions leading to submucosal injury, inflammation, and ulcer formation. *Helicobacter pylori* isolates produce cytotoxins; purified cytotoxins with a molecular weight of 128 and 82 kd demonstrate vacuolizing activity in different cell lines.[18] This activity was abolished by heat and proteases. This cytotoxic activity was more common in bacteria isolated from patients with duodenal ulcer than in those with gastritis only.[68] Antibodies against these cytotoxins were also identified in patients with ulcer disease.[18] The bacterial toxin demonstrates also some homology to ion channel proteins. *Helicobacter pylori* produced also lysates that are cytotoxic to Chinese hamster ovary cells.[19] The enzyme urease that allows the bacteria to survive in the stomach is also acting as an injurious factor, either directly or through the ammonia that is produced from urea. Several reports demonstrated the toxic effect of ammonia to the gastric mucosa.[127] Ammonia impairs mitochondrial and cell respiration, thus decreasing cell viability. In addition, it disturbs the ionic integrity of the gastric mucus, which allows back diffusion of H^+, resulting in cell injury.

Other bacterial enzymes that may affect the mucus layer are a protease named *mucinase*, lipase, and phospholipase. These three enzymes degrade the mucus by their activity on the protein or lipid constituents of the mucus.[109]

Several strains of *H pylori* produce hemolysin. Hemolysin is cytotoxic and has a potential to damage gastric cells.[136]

Helicobacter pylori, like other bacteria, can induce an inflammatory process in the tissue by several mechanisms. Occasionally the organism was demonstrated in the lamina propria, a fact that indicates the possible ability of the bacteria to invade the gastric mucosa. This rare phenomenon may explain also the escape of the organism from eradication. Other putative mediators of inflammation possessed by the bacteria are chemotoxin for neutrophils, proteins that induce the expression of interleukin (IL)-2 receptors, IL-1, TNF, and oxidative radicals by monocytes and macrophages.[83] Luekotriene B4, leukocyte migration inhibition factor, and platelet-activating factor are also increased in tissue infected with *H pylori*.[25, 43]

Helicobacter pylori infection may stimulate the formation of antibodies that cross-react with human antral gastric antigens. Dunn and colleagues have demonstrated cross-antigenicity between 65-kd heat shock proteins of the bacteria and antigens of gastric epithelial cells.[32]

McGovern and co-workers have reported increased infiltration of eosinophils in *H pylori*-associated antral gastritis.[28] Karttunen and colleagues have reported a similar phenomenon but in relation to accumulation of lymphocytes.[72] Lymph follicles commonly are observed in biopsies of *H pylori*-infected individuals.[44]

All the previously mentioned observed inflammatory markers suggest an important role for the inflammation in the process of damage to mucosal integrity and viability.

Another theory to explain the mucosal injury was introduced by Levi and co-workers, who reported for the first time the increased gastrin levels in patients infected with *H pylori*.[80] The explanation for the hypergastrinemia as proposed by Levi and co-workers is that the ammonia produced by the organism interferes with the normal feedback inhibition of gastrin release by intraluminal acid. Perwett and colleagues abolished the hypergastrinemia by eradication of the bacteria.[108] In contrast with this theory, however, significant differences in basal and peak acid output could not be demonstrated by other investigators.

Queiroz and co-workers observed significant lower histamine concentration in mucosal samples of children infected with *H pylori* relative to those who were uninfected. This observation suggests increased histamine mobilization in infected patients due to the effect of chronically elevated gastric acid secretion.[114]

In addition to the demonstrated hypergastrinemia, increased levels of pepsinogen I were detected in sera of children infected with *H pylori* by Oderda and colleagues.[104] Cave and Cave were able to stimulate pepsinogen secretion from isolated rabbit gastric glands by *H pylori* sonicates.[12]

PATHOLOGIC SPECTRUM OF *HELICOBACTER PYLORI* INFECTION

Helicobacter pylori resides exclusively in gastric mucosa; however, it can be found in remote areas that underwent metaplastic changes in which gastric epithelial cells are present, such as the esophagus, duodenum, or Meckel's diverticulum. The highest concentration of the bacteria is found in the antral area. The demonstration of the organism in the mucosa was almost always associated with evidence of inflammation. This is true for adults and children.[109] In contrast, the inflammation caused by *H pylori* is not always evidenced macroscopically by endoscopy.

Proof that *H pylori* is a primary cause for gastric inflammation rather than a secondary colonizer of inflamed tissue was evidenced by the fact that the inflammation could be induced by challenging animals and humans by oral administration of the bacteria.[99] In addition, it is unusual to identify the bacteria in cases of secondary gastritis, such as Crohn's disease, alcoholic gastritis, eosinophilic gastritis, or NSAID- and steroid-associated gastritis.[31]

Helicobacter pylori infection is usually characterized by chronic type B gastritis. In contrast with adults, in whom the active components of the inflammation are neutrophils, in children it is the lymphocytes.[28, 62] Nodularity of the antral mucosa was documented in many reports dealing with *H pylori* infection in children. The percentage of patients who demonstrate nodular gastritis ranges between 30% and 100%.[10, 11, 28, 65, 96, 113] This frequency differs from the one found in adults. Mitchell and co-workers reported 50% nodularity in children and only 15.8% in adults.[96] Most of the reports on adults do not mention the existence of nodularity. The initial observation that nodularity is accompanied by an increased number of lymphoid follicles in the gastric mucosa was confirmed by several other reports dealing with children.[10, 44, 113] The association of *H pylori* and gastric and duodenal ulcer in adult patients ranges from 70% to 100%.[110] In children, peptic ulcer disease is quite rare. Most of the gastric ulcers in children are secondary rather than primary. The demonstration of *H pylori* infection in children with peptic ulcer differs from report to report. Prieto and colleagues, who investigated endoscopically 270 pediatric patients, detected *H pylori* in 91 (38.7%) cases. Gastric ulcer was found in 12 patients, of which 9 (75%) had *H pylori* infection. Duodenal ulcer was diagnosed in 11 patients, of which 10 (90.9%) were positive for *H pylori*.[113]

Mitchell and colleagues from Australia, who investigated 227 patients, found 12 (5.3%) cases of ulcer. In the group of the nine cases with duodenal ulcer, three (30%) were infected with *H pylori*. Gastric ulcer was diagnosed in three patients, and only one (30%) was positive for *H pylori*.[96] The fact that ulcers are recorded infrequently in children makes the exact estimation of association of *H pylori* infection and ulcer disease in this age group difficult.

In contrast with the common acceptance that *H pylori* colonization is almost always associated with gastric mucosal pathology, several investigators report cases with normal histology. Hill and colleagues found normality in 33%; Cadranel and colleagues, in 12.5%; and Prieto and colleagues in 6.64%.[11, 65, 113] There may be a sample error, however, and the inflammation may have been missed.

SYMPTOMS AND *HELICOBACTER PYLORI* INFECTION IN CHILDREN

There are conflicting reports on the association of *H pylori* gastritis and abdominal pain or other gastrointestinal symptoms in children. Large studies, such as those performed by Fiedorek and co-workers in Arkansas or Blecker and colleagues in Belgium, demonstrated a high prevalence of *H pylori* colonization in asymptomatic children.[6, 42] Other investigators such as Glassman, Mahony, and Reifen were unable to demonstrate differences in the pattern of gastrointestinal symptoms between children with and without *H pylori* infection.[47, 82, 117]

Studying specifically groups of children with recurrent abdominal pain, Fiedorek and colleagues and Van der Meer and co-workers failed to demonstrate a close relation between *H pylori* seropositivity, positive 13_c-urea breath test, and gastric biopsy and the entity of recurrent abdominal pain.[40, 131]

Oderda and co-workers found resolution of symptoms in children with *H pylori* gastritis presenting with recurrent abdominal pain (RAP) after treatment with bismuth and ampicillin; however, recurrence of *H pylori* infection resulted in only a minor degree of symptomatic recurrence.[102]

Drumm and co-workers treated 15 children with *H pylori*–associated gastritis, 10 of whom had duodenal ulcer with bismuth subsalicylate and ampicillin. The effect of the treatment was resolution of symptoms in the patients with ulcers but poor response in those who had gastritis alone.[30]

Except for dyspeptic symptoms, *H pylori* infection was described with a similar clinical picture of Ménétrier's disease, including protein-losing gastropathy. This pathology disappeared after the eradication of bacteria.[17]

EPIDEMIOLOGY

The prevalence of *H pylori* infection depends on the patient's residence in a socioeconomically developed or underdeveloped country, his or her socioeconomic status, and age.[41, 56, 93, 97, 107] In Western countries, *H pylori* infection is rare in patients fewer than 5 years of age. After the age of 50 years, more than 50% of patients have serologic evidence of infection. Prieto and coworkers in Spain reported 91 cases of *H pylori*, of whom 9 (10%) were under the age of 5 years.[113] In France, 3.5% of patients are infected in the first decade. In contrast, in countries such as Algeria, Ivory Coast, and Gambia, 45% to 90% of children are infected during the first 10 years of life.[113]

The study of Fiedorek and colleagues in Arkansas demonstrated the relationship between the infection rate with *H pylori* and the socioeconomic condition of the families of the investigated children. A clear association between the family income and the prevalence of *H pylori* infection was present. Blacks were more likely to be infected than whites.[41] The same pattern of increased colonization in lower social classes was found in adults also. Mitchell and colleagues investigated the prevalence of *H pylori* in southern China using ELISA. The study was performed in Guandong province, in Guangzhou City, and in three rural areas. The prevalence of *H pylori* infection in the city (52.4%) was significantly higher than that in the rural area (38.6%).[97]

This study established a significant positive correlation between the role of *H pylori* infection and density of living and age. The prevalence of infection increased with age. By the age of 5 years, 23% of all children living in southern China were infected with *H pylori*. In children more than 5 years of age, in both urban and rural areas, the difference in seroprevalence of *H pylori* for each age group increased by approximately 1% per year.[97]

Person-to-person transmission of *H pylori* was implicated to be the most likely mode of disease spread, but the actual rate of transmission is still controversial.

Chewing of food by the mother before or eating from communal bowls could be a potential mechanism of transmission in developing countries. Fecal-oral route was also suggested to explain the bacterial spread. Klein and colleagues propose water contamination with fecal material as an important source of infection.[75]

Recently, Kelly and co-workers were able to isolate the bacteria from the feces of 12 (48%) of 25 subjects colonized with *H pylori*. The high success rate of isolation relative to previous studies was attributed to the method of using supernatant achieved after the centrifugation of stool rather than direct culture of the stool sample. This study can serve as proof of fecal-oral transmission.[73]

Few groups also have demonstrated intrafamilial clustering of *H pylori* infection. Drumm and co-workers found positive serology in more than 80% of siblings of children colonized with *H pylori* in comparison with 13% of age-matched controls.[29] Malaty and colleagues also provided data demonstrating increased prevalence of colonized children of infected parents relative to those who were not.[84] Clustering of *H pylori* also was documented within institutions for patients who were mentally challenged.[5]

Langenberg and colleagues reported the risk of transmission of *H pylori* by endoscopy.[77]

In addition to the environmental factors contributing to the transmission, some researchers have suggested that host factors may have a role in the rate of infection and pathology induced by the organism. Boren and colleagues reported the involvement of Lewis blood group antigen in the attachment of *H pylori* to gastric mucosa.[8] It was also reported that HLA-DQAI gene contributes to the host response against *H pylori*.[3] These findings suggest that the host's genetic factors contribute to the susceptibility or resistance to *H pylori* infection.

DIAGNOSIS OF *HELICOBACTER PYLORI*

Various diagnostic tests are available for the detection of *H pylori* (Table 1). They can be categorized into direct or indirect methods. Identification of the organism in the gastric mucosa using microbiologic techniques, such as culture, PCR, and histology, provide direct evidence of its presence. Indirect evidence is based on biochemical properties of the bacteria, particularly its ability to hydrolyze urea (e.g., urea breath tests or urease tests). Serologic tests are considered ineffective because they cannot provide proof of an existing infection. The availability of the vast variety of tests could be problematic for the clinician who is selecting the optimal test to be used. The diagnostic test should be adjusted to the individual patient, but the choice is necessarily based on the methods available to each clinician. No ideal evaluation has yet emerged, and, in most cases, accurate diagnosis relies on a combination of tests. Furthermore, those tests used for primary detection are not necessarily suitable for follow-up, in which less invasive and more quantitative methods are indicated.

Culture

Identification of *H pylori* by culture from antral mucosa obtained by endoscopy is considered the most accurate method. It has the advantage

Table 1. DIAGNOSTIC TESTS FOR THE DETECTION OF *H PYLORI*

Method	Specimen	Sensitivity	Specificity	Comments
Culture	Mucosa	+	+ + +	Technically complicated; time-consuming. Provides antibiotic sensitivity information.
Culture	Stools	±	+ + +	Not for routine clinical use.
Histology	Mucosal biopsy	+ +	+ +	Specimen can be re-examined, provides a permanent record.
Urease test	Mucosal biopsy	+ +	+ +	Rapid, simple, and reliable diagnosis; one-step test; provides instant results.
PCR	Gastric mucosa, stool, secretion	+ +	+ +	Experimental at present.
Urea breath test	Breath	+ +	+ +	^{13}C has no radiation but is costly; ^{14}C has low radiation, is simpler and less expensive, not recommended for children.
ELISA—laboratory	Serum	+ +	+	Provides titer; IgG is preferred.
ELISA—office	Serum	+ +	±	Performed in 10 min.; not quantitative; used only for excluding.
ELISA—office	Saliva	+	±	Rapid results; not quantitative.

of providing an antibiogram, which is important for patients who are allergic to antibiotics, previously experienced therapy failure, or live in countries where rates of antibiotic resistance to *H pylori* are high. Unfortunately, culturing has several limitations. The procedure is technically difficult and time-consuming, usually taking 3 to 6 days to grow the bacteria. In addition, even in experienced laboratories, an isolation rate of only 75% to 90% can be achieved, making this a highly specific test but of limited to moderate sensitivity.[52] Biopsied material for culture should be kept moist in a minimal amount of saline and plated within 2 hours of retrieval. Homogenized or minced tissue is transferred to chocolate or brain-heart infusion blood agar plate incubated in 10% CO_2 or in a Campy Pak (BBL Microbiology Systems, Beckton & Dickinson, Cockeysville, MD) atmosphere at 37°C. Identification of the organism is made by the presence of gram-negative curved bacteria, with positive urease catalase and oxidase reactions.[52, 92] If culture cannot be performed close to the time of endoscopy, the specimen should be stored on dry ice in a skim-milk (17%) glycerol mixture.[60] Many factors have been implicated in unsuccessful growth of *H pylori*, including (1) culturing the part of a specimen containing no bacteria (due to uneven distribution of the organism)[98]; (2) ingestion of topical anesthetic during endoscopy;

(3) contamination of the biopsy forceps with glutaraldehyde or with other organism; and (4) recent use of antibiotics or H_2 antagonist. Not only recent use of antibiotics but also of bismuth-containing medications or omeprazole can inhibit bacterial growth.[22] Finally, although *H pylori* is usually cultured from gastric mucosa obtained by endoscopy, isolation of *H pylori* was recently reported in human feces after concentration of fecal bacteria by centrifugation in a microaerophilic atmosphere. This potentially noninvasive method needs further enhancement for routine use because it detects only approximately 50% of cases of proven gastric colonization.[126]

Histology

Histology, another direct method, can provide information about tissue morphology (e.g., gastritis or appearance of nodular gastritis that was reported by these authors[10] and confirmed by others[62] to be specific for *H pylori* infection in children). Besides being a highly sensitive test, it has the advantages that specimens can be re-examined, used for different staining techniques, and preserved to provide a permanent record. Furthermore, although the tissue can be used for Gram staining, this method almost has been abandoned owing to its low yield. Although in some cases the organism can be demonstrated on standard hematoxylin and eosin stain, this is not considered a reliable method.[137] Although no specific stain exists for *H pylori*, two common staining methods are the most applicable. The Whartin-Starry silver stain is a preferable technique. Despite its cost and technical demands, this stain became popular because of its effectiveness. Giemsa stain is less expensive and was found by some investigators to be equivalent in quality to silver stain.[58] The characteristic histologic appearance of *H pylori* is a 3.0 $\times$ 0.5 μM spiral rod located at the gastric mucosa adjacent to the gastric epithelium.[58, 86, 137]

Besides regular histologic tests, immunochemical and immunofluorescent methods exist.[121] They require the use of a fluorescent microscope and fluorescent antibodies, making the system more expensive without contributing any further information to the findings from standard histology methods. Therefore, they are not routinely used in most laboratories.

Rapid Urease Test

At endoscopy, after retrieving a biopsy, the simplest and least expensive method of diagnosis is the rapid urease test.[90, 92] Its main advantage is providing quick results within hours or even minutes. The test is based on an almost unique characteristic of *H pylori*, its ability to produce urease. Urease converts urea to ammonia and bicarbonate, and in this way increases the pH of the surrounding medium, which can be detected by a change in color on a pH indicator (e.g., phenol red). Currently, mostly commercial kits are used, such as the CLO test (Delta-West Ltd, Perth, Australia) or CM test (Pemmler Pharma GmbH, Marburg, Germany), which consists of a pellet of modified Christensen's agar and a mounted indicator.[125] This is a one-step test, and the specimen does not require any special handling; it is put into the tube and cultured at room temperature, with the results indicated by changing of the contents' color. Its specificity is comparable to that of histology, although its sensitivity is slightly lower because this test depends on the density of the bacteria and because urease-negative bacteria can cause false-negative results. There are reports of lower sensitivity of this test in children, probably because of the lower bacteria content in the tissue.[27]

Polymerase Chain Reaction

Polymerase chain reaction (PCR) is another method of direct detection of the presence of the organism but without the need to grow it.[14] Furthermore PCR does not require the use of tissue with the highest degree of contamination, such as gastric mucosa, because sources such as feces or saliva can replace endoscopic materials.[73, 85] Polymerase chain reaction permits rapid detection of H pylori from fresh gastric biopsy specimens, and it also can detect H pylori from paraffin-wax–embedded biopsy specimens. The primer is derived from the nucleotide sequence of the urease A gene of H pylori[14, 15]; another primer used is nucleotides derived from H pylori 16S rRNA.[35, 66] These primers are specific to all strains of H pylori and are not detected in other bacterial species, making PCR highly specific.[15] Moreover, PCR is the most sensitive procedure compared with the rapid urease test, culture, and histology.[38, 130] Some insidious factors, however, can influence this high sensitivity and specificity. The endoscope and the biopsy forceps need extensive cleaning and disinfection to avoid "DNA contamination."[109] Other reports of reduced sensitivity blame patchy colonization of the bacteria in gastric mucosa or the presence of inhibitors to PCR.[34] Nested PCR might be a potential method affording higher sensitivity.[111]

Serology

Serodiagnosis of H pylori is noninvasive and indirect. It should not be used as the primary diagnostic test unless used in combination with other tests. It is most effective by itself for epidemiologic or screening evaluations. The basis for all of the various serologic tests is the ability of H pylori to elicit both a local and a systemic immune response. The antibodies to H pylori can be detected by bacterial agglutination, complement fixation, and ELISA. Of these three methods, ELISA is the technique of choice because it is simple, quick, inexpensive, and sensitive.[7]

Two types of ELISA are currently available. The "rapid office test" (using commercial kits) can be performed not only on serum but also on saliva or gingival secretion, making it particularly appropriate for children.[69] This is not a quantitative test, and the results are expressed either as positive or negative. The main disadvantage of this test is the high rate of false-positive results. As a result, the rapid and sensitive qualities of this test can be used more advantageously for exclusion, whereas positive results need to be supplemented by another confirmatory method. The "machine-read, laboratory-based serology tests" are more accurate and provide quantitative results.

Factors that affect the accuracy of the ELISA include the nature of the *H pylori* antigen preparation, the class of antibody against which the antibody to human serum is directed, and the cutoff point selected for a positive result that inversely influences the specificity and sensitivity. ELISA, based on whole-cell antigen extract, can cross-react with sera containing antibodies to *Campylobacter jejuni,* which shares common epitopes with *H pylori* and can produce false-positive results.[127] Therefore, second-generation ELISA tests were developed based on more purified antigens of *H pylori*, such as cell-associated and outer membrane proteins, or on the "sandwich principle," which uses a combination of a urease fraction together with a structural protein.[7] Alternatively, by using immunoblotting, both sensitivity and specificity can be enhanced, but at the expense of being more complex, time-consuming and costly, making it less practical for routine use and more suitable for research purposes or as a confirmatory test. The value of using IgA or IgM for *H pylori* detection is controversial; however, neither was found to be an effective indicator in pediatric populations, and only ELISA based on IgG is recommended for children.[21] The cutoff point is higher in adults than in children; therefore, the accepted positive result in adults (defined as an optical density greater than 2 SD above the mean value obtained for noncolonized individuals) is not applicable to children. Thus, ELISA used to diagnose *H pylori* in children should be standardized with controls of children's sera.[20]

In conclusion, serology tests in children are attractive because they are noninvasive and simple. Moreover, because there are fewer infected children than adults, positive findings are more diagnostic for the pediatric population.[102] Children, unlike adults, demonstrate a correlation between the magnitude of the IgG antibodies and the bacterial load or the histologic severity of the gastritis.[21] Nonetheless, serology cannot be the only diagnostic test used, nor can it monitor immediate effects of antibacterial therapy because of the delay between bacterial eradication and the decline in antibodies. On the other hand, it is the ideal test for screening. Serologic testing for *H pylori* antibodies in children with recurrent abdominal pain identifies those who warrant further investigation and also avoids unnecessary invasive procedures in seronegative children.[20, 127]

Breath Tests

The urea breath test is a noninvasive and indirect test for *H pylori*. It takes advantage of the specific characteristic that high urease activity is liberated by *H pylori*. Urea that has been labeled with a carbon isotope ^{13}C is taken orally with a meal to delay gastric emptying and to enhance the exposure of the urea to gastric mucosa. In infected patients, the urea is hydrolyzed by the bacterial urease to ammonia and labeled bicarbonate, which diffuse into the blood, whereby the latter is excreted by the lungs and can be identified in the expired breath as labeled CO_2. The labeled carbon can then be quantified. A variety of modifications exist in the methodology of this test in terms of (1) the dose of the labeled urea used; (2) types (or absence) of standard meals given at the onset of testing; (3) the amounts (or none) of the nonradioactive carrier added to the labeled urea; (4) the intervals and length of the test; and (5) the method of expressing results.[54] In general, by adding nonlabeled urea and concomitant administration of a meal, the amount of labeled urea can be reduced.[115] The duration of the study ranges from 30 to 180 minutes. In most centers, either a single sample is collected at 20 minutes after ingestion[89] or two measurements are performed at 30 and 60 minutes.[2, 54]

The urea is labeled either with ^{13}C or ^{14}C. The latter is more commonly used in adults than in children because it is an inexpensive isotope and can be measured easily using a scintillation counter. Because ^{14}C does not occur naturally, it has an intrinsic advantage over ^{13}C as an isotopic label. The required amount of radioactivity is extremely low, especially when "cold" ^{12}C urea is added. It was estimated that a single upper gastrointestinal series produces more exposure than 1000 ^{14}C urea breath tests.[115] Although ^{14}C has a physical half-life of approximately 5000 years, it has a rapid excretion in breath and urine.[64] Still, concern has been expressed about its safe use in children and in pregnant woman. Therefore, ^{13}C has been recommended in the pediatric population; ^{13}C, however, is significantly more expensive and requires a gas isotope ratio mass spectrometer for quantification. The accuracy of the test can be influenced by several factors. The most common reason for false-negative results is breath testing too soon after a course of antibiotics, bismuth salt, or omeprazole.[1, 2] Breath tests should not be performed until at least 1 month after completing such a treatment. False-negative findings also can emerge in conditions with rapid emptying of urea from the stomach or with sampling carried out too late.[89] False-positive results are possible if other urease-producing bacteria are present in the stomach or from urease activity of oral bacteria. The latter can be avoided by not sampling too early and by rinsing the mouth. The urea breath test can semiquantitatively assess the bacterial load that correlates with the amount of expired ^{14}C.[64] This, together with the fact that it is the most reliable of the noninvasive tests, has established the urea breath test as the ideal test in situations when knowledge of *H pylori* status alone is needed, such as for follow-up after attempted *H pylori* eradication. Although the breath test provides information about existing *H pylori*, it does not distinguish *H pylori*-infected children with peptic ulcer disease from those with nonulcer dyspepsia or abdominal pain.[133] Therefore, this indirect test cannot replace upper gastrointestinal endoscopy in the initial evaluation of children and adolescents with symptoms associated with the upper gastrointestinal tract. Thus, it became the authors' practice that, after *H pylori* is diagnosed by endoscopy (either via histology or by the rapid urease test before treatment is started), the authors perform a urea breath test that provides a quantitative baseline. It is repeated at 4 weeks after treatment is completed and when relapse is suspected and endoscopy is not necessarily indicated.

Radiology

Upper gastrointestinal barium series is not an effective tool in diagnosis of either peptic ulcer disease or gastritis, particularly in children. In the authors' experience, however, a typical appearance of nodular gastritis is highly suggestive of *H pylori* infection, especially in the pediatric population.[10] Such findings almost always correlate with an endoscopic picture of antral nodularity, and *H pylori* infection should be confirmed by one of the other diagnostic tests.

TREATMENT

The National Institute of Health Consensus Development Conference on *Helicobacter pylori* in Peptic Ulcer Disease published a consensus statement that ulcer patients with *H pylori* infection require treatment with antimicrobial agents in addition to antisecretory drugs whether on first presentation with the illness or on recurrence.[101] The value of treating of nonulcer dyspepsia patients with *H pylori* infection remains to be determined.

In contrast with the recommendation for adult patients, no consensus exists for the treatment for children with *H pylori*-associated gastroduodenal disease.

Eradication of *H pylori* infection reduces the recurrence of primary duodenal ulcers in children.[70, 135, 136] Therefore, compelling evidence now supports eradication therapy in *H pylori*-infected children and adolescents with endoscopically proven peptic ulcer disease. Because most children with *H pylori* infection have no clinical symptoms and no convincing evidence suggests that *H pylori* infection causes symptoms in the absence of mucosal ulceration, the authors concur with Sherman and colleagues[122, 132] that there is no justification for treating all children infected with this pathogen.

In the *H pylori* infection meeting held in Houston in October 1994, Graham concluded that "today we have therapies that are well tolerated and effective for curing most *H pylori* infections." The most widely used protocols for adult patients are triple and dual therapies employing bismuth or H_2 blockers and one or two antimicrobial agents.[4, 9, 52, 53, 55] The large variety of treatment protocols suggests that no single ideal option exists.

Recurrence rates of duodenal ulcers are as high as 79% after 1 year in those patients in whom the organism is not eliminated totally, compared with rates of 27% in those treated successfully.[59]

Although H_2 blockers are effective in healing duodenal and gastric ulcers, the relapse rate after therapy is very high. Underlying gastritis is probably not affected by acid-suppression therapy.

Recently Graham and co-workers reported that 84% of 105 H pylori-positive patients experienced resolution of their duodenal ulcer after 8 weeks of H_2-blocker therapy and only 14% required antimicrobial treatment.[55]

Helicobacter pylori seems to be resistant to cimetidine, sucralfate, and antacids.[4, 74, 112] Recently, omeprazole, a proton pump inhibitor used in treatment for peptic-ulcer disease, has been found to have anti-Helicobacter activity[67]; however, its role in the treatment of Helicobacter-positive patients remains to be determined.

Kilbridge and colleagues[74] reported that treatment with H_2-receptor blockers, although effective in promoting initial clinical improvement in 80% of children infected with H pylori, resulted in a high rate of symptom recurrence and reinfection (68%) after 2 years. Glassman and co-workers[46] found that only 53% of H pylori-positive children were asymptomatic 6 years after therapy with H_2-receptor antagonists.

Bismuth salts remain the most effective single agent in eradicating H pylori.[78] The mechanism of action seems to include inhibition of the production of the enzymes elaborated by the organism and disruption of its outer membrane.[123]

Bismuth subcitrate alone is superior to H_2 blockers and has cleared the infection in 10% to 30% of adult patients. Antibiotics alone show poor results, although a combination of amoxicillin and bismuth showed clearance of H pylori in 30% to 50% of patients 1 month after treatment. There was, however, a high relapse rate after discontinuation of medication. A combination of metronidazole and bismuth yielded 74% clearance, and the addition of tetracycline cleared the organism in 94% of cases, with sustained remission at 18 months. Treatment programs range from 7 to 28 days.

Triple therapy with two antimicrobials and bismuth salts is no more effective in eradication of gastric H pylori or promoting healing of the inflammatory lesion but reduces the rate of relapse from 74% to 19%.[16, 79, 87, 88] Antimicrobial agents, including penicillin G, erythromycin, tetracycline, tinidazole, metronidazole, and gentamicin, have been used successfully in patients infected with H pylori.[48, 111]

The results of clinical trials using a single antibiotic for gastric Helicobacter infection have also been disappointing. De Giacomo and co-workers[24] found that children given amoxicillin had no improvement of symptoms, and Oderda and colleagues[108] reported a recurrence rate of

75% in 30 children who initially responded to 4 weeks of amoxicillin. Drumm and colleagues[29] used bismuth subsalicylate and amoxicillin to treat 16 children who had failed initial therapy with H_2-receptor antagonists. They documented both eradication of *Helicobacter* and resolution of gastritis in 75% of their patients. In a later study, Oderda and colleagues[103] reported that therapy with amoxicillin and tinidazole resulted in resolution of symptoms in 94% and healing of gastritis in 84% of the children examined. The recurrence rate in this study was 16.64% after 6 months. Similar results were reported by De Giacomo and colleagues,[23] who found that after 4 weeks of amoxicillin and bismuth subcitrate administration, *Helicobacter* was eradicated and gastritis had healed in 68% of 19 adolescents.

There is a continuing search for new therapies. Much work is currently directed toward evaluation of dual therapies using a proton pump inhibitor and an antimicrobial agent.[13, 45, 71, 76, 81, 116, 123] The most commonly used antibiotic in these studies is amoxicillin. Excellent results have not been universally obtained. The best results have been obtained with omeprazole (20 mg twice a day) and amoxicillin (1 g three times a day), but cure rates probably average 50% to 60%, with cures over 80% being rare. An alternate therapy is to combine a proton pump inhibitor and several antibacterials.

Metronidazole resistance has become an increasing problem that may severely limit the usefulness of the original triple therapy, especially in developing countries.[118] Effective therapies not requiring metronidazole are needed. Clarithromycin is a new macrolide with good anti-*H pylori* activity in vitro[61, 100] and has proven to be relatively effective when used as monotherapy and highly effective in combination with omeprazole and other antimicrobials.[1, 81] It was found to be an effective therapy, replacing metronidazole in the traditional triple therapy.[1] It is also a good alternative for patients who are allergic to penicillin. Most of the protocols using clarithromycin were of short duration, between 7 and 14 days.

When deciding on the regime of treatment in children, one should consider different possible obstacles and complications. Prescribing too many drugs for long periods may raise low compliance. The different antimicrobials may expose the child to different adverse effects of the drugs. Bismuth subsalicylate treatment raises the possibility of complications stemming from the bismuth and the salicylate moieties.

Several authors have argued that the epidemiologic data associating the acquisition of *H pylori* infection in childhood with the development of gastric cancer in adulthood justify the eradication of *H pylori* in every infected child or adolescent. Against this rationale stands the fact that gastric cancer is very rare, whereas *H pylori* infection is relatively common. Future cost–benefit analyses and results of interventional studies may supply the answer to this question. It is also possible that the research on different strains of *H pylori*, especially those with cytopathic effect, will provide the necessary information for decision.

Another issue that needs further evaluation is the rate of reinfection in the pediatric population. This information will provide the knowledge of whether sequential follow-up of patients is necessary.

The method of choice to demonstrate bacterial eradication after treatment is, at present, the breath test. The usefulness of serology is still debatable. Further studies of the latter method using different bacterial antigens may increase the value of the method.

SUMMARY

As in adults, the data accumulated in past years on peptic disease in children demonstrate the specific association between the disease and *H pylori* colonization in the gastric mucosa. In addition, evidence suggests that the treatment of peptic ulcer by combinations that eradicate the bacteria changes the natural history of peptic ulcer, thus diminishing significantly the recurrence of the disease. The diagnosis of *H pylori* infection relies on the combination of direct and indirect methods. The direct methods include different staining methods, and culture of the bacteria from endoscopic specimens. Urease tests, serology, and ^{13}C, 14C-breath tests are used as indirect methods, mainly for follow-up and as evidence for the success of treatment.

At the present time, no evidence shows that *H pylori* infection is associated with a specific clinical picture. The attempt to associate *H pylori* gastritis with the entity of RAP did not gain enough support. Children with *H pylori* colonization are often asymptomatic. Several regimens of treatment were used to eradicate *H pylori* in children. The treatment is usually based on combinations that include H_2 blockers or a bismuth salt and antibacterial agents, such as amoxicillin and metronidazole. Recently, omeprazole and clarithromycin were shown also to be efficient for the purpose. Treatment schedules of 4 weeks and more have recently been reduced to 1 week. In general, the authors' impression is that pediatricians tend to overtreat *H pylori* infection. Is this policy justified? Future research will provide the answer. Epidemiologic studies demonstrate that environmental and genetic factors determine the susceptibility toward colonization with *H pylori*.

Future research will provide the knowledge of possible reservoir of the organism, better treatment modalities, the possible role of the organism in development of gastric malignancies, and host factors that are important in the evolution of *H pylori* infection.

References

1. Al-Assi MT, Ramirez FC, Lew GM, et al: Clarithromycin, tetracycline and bismuth: A new non-metronidazole therapy for *Helicobacter pylori* infection. Am J Gastroenterol 89:1203, 1994
2. Atherton JC, Spiller RC: The urea breath test for *Helicobacter pylori*. Gut 35:723, 1994

3. Azuma T, Konishi J, Tanaka Y, et al: Contribution of HLA DQA gene to host's response against *Helicobacter pylori*. Lancet 343:542, 1994
4. Barbara L, Biasco G, Capurso L, et al: Effects of sucralfate and sulglycotide treatment on active gastritis and *Helicobacter pylori* colonization of the gastric mucosa in non-ulcer dyspepsia patients. Am J Gastroenterol 85:1109, 1990
5. Berkowicz J, Lee A: Person to person transmission of *Campylobacter pylori*. Lancet 11:680, 1987
6. Blecker U, Hauser B, Lanciers S, et al: The prevalence of *Helicobacter pylori*-positive serology in asymptomatic children. J Pediatr Gastroenterol Nutr 16:252, 1993
7. Blecker U, Lanciers S, Hauser B, et al: Diagnosis of *Helicobacter pylori* infection in adults and children by using the Malakit *Helicobacter pylori*, a commercially available enzyme linked immunoadsorbent assay. J Clin Microbiol 31:1770, 1993
8. Boren T, Falk P, Roth KR, et al: Attachment of *Helicobacter pylori* to human gastric epithelium radiated by blood group antigens. Science 262:1892, 1993
9. Borsch GM, Graham DY: *Helicobacter pylori*. *In* Collen MJ, Benjamin SB (eds): Pharmacology of Peptic Ulcer Disease, Handbook of Experimental Pharmacology, Vol 99. Berlin, Springer-Verlag, 1991, pp 107–148
10. Bujanover Y, Konikoff F, Baratz M: Nodular gastritis and *Helicobacter pylori*. J Pediatr Gastroenterol Nutr 11:41, 44, 1990
11. Cadranel S, Goosens H, De Boeck M, et al: *Campylobacter pyloridis* in children. Lancet 1:735, 1986
12. Cave TR, Cave DR: *Helicobacter pylori* stimulates pepsin secretion from isolated rabbit gastric glands. Scan J Gastroenterol 26(suppl):181, 1987
13. Cellini L, Marzio L, Di girolamo A, et al: Enhanced clearing of *Helicobacter pylori* after omeprazole plus roxithromycin treatment. FEMS Microbiol Lett 68:255–257, 1991
14. Clayton C, Kleanthous K, Tabaqchali S: Detection and identification of *Helicobacter pylori* by the polymerase chain reaction. J Clin Pathol 44:515, 1991
15. Clayton CL, Kleanthous PJ, Coates DD, et al: Sensitive detection of *Helicobacter pylori* by polymerase chain reaction. J Clin Microbiol 30:192, 1992
16. Coghlan JG, Gilligan D, Humphries H, et al: *Campylobacter pylori* and recurrence of duodenal ulcer: A 12-month study. Lancet 2:1109–1111, 1987
17. Cohen HA, Shapiro RP, Frydman M, et al: Childhood protein losing enteropathy associated with *Helicobacter pylori* infection. J Pediatr Gastroenterol Nutr 13:201, 1991
18. Cover TL, Blaser MJ: Purification and characterization of the vacuolating toxin from *Helicobacter pylori*. J Biol Chem 87:1554, 1992
19. Cover TL, Dooley CP, Blaser MJ: Characterization of and human serologic response to proteins in *Helicobacter pylori* broth culture supernatants with vacuolizing cytotoxin activity. Infect Immunol 58:603, 1990
20. Crabtree JE, Mahony MJ, Taylor JD, et al: Immune response to *Helicobacter pylori* in children with recurrent abdominal pain. J Clin Pathol 44:768, 1991
21. Czinn SZ, Carr HS, Speck WT: Diagnosis of gastritis caused by *Helicobacter pylori* in children by means of ELISA. Rev Infect Dis 13(suppl 8):700–703, 1991
22. Daw MA, Deegan P, Leen E, et al: The effect of omeprazol on *Helicobacter pylori* and associated gastritis. Aliment Pharmacol Ther 5:435, 1991
23. De Giacomo C, Fiocca R, Villani L, et al: *Helicobacter pylori* infection and chronic gastritis: Clinical, serological, and histologic correlations in children treated with amoxicillin and colloidal bismuth subcitrate. J Pediatr Gastroenterol Nutr 11:310–316, 1990
24. De Giacomo C, Maggiore G, Licardi G, et al: Effects of antibacterial treatment of *Campylobacter pylori*-associated gastritis in children. *Gastroenterology* 95:1699, 1988
25. Denizot Y, Sohhami I, Rambaud JC, et al: Paf acether synthesis by *Helicobacter pyleri*. Gut 31:1242, 1990
26. Doenges JL: Spirochates in the gastric glands of macacus rhesus and in humans without definitive history of related disease. Proc Soc Exp Biol Med 38:536–538, 1938
27. Doenges JL: Spirochetes in the gastric glands of macacus rhesus and of man without related disease. Arch Pathol Lab Med 27:469, 1939
28. Drumm NB: *Helicobacter pylori* in the pediatric patient. Gastro Clin North Am 22:169, 1993

29. Drumm B, Perez-Perez GI, Blaser MJ, et al: Intrafamilial clustering of *Helicobacter pylori* infection. N Engl J Med 322:359, 1990
30. Drumm B, Sherman P, Chiasson D, et al: Treatment of *Campylobacter pylori*-associated antral gastritis in children with bismuth subsalicylate and ampicillin. J Pediatr 113:908, 1988
31. Drumm NB, Sherman P, Cutz E, et al: Association of *Campylobacter pylori* on the gastric mucosa with antral gastritis in children. N Engl J Med 326:1557, 1987
32. Dunn BE, Roop RM, Sung CC, et al: Identification and purification of a cpn 6a heat shock protein homolog from *Helicobacter pylori.* Infect Immun 60:1946, 1992
33. Eaton KA, Morgan DR, Krakowka S: *Campylobacter pylori* virulence factors in gnotabiotic piglets. Infect Immun 57:1119, 1989
34. El Zaatari FAK, Naguyen AH, Genta MR, et al: Determination of *Helicobacter pylori* status by reverse transcription polymerase chain reaction, comparison with urea breath test. Dig Dis Sci 40:109, 1995
35. Engastrand L, Nguyen AMH, Graham DY, et al: Reverse transcription and polymerase chain reaction rRNA for detection of helicobacter species. J Clin Microbiol 30:2295, 1992
36. Evans DG, Evans DJ, Moulds JJ, et al: N-acetylneuraminyl lactose bindings fibrillar hemaglutinin of *Campylobacter pylori:* A putative colonization factor antigen. Infect Immun 56:2896, 1988
37. Evans DJ, Evans DG, Kirkpatrick SS, et al: Characterization of the *Helicobacter pylori* urease and purification of its subunits. Microb Pathol 10:15, 1991
38. Faber R, Sobhani I, Laurent Puig P: Polymerase chain reaction assay for the detection of *Helicobacter pylori* in gastric biopsy specimens: Comparison with culture, rapid urease test, and histopathologic tests. Gut 35:905, 1994
39. Fauchere JL, Blaser MJ: Adherence of *Helicobacter pylori* cells and their surface components to HeLa membranes. Microb Pathog 9:427, 1990
40. Fiedorek SC, Casteel HB, Pumphrey CL, et al: The role of *Helicobacter pylori* in recurrent functional abdominal pain in children. Am J Gastroenterol 87:347, 1992
41. Fiedorek SC, Evans DG, Evans DJ, et al: *H pylori* infection epidemiology in children: Importance of socioeconomic status, age gender and race. Gastroenterology 98:A44, 1990
42. Fiedorek SC, Malaty HM, Evans OL, et al: Factors influencing the epidemiology of *Helicobacter pylori* infection in children. Pediatrics 88:578, 1991
43. Fukuda T, Kimura S, Arakawa T, et al: Possible role of leukotrienes in gastritis associated with *Campylobacter pylori.* J Clin Gastroenterol 12(suppl 1):131, 1990
44. Genta RM, Hamner HW, Graham DY: Gastric lymphoid follicles in *Helicobacter pylori* infection: Frequency, distribution and response to triple therapy. Hum Pathol 24:577, 1993
45. George LL, Borody TJ, Andrews P, et al: Cure of duodenal ulcer after eradication of *Helicobacter pylori.* Med J Aust 153:145–149, 1990
46. Glassman MS: *Helicobacter pylori* infection in children: A clinical overview. Clin Pediatr 8:481–487, 1992
47. Glassman MS, Schwartz SM, Medow MS, et al: *Campylobacter pylori* related gastrointestinal disease in children. Incidence and clinical findings. Dig Dis Sci 34:1501, 1989
48. Glupczynski Y, Burette A: Drug therapy of *Helicobacter pylori* infection: Problems and pitfalls. Am J Gastroenterol 85:1545–1551, 1990
49. Goodwin CS: Duodenal ulcer, *Campylobacter pylori* and the "leaking roof" concept. Lancet 2:1467, 1988
50. Goodwin CS, Armstrong JA: Microbiological aspects of *Helicobacter pylori (Campylobacter pylori).* Eur Clin Microbiol Infect Dis 9:1, 1990
51. Goodwin CS, Armstrong JA, Chilvers T, et al: Transfer of *Campylobacter pylori* and *Campylobacter mustelae* to helicobacter gen. nov. as *Helicobacter pylori* comb. nov. and *Helicobacter mustelae* comb. nov. respectively. Int J Syst Bacteriol 39:397, 1989
52. Goodwin CS, Blincow ED, Warren JR, et al: Evaluation of culture techniques for isolating *Campylobacter pyloridis* from endoscopic biopsies of gastric mucosa. J Clin Pathol 38:1127, 1985

53. Graham DY, Borsch GM: The who's and when's of therapy for *Helicobacter pylori*. Am J Gastroenterol 85:1552, 1990
54. Graham DY, Klein PD: What you should know about the methods, problems, interpretations and uses of urea breath test. Am J Gastroenterol 86:118, 1991
55. Graham DY, Lew GM, Evans DG, et al: Effect of triple therapy on duodenal ulcer: A randomized controlled trial. Ann Intern Med 115:266, 1991
56. Graham DY, Malaty HM, Evans DG, et al: Epidemiology of *Helicobacter pylori* in an asymptomatic population in the United States. Gastroenterology 100:1495, 1991
57. Graham DY, Opekun AR, Klein PD: Clarithromycin for the eradication of *Helicobacter pylori*. J Clin Gastroenterology 14:292, 1992
58. Gray SF, Wyatt JI, Rathbone BJ: Simplified techniques for identifying *Campylobacter pyloritis*. J Clin Pathol 39:1279, 1986
59. Gryboski JD: Peptic ulcer disease in children. Pediatr Rev 12:15, 1990
60. Han SW, Flamm R, Hachmen CY, et al: Transport and storage of gastric biopsies and cultures containing *Helicobacter pylori*. Gastroenterology 106:A89, 1994
61. Hardy DI, Hanson CW, Hensey DM, et al: Susceptibility of *Campylobacter pylori* to macrolides and fluoroquinolones. J Antimicrob Chemother 22:631, 1988
62. Hassall E, Dimmick JE: Unique features of *Helicobacter pylori* disease in children. Dig Dis Sci 36:417, 1991
63. Hazell SL, Evans DJ Jr, Graham DY: *Helicobacter pylori* catalase. J Gen Microbiol 137:57, 1991
64. Hilker E, Stool R, Domechke W: Quantitative assessment of *Helicobacter pylori* colonization of the gastric mucosa by ^{13}C-urea breath test. Gastroenterology 106:A93, 1994
65. Hill R, Perman J, Worthy P, et al: *Campylobacter pyloridis* and gastritis in children. Lancet 1:338, 1986
66. Ho SA, Hoyle JA, Lewis FA, et al: Direct polymerase chain reaction for detection of *Helicobacter pylori* in humans and animals. J Clin Microbiol 29:2543, 1991
67. Hui WM, Lam SK, Ho J, et al: Effect of omeprazole on duodenal ulcer-associated antral gastritis and *Helicobacter pylori*. Dig Dis Sci 36:577, 1991
68. Hupertz V, Czinn S: Demonstration of a cytotoxin from *Campylobacter pylori*. Eur J Clin Microbiol Infect Dis 7:576, 1988
69. Hussan MO, Gottrand F, Turck D, et al: Detection of *H. pylori* in saliva using monoclonal antibody. J Med Microbiol Virol Parasitol 279:466, 1993
70. Israel DM, Hassall E: Treatment and long-term follow-up of *Helicobacter pylori* associated duodenal ulcer disease in children. J Pediatr 123:53, 1993
71. Iwahi T, Satoh H, Nakao M, et al: Lansoprazole, a novel benzimidazole proton pump inhibitor and its related compounds have selective activity against *Helicobacter pylori*. Antimicrob Agents Chemother 35:490–496, 1991
72. Karttunen T, Niemela S, Lehtola J: *Helicobacter pylori* in dyspeptic patients: Quantative association with severity of gastritis intragastric pH and serum gastrin concentration. Scan J Gastroenterol 186(suppl):124, 1991
73. Kelly SM, Pitcher MCL, Farmery SM, et al: Isolation of *Helicobacter pylori* from feces of patients with dyspepsia in the United Kingdom. Gastroenterology 107:1671, 1994
74. Kilbridge PM, Dahms BB, Czinn SJ: *Campylobacter pylori*-associated gastritis and peptic ulcer disease in children. Am J Dis Child 142:1149, 1988
75. Klein PD, Graham DY, Gaillour, et al: Water source as risk factor for *Helicobacter pylori* infection in Peruvian children. Lancet 337:1503, 1991
76. Labenz J, Gyenes E, Ruhl GH, et al: Short term therapy with high dosage omeprazole and amoxicillin for *Helicobacter pylori* eradication: A pilot study. Med Klin 87:118–119, 1992
77. Langenberg W, Rauws EAJ, Oudbrier JK, et al: Patient to patient transmission of *Campylobacter pylori* infection by fiberoptic gastroduodenoscopy and biopsy. J Infect Dis 161:507, 1990
78. Lanza FL, Skoglund ML, Rack MF, et al: The effect of bismuth sub-salicylate on the histological gastritis seen in *Campylobacter pylori*: A placebo-controlled study. Am J Gastroenterol 84:1060–1064, 1989
79. Lee FI, Samolff IM, Hardman M: Comparison of tri-potassium di-citrato and bis-

muthate tablets with ranitidine in healing and relapse of duodenal ulcers. Lancet 1(8441):1209–1302, 1985

80. Levi S, Beardshall K, Haddad G, et al: *Campylobacter pylori* and duodenal ulcers: The gastric link. Lancet 1:1167, 1989
81. Logan RP, Gummett PA, Hegarty BT, et al: Clarithromycin and omeprazole for *Helicobacter pylori* (letter). Lancet 340:239, 1992
82. Mahony MJ, Wyatt JI, Littlewood JM: Management and response to treatment of *Helicobacter pylori* gastritis. Arch Dis Child 67:940, 1992
83. Mai UEH, Perez-Perez GI, Wahl LM, et al: Soluble surface proteins from *Helicobacter pylori* activate monocytes/macrophages by lipopolysaccharide independent mechanisms. J Clin Invest 87:894, 1991
84. Malaty HM, Graham DY, Klein PD, et al: Transmission of *Helicobacter pylori* infection. Scand J Gastroenterol 26:927, 1991
85. Maostone NP, Lynch DAF, Lewis AF, et al: Identification of *Helicobacter pylori* DNA in the mouths and stomachs of patients with gastritis using PCR. J Clin Pathol 46:540, 1993
86. Marshall BJ, Warren JR: Unidentified curved bacillus on gastric epithelium in active chronic gastritis. Lancet 1:1273, 1983
87. Marshall BJ, Goodwin CS, Warren JR, et al: Long-term healing gastritis and low duodenal ulcer relapse after eradication of Campylobacter pyloroides. A prospective double-blind study. Gastroenterology 92:A1518, 1987
88. Marshall BJ, Goodwin CS, Warren JR, et al: Prospective double-blind trial of duodenal relapse after eradication of *Campylobacter pylori*. Lancet 2:1437–1441, 1988
89. Marshall BJ, Plankey MW, Hopffman SR, et al: A 20 minute breath test for *H. pylori*. Am J Gastroenterology 86:438, 1991
90. Marshall BJ, Warren JR, Francis SR, et al: Rapid urease test in the management of *Campylobacter pyloridis* associated gastritis. Am J Gastroenterol 82:200, 1987
91. McGovern TW, Talley NJ, Kephart GM, et al: Eosinophil infiltration and degranulation in *Helicobacter pylori* associated chronic gastritis. Dig Dis Sci 26:435, 1991
92. McNulty CAM, Dent JC, Uff JS: Detection of *Campylobacter pylori* by the biopsy urease test: An assessment in 1445 patients. Gut 30:1058, 1989
93. Megraud F: Epidemiology of *Helicobacter pylori* infection. Gastro Clin North Am 22:73, 1993
94. Megraud F: Microbiological characteristics of *Campylobacter pylori*. Eur J Gastroenterol Hepatol 1:5–12, 1989
95. Megraud F, Brassens Robbe MP, Denis F, et al: Seroepidemiology of *Campylobacter pylori* infection in various populations. J Clin Microbiol 27:1870, 1989
96. Mitchell HM, Bohane TD, Tobias V, et al: *Helicobacter pylori* infection in children: Potential clues to pathogenesis. J Pediatr Gastroenterol Nutr 161:120, 1993
97. Mitchell WM, Li YY, Hu PJ, et al: Epidemiology of *Helicobacter pylori* in Southern China: Identification of early childhood as the critical period for acquisition. J Infect Dis 166:149, 1992
98. Morris A, Ali MR, Brown P, et al: *Campylobacter pylori* infection in biopsy specimens of gastric antrum: laboratory diagnosis and estimation of sampling error. J Clin Pathol 42:727, 1989
99. Morris AJ, Ali MR, Nicholson GI, et al: Long term follow up of voluntary ingestion of *Helicobacter pylori*. Ann Intern Med 114:662, 1991
100. Nagata T, Numata K, Hanada K, et al: The susceptibility of *Campylobacter pylori* to antiulcer agents and antibiotics. J Clin Gastroenterol 12(suppl 1):135, 1990
101. NIH Consensus conference: *H. pylori* in Peptic Ulcer Disease. JAMA 272:65–69, 1994
102. Oderda G, Dell'Olio D, Morra I, et al: *Campylobacter pylori* gastritis: Long term results of treatment with amoxycillin. Arch Dis Child 64:326, 1989
103. Oderda G, Holton J, Altare F, et al: Anoxicillin plus tinidazole for *Campylobacter pylori* gastritis in children: Assessment by serum IgG antibody, Pepsinogen I and gastrin level. Lancet 1:690, 1989
104. Oderda G, Vaira P, Dell'olio D, et al: Serum pepsinogen and gastrin concentrations in children positive for *Helicobacter pylori*. J Clin Pathol 43:762, 1990

105. Oderda G, Vaira D, Holton J, et al: *Helicobacter pylori* in children with peptic ulcer and their families. Dig Dis Sci 36:572, 1991
106. Perez-Perez GI, Blaser MJ: Conservation and diversity of *Campylobacter pyloridis* major antigens. Infect Immun 55:1256, 1987
107. Perez-Perez GI, Davorkin BM, Chodos JE, et al: *Campylobacter pylori* antibodies in humans. Ann Intern Med 109:11, 1988
108. Perwett EJ, Smith JTL, Nwokolo CU, et al: Eradication of *Helicobacter pylori* abolishes 24 hour hypergastrinema: A perspective study in healthy subjects. Aliment Pharm Ther 5:283, 1991
109. Peterson WL: *Helicobacter pylori* and peptic ulcer disease. N Engl J Med 324:1043, 1991
110. Peterson WL, Graham DY, Marshall BJ, et al: Clarithromycin as monotherapy for eradication of *Helicobacter pylori*: A randomized, double-blind trial. Am J Gastroenterol 88:1860, 1993
111. Pierre C, Lecossier D, Boussougant Y, et al: Use of reamplification protocol improves sensitivity of detection of *Mycobacterium* tuberculosis in clinical samples by amplification of DNA. J Clin Microbiol 28:712, 1991
112. Price AB, Levi J, Dolby JM, et al: *Campylobacter pyloridis* in peptic ulcer disease: Microbiology, pathology and scanning electron microscopy. Gut 26:1183–1188, 1985
113. Prieto G, Polanco I, Larraui J, et al: *Helicobacter pylori* infection in children: Clinical endoscopic and histologic correlations. J Pediatr Gastroenterol Nutr 14:420, 1992
114. Queiroz DMM, Mendes EN, Rocha GA, et al: Histamine concentration of gastric mucosa in *Helicobacter pylori* positive and negative children. Gut 32:464, 1991
115. Raju GS, Smith MJ, Morton D, et al: Mini dose ^{14}C-urea breath test for the detection of *Helicobacter pylori*. Am J Gastroenterol 89:1027, 1994
116. Rauws EA, Tytgat GN: Cure of duodenal ulcer associated with eradication of *Helicobacter pylori*. Lancet 335:1233–1235, 1990
117. Reifen R, Rassoly I, Drumm B, et al: Symptomatology and demographic features of *Helicobacter pylori* infection in children. Isr Med Sci 161(suppl):25, 1992
118. Results of multicentric European survey in 1991 of metronidazole resistance in *Helicobacter pylori*: European Study Group on Antibiotic Susceptibility of *Helicobacter pylori*. Eur J Clin Microbiol Infect Dis 11:1771, 1992
119. Roosendaal R, Kuipers EJ, Brule AJC, et al: Importance of the fiberoptic endoscopic cleaning procedure for detection of *Helicobacter pylori* in gastric biopsy specimens by PCR. J Clin Microbiol 32:1123, 1994
120. Sarosiek J, Bilski J, Murty VLN, et al: Colloidal bismuth subcitrate (De nol) inhibits degradation of gastric mucus by *Campylobacter pylori* protease. Am J Gastroenterol 84:506, 1989
121. Schaber EF, Umlauft G, Stoffler F, et al: Indirect immunofluorescence test and enzyme linked immunoadsorbent assay for detection of *Campylobacter pylori*. J Clin Microbiol 27:327, 1989
122. Sherman PM: Peptic ulcer disease in children: Diagnosis, treatment, and the implication of *Helicobacter pylori*. Gastroenterol Clin North Am 23:707, 1994
123. Slomiany BL, Kasinathan C, Slomiany A: Lipolytic activity of *Campylobacter pylori*: Effect of colloidal bismuth sub-citrate (De-Nol). Am J Gastroenterol 84:1273–1277, 1989
124. Stubbs JB, Marshall BJ: Radiation dose estimates for the carbon 14 labeled urea breath test. J Nucl Med 34:821, 1993
125. Thillainayagam AV, Arvind AS, Cook RS, et al: Diagnostic efficiency of an ultra rapid endoscopy room test for *Helicobacter pylori*. Gut 32:467, 1991
126. Thomas JE, Gibson GR, Darboe MK, et al: Isolation of *Helicobacter pylori* from human feces. Lancet 340:1194, 1992
127. Thomas JE, Whatmore AM, Barer MR, et al: Serodiagnosis of *Helicobacter* infection in children. J Clin Microbiol 28:2641–2646, 1990
128. Triebling AT, Korsten MA, Dlugosz JW, et al: Severity of helicobacter induced gastric injury correlates with gastric juice ammonia. Dig Dis Sci 76:1089, 1991
129. Unge P, Gad A, Gnarpe H, et al: Does omeprazole improve antimicrobial therapy directed toward gastric *Campylobacter pylori* in patients with antral gastritis? A pilot study. Scand J Gastroenterol 167(suppl):49–54, 1989

130. Valentine JL, Arthur RR, Mobley HLT, et al: Detection of *Helicobacter pylori* by using the polymerase chain reaction. J Clin Microbiol 29:989, 1991
131. Van der Meer SB, Forget PP, Loffeld RJLF, et al: The prevalence of *Helicobacter pylori* serum antibodies in children with recurrent abdominal pain. Eur J Pediatr 151:799, 1992
132. Van Zanten S, Sherman PM: Indications for treatment of *Helicobacter pylori* infection: A systematic overview. Can Med Assoc J 150:189, 1993
133. Vandenplas Y, Blecker U, Devreker T, et al: Contribution of the ^{13}C-urea breath test to the detection of *Helicobacter pylori* gastritis in children. Pediatrics 90:608, 1992
134. Vargas M, Lee A, Fox JG, et al: Inhibition of acid secretion from parietal cells by non human infecting helicobacter species: A factor in colonization of gastric mucosa? Infect Immun 59:3694, 1991
135. Westblom U, Madan E, Gudipati S, et al: Diagnosis of *Helicobacter pylori* in adult and pediatric patients by using Pyloriset, a rapid latex agglutination test. J Clin Microbiol 30:96, 1992
136. Wetherall BL, Johnson AM: Haemolytic activity of *Campylobacter pylori.* Eur J Clin Microbiol Infect Dis 8:706, 1989
137. Yardley JH, Paull H: *Campylobacter pylori:* A newly recognized infectious agent in the gastrointestinal tract. Am J Surg Pathol 12(suppl):89, 1988
138. Yeung CK, Fu KH, Yeun KY, et al: *Helicobacter pylori* and associated duodenal ulcer. Arch Dis Child 65:1212, 1990

Address reprint requests to

Yoram Bujanover, MD
Dana Children's Hospital
Sourasky-Tel Aviv Medical Center
6 Weizman Street
Tel Aviv
Israel

0031–3955/96 $0.00 + .20

ULCERATIVE COLITIS IN CHILDREN

Barbara S. Kirschner, MD

Since chronic inflammatory bowel disease (IBD) in children was last reviewed in the *Pediatric Clinics of North America*,[44] much new information has accumulated. In particular, the areas of genetic predisposition and alteration in the mucosal immune response have gained from intense research regarding the basic pathogenetic mechanisms of these disorders. Patients have benefited from recent drug trials that have expanded the therapeutic armamentarium available for treating IBD. This article describes recent advances in the field and summarizes the clinical presentation, diagnostic evaluation, and management of children with chronic ulcerative colitis (UC).

EPIDEMIOLOGIC ASPECTS

In parts of the world where health data of the entire population are recorded for epidemiologic purposes, several reports have shown an increasing incidence of IBD in recent decades. With regard to children, a comprehensive study from Scotland demonstrated a threefold rise in newly diagnosed Crohn's disease (CD) between 1968 and 1983, which further increased to 4.4-fold from 1968 to 1988.[5, 16] In contrast, UC showed annual fluctuations but not a consistent upward trend during the same period.[5] The importance of familial predisposition is illustrated in a multicenter international study that compared 499 children with IBD (302 CD and 197 UC) with 998 healthy controls. It showed that a

From the Departments of Pediatrics and Medicine, Pritzker School of Medicine, University of Chicago; and the Section of Pediatric Gastroenterology, Hepatology and Nutrition, Wyler Children's Hospital, Chicago, Illinois positive family history was the most consistent risk factor for children with IBD (odds ratio 5.6).[21] Other potential factors that might influence the development of UC in children, such as breast-feeding versus formula-feeding, predisposition to infantile gastroenteritis or food intolerance, and stressful life events (e.g., parental death, divorce, or poverty), were not statistically different between the patient and control groups in that study. Twin studies also demonstrate an increased likelihood for UC when one twin has UC; however, the influence is much less than that observed for CD.[108] The prevalence of IBD is increased in Jewish people, especially Ashkenazi and those in the United States in contrast with those in Israel.[80] Interestingly, South Asians who move from India to England also show a higher incidence, suggesting that environmental factors may influence the development of IBD.[75] The recognition that nonsmokers are more likely to develop UC and that smoking may improve symptoms also supports a role for exogenous influences in modulating the activity of UC.

GENETIC STUDIES

The familial and ethnic predisposition to IBD has led to intense investigation of genetic associations. Toyota and colleagues reported that patients with UC were more likely to have the HLA-DR2 allele (in contrast with HLA-DR1/Dqw5 alleles in patients with CD).[102] However, genetic heterogeneity of patients with UC is demonstrated by the presence of perinuclear anticytoplasmic antibody (p-ANCA) in the majority (66%–83%), but not all, affected patients.[12, 76, 91, 114, 115] The presence of p-ANCA seems to identify a subgroup of patients with UC who are at risk for developing primary sclerosing cholangitis (PSC) and chronic inflammation of the ileoanal reservoir (i.e., "pouchitis") in those patients who have undergone colectomy and creation of an ileal pouch.[12, 91]

ETIOPATHOGENESIS

Although the pathogenesis of UC is unknown, current hypotheses include a genetic predisposition that is reflected in an altered immunologic response within the intestinal mucosa.[58, 86, 102, 115] Recent studies have used knock-out gene techniques to produce experimentally induced enterocolitis in interleukin (IL)-10–deficient mice[51] and colitis in IL-2–deficient mice.[83] Intestinal microflora are necessary in triggering and perpetuating IBD in both animal models. When these animals are raised in germ-free environments, either they remain disease-free or an attenuated form of the disease develops. Disease in the IL-2–deficient mouse seems to represent a model for UC in humans. In 100% of those animals that survive the first 9 weeks of life, IBD that is clinically and histologically similar to UC develops. The small intestine is not affected in this model. Mombaerts and colleagues described a condition resembling UC in humans in T-cell receptor (i.e., TCRα, TCRβ, TCRβχδ) mutant mice.[65] These authors suggested that UC may originate from the lack of αβ T-cell–mediated suppression of B cells. This would be consistent with studies of human mucosa in UC that have shown enhanced immunoglobulin production, especially subclass IgG1, in UC.[58] Differing genetic predisposition [i.e., permissive strains (129/Sv and C3H/Hc)] and less permissive strains (BALB/c) of the mouse mutants were observed.

Although in the past, investigators have searched for a specific etiologic (i.e., infectious) agent as a cause of UC, it now seems that several infectious agents may trigger the initial presentation or a relapse of UC.[48, 86, 88] Knowledge concerning the role of cytokines in UC may provide the basis for more targeted and specific therapies in human disease.[68, 86]

CLINICAL FEATURES OF IBD IN CHILDHOOD

Ulcerative colitis tends to run a more complicated course in children than in adults. There is a greater likelihood of pancolonic versus limited colonic involvement, increased chance for proximal extension of initially localized disease, and an enhanced rate of colectomy.[64] Diagnosis generally occurs when the patient is between 5 and 16 years of age, but onset during infancy has been described.[11, 33, 34] Variability in the age of onset, extent of intestinal involvement, severity of intestinal symptoms, and extraintestinal manifestations result in diverse patterns of clinical presentation that necessitate individualized approaches to therapy.

Most pediatric gastroenterologists have thought that young children with pancolitis were subject to a particularly difficult course; however, Gryboski reported contrasting results in a group of 38 children with UC who were diagnosed at fewer than 10 years of age.[33] Although 71% of these children had pancolitis, the majority had clinically mild (53%) or moderate (37%) disease. Only 2 children underwent colectomy during a 6.7-year follow-up period.

Michener and colleagues observed that the frequency of colectomy in children with UC has decreased significantly during the past two decades.[63] Although 48.9% of children with UC underwent colectomy between 1955 and 1965, the rate fell to 26.2% between 1965 and 1974. This change undoubtedly reflects improved medical therapies (e.g., intravenous nutritional support, broad-spectrum antibiotics, and immunosuppressive drugs). In addition, the use of colonoscopy for cancer surveillance rather than performing "prophylactic colectomy" has become standard practice in many centers for children whose disease improves with medical therapy.

Presenting Signs and Symptoms

The most consistent features of UC are stools mixed with blood and mucus and lower abdominal cramping that is most intense during defecation. Episodes are characterized as mild, moderate, or severe, depending on stool frequency, amount of abdominal tenderness, fever, and hemoglobin and albumin concentrations.[106, 112]

Systemic and Extraintestinal Features

Although the sight of blood mixed with stool usually alerts parents to the presence of a condition needing medical attention, at times the initial signs and symptoms of UC may be subtle. In these cases, systemic and extraintestinal manifestations may precede and overshadow the intestinal ones, causing errors in diagnosis and delays in the recognition of UC.[36, 44] Mistaken diagnoses can include acute infectious colitis (especially when an enteric pathogen is isolated concurrently with the onset of UC), iron deficiency anemia, juvenile rheumatoid arthritis, eating disorders, and growth problems attributed to endocrine causes.[36, 44, 66, 88]

Weight Loss

Unexpected weight loss or failure to maintain a normal velocity of weight gain may occur during the prodromal phase prior to the signs of overt UC. In the author's patient population, 68% of children have lost weight (mean, 4.1 kg) at the time of diagnosis. [44]

Arthralgias and Arthritis

Arthralgias and arthritis are among the most frequent extraintestinal complaints of children with UC.[55, 72] In general, joint involvement is pauciarticular, affecting large joints, such as knees, ankles, and hips. Joint complaints often coincide with disease activity and improve with medical treatment that decreases the underlying intestinal inflammation. Joint deformity is not a feature of UC-associated joint disease. Refractory joint symptoms may require nonsteroidal anti-inflammatory therapy, although this should be limited in duration because of the possibility of causing disease exacerbation.[20] The presence of ankylosing spondylitis is more consistent with a diagnosis of CD, especially in those patients who are positive for HLA-B27.[72]

Delayed Growth and Sexual Maturation

Growth delay in children with UC may occur prior to the recognition of UC and independent of corticosteroid medications. Its presence is suggested by either reduced growth velocity (cm/yr) for age or a fall from the child's previous height channel. A growth rate of fewer than 5 cm/yr prior to sexual maturation should prompt an assessment to determine whether growth is being suppressed.[69] Interference with growth is more common in patients with CD (35% to 88%) than in those with UC (6% to 12%).[38, 40, 66] Estimating skeletal age with a radiograph of the wrist detects delayed skeletal maturation in children without prior growth records.

The cause of growth failure in children with UC is multifactorial. Fasting and provocative growth hormone levels are normal in most growth-impaired children with IBD, although most studies have described children with CD rather than UC.[23, 39, 41, 98] In children who have been investigated, chronic undernutrition, reduced levels of growth-promoting peptides [i.e., insulin-like growth factor (IGF)-1 or somatomedin C], or possibly elevation in circulating cytokines is thought to be responsible for this complication.[39, 43, 68, 99, 100]

Malabsorption

Generalized malabsorption is not a feature of UC because the small intestine is not involved in this condition. Lactose malabsorption may occur and cause gaseousness, bloating, abdominal cramps, or diarrhea. It should be suspected in patients whose ethnicity places them at risk for lactose deficiency (e.g., Jews, African Americans, and Asians) and should be addressed if it causes symptoms.[42] Protein-losing enteropathy results from leakage of proteins through the inflamed colon and can be quantified when indicated by measuring fecal α_1-antitrypsin either in random specimens or as a clearance.[29]

Nutritional Deficiency

As described earlier, reduced calorie intake has been documented in children with CD and growth failure who ingest 1764 kJ/d (420 kcal/d) less than do healthy matched controls.[100] Protein requirements may increase above that normally recommended when there is extensive enteric protein loss.[29] Iron deficiency anemia frequently is observed in children with UC, and affected patients should receive therapeutic doses of iron (5 mg/kg/d) until the anemia is corrected. Several preparations may need to be tried before a form that is tolerated by the patient is found. Patients not responding to oral supplementation may require parenteral administration. The author has used intravenous iron dextran complex in highly selected children with chronic anemia. Test doses are mandatory to identify hypersensitivity and decrease the risk of serious reactions. Zinc deficiency that may accompany excessive enteric albumin loss should be treated with oral zinc sulfate supplementation (200 mg/d) for 2 to 4 weeks.

Delayed Sexual Maturation

Pubertal development may be delayed or arrested in patients with active UC.[36, 46] Because the adolescent growth spurt is linked to pubertal stage, the interference with sexual progress is often distressing to patients with UC. The author's studies show that when menarche does occur, it does not necessarily herald the cessation of linear growth.[47]

Growth after menarche is influenced by the age of menarche in girls with IBD. Girls whose menarche began prior to 13 years of age grew an average of 10.6 cm following menarche, whereas those with menarche after age 16 years grew only 2.3 cm.

Mucocutaneous Lesions

Clusters or large oral ulcers (i.e., aphthous stomatitis) are frequently present during the initial attack or relapse of UC. Cutaneous extraintestinal signs of UC include erythema nodosum, pyoderma gangrenosum, and diffuse papulonecrotic eruptions. Resolution usually coincides with improvement of the colonic disease, although pyoderma gangrenosum may be refractory and require intensive local and systemic therapy. The association of recurrent oral ulcers and colitic symptoms with genital ulcers should alert the physician to the possibility of Behçet's syndrome.

Renal Disease

Renal caliculi develop in approximately 6% of patients as predominately uric acid in UC and oxalate in CD. Overt disease may be preceded by a period of asymptomatic microscopic hematuria. Secondary amyloidosis has been reported in pediatric patients with CD, but the author is not aware of its occurrence in UC.

Hepatobiliary Disease

Disease involving the liver and biliary tract is uncommon, occurring in as few as 4% of children with IBD.[56] The most frequently described hepatic complication, PSC, occurs almost exclusively in children with UC. Interestingly, many of reported pediatric cases have had clinical signs or laboratory features of hepatobiliary disease prior to showing intestinal signs of UC. Most cases are identified because of an elevated alkaline phosphatase or γ-glutamyltransferase noted during routine hematologic monitoring. Pruritus may not be present early during the course. Recently, the association of p-ANCA with PSC has led to the concept that it may be a marker of genetic susceptibility for this complication.[12, 91] An endoscopic retrograde cholangiogram is necessary to document PSC. Whether ursodeoxycholic acid increases bile flow sufficiently to reduce or prevent the progression of biliary narrowing is unknown; however, because of the serious implications of PSC and the relative safety of ursodeoxycholate, many pediatric gastroenterologists use this drug at a dosage of 15 to 25 mg/kg/d for children with PSC.[8a] Other causes of chronic liver disease, especially autoimmune hepatitis, should be excluded by appropriate serologic tests and liver biopsy when liver function is persistently abnormal.

Ocular Complications

Ophthalmologic complications may be a sign of IBD or IBD that is secondary to corticosteroid therapy.[36] Uveitis, iritis, and episcleritis are rare, occurring in less than 1% of affected patients. Corticosteroids increase the frequency of posterior subcapsular cataracts and raise intraocular pressure (IOP). The author investigated the role of corticosteroid therapy on the development of these complications in children with IBD[104, 105] and found that individual susceptibility to corticosteroids rather than the cumulative steroid dosage seemed to affect the frequency of lenticular opacities and IOP. Intraocular pressure of more than 20 mm Hg was seen in 22% of steroid-treated children but in none of the controls. Fortunately, lowering the prednisone to less than 10 mg/d reduced IOP to the normal range in most children. Posterior subcapsular cataracts (i.e., grade 1, which did not interfere with visual acuity) were observed in 20.7% of children; however, only 5.2% of patients had both raised IOP and cataracts, suggesting different individual susceptibility for these eye lesions. In view of these findings, ophthalmologic evaluation should be performed at 6-month intervals in children receiving long-term corticosteroid therapy.

DIAGNOSING ULCERATIVE COLITIS IN CHILDREN

For details on establishing the diagnosis of UC in children and adolescents, see Table 1.

General Considerations

Children with UC may not have experienced serious health problems prior to their diagnosis. Thus, the emotional impact of intrusive diagnostic studies, such as rectal examinations, barium radiographs, and endoscopy, may be considerable. Reassuring the child that his or her comfort is important and allowing him or her the option of the presence of a parent during examinations whenever possible help to establish trust in the physician.

Excluding Intestinal Pathogens

Probably the most important aspect of diagnosing UC is the exclusion of enteric infection. Pathogens that may mimic UC include *Salmonella*, *Shigella*, *Campylobacter*, *Aeromonas*, *Plesiomonas*, *Yersinia*, *Escherichia coli* 0157:H7, *Clostridium difficile*, and *Entamoeba histolytica*. In some cases, acute bacterial gastroenteritis may be associated with or trigger the first episode of IBD.[48, 88] Histologic features have been described that differentiate acute infectious colitis from IBD[95]; however, based on this

Table 1. ESTABLISHING THE DIAGNOSIS OF ULCERATIVE COLITIS IN CHILDREN AND ADOLESCENTS

History	Abdominal cramping
	Blood mixed with stools
Physical Examination	Anthropometrics (Ht and Wt)
	Abdominal tenderness
	Pubertal stage for age
Hematologic Tests	
CBC, Differential	Leukocytosis, bandemia
	Anemia, microcytic indices
Platelet Count	Thrombocytosis
Acute Phase Reactants	Elevated or normal
Erythrocyte Sedimentation Rate	
C-Reactive Protein; Orosomucoid	
Serum Albumin	Often reduced ($<$ 3.3 g/dL)
Serum Electrolytes	Watch for low potassium, calcium, magnesium
Stool Examinations	
Occult Blood and Leukocytes	Usually present
Stool Culture	Exclude bacterial pathogens*
Ova and Parasites	Negative
Endoscopic Evaluation	Colonoscopy with biopsies†
Radiologic Studies	Baseline abdominal film to assess colon diameter
	Upper GI/SB follow-through if diagnosis unclear
	Barium enema (double contrast)† (rarely indicated)

*Routine cultures plus tests for *Yersinia*, *Escherichia coli* H7:0157, and *Clostridium difficile*.
†Limit air insufflation by barium enema or colonoscopy in patients with severe disease to reduce the likelihood of inducing toxic megacolon.

author's experience and reports in the literature, it may not always be possible to accurately distinguish an acute infectious process from UC early in the course of disease, even with an assessment of biopsy material.[60]

Laboratory Tests

As a first stage, screening tests should include the stool examinations for enteric pathogens, occult blood and fecal leukocytes, and selected blood tests. The blood tests the author uses for screening children for UC include complete blood count (with attention to detecting a reduced mean corpuscular volume and elevated band count, with or without leukocytosis), platelet count, serum albumin, erythrocyte sedimentation rate, and C-reactive protein.[10, 35, 44] Holmquist and colleagues noted that thrombocytosis, hypoalbuminemia, and high serum orosomucoid correlate best with histologic inflammation of the colon in UC.[35] Important to note, however, is that 36% of their pediatric patients had no abnormal blood test results. Acute phase reactants (e.g., erythrocyte sedimentation rate, C-reactive protein, or orosomucoid) are more likely to be elevated in patients with CD than in those with UC.[10, 35, 44] Radiologic assessment of skeletal age is indicated in children with unexplained short stature to determine whether delayed maturation is present.

Endoscopic Evaluation

Endoscopic assessment with biopsies in most instances establishes the diagnosis of UC.[35, 44, 60, 79, 95, 106] In some cases of colitis, the endoscopic and histologic features are atypical for either UC or CD. These children are categorized as having indeterminate colitis. In addition, as alluded to earlier, early in the course of UC, the histologic features may not allow a pathologist to unequivocally assign the diagnosis of UC. Markowitz and colleagues noted that 5 of 12 children who subsequently required a colectomy for UC initially had atypical histology consisting of patchy or absent inflammation in the rectum and sigmoid.[60] Children with severe active disease should not be subjected to air insufflation with either barium enema or extensive colonoscopy to avoid precipitating toxic megacolon.

Sedation

Pediatric gastroenterologists generally use conscious sedation when performing endoscopy in children.[2, 79] The relaxation induced increases patient compliance and reduces fear for subsequent studies, thereby ensuring a more thorough examination. In the author's center, midazolam (0.1 mg/kg) and meperidine (1.0 mg/kg) are usually given intravenously as the initial sedation. Subsequent incremental doses are given as needed to a maximum cumulative midazolam dose of 0.3 mg/kg, and 2.0 mg/kg of meperidine. Adequate monitoring of transcutaneous O_2 saturation, heart rate, and blood pressure must be maintained. Intravenous fentanyl or other drugs are used in some centers. General anesthesia with tracheal intubation is reserved for those children who are unable to tolerate endoscopy or who have underlying conditions that may cause greater degrees of hypoxemia during sedation, such as cyanotic heart disease or severe pulmonary or neurologic disease.

Radiologic Studies

Since the advent of endoscopy, barium enema generally is not initially used to diagnose UC. If doubt exists as to the form of colitis (UC versus CD) after flexible sigmoidoscopy or colonoscopy, then an upper gastrointestinal radiograph with small bowel follow-through is indicated to determine whether radiologic features of CD are present. In some cases, upper gastrointestinal endoscopy is used to exclude CD in the esophagus, stomach, or duodenum.

Goals of Therapeutic Intervention

Medical intervention should address control of gastrointestinal complaints, provision of adequate nutritional intake for normal linear growth and weight gain, alleviation of extraintestinal symptoms (e.g., arthralgia and arthritis or anemia), and assessing the impact of the disease as reflected by impaired social activities and school absences. School activities (e.g., gym and bathroom privileges) may need to be modified. Emotional support should include special attention to anxiety, depression, and low self-esteem, all of which have been reported in children with active IBD.[14, 92] Discussing public figures who have achieved success despite IBD encourages patients to participate more fully in extracurricular activities.

ULCERATIVE COLITIS

Medical Management

For details on medical management of UC, see Table 2.

Mild Disease

The standard therapy for children with mildly active UC is sulfasalazine (SASP) or one of the newer 5-aminosalicylate (5-ASA; mesalamine) preparations either alone or in combination with topical enemas

Table 2. MEDICATION DOSES FOR CHILDREN WITH ULCERATIVE COLITIS

Aminosalicylates	
Oral sulfasalazine	50–75 mg/kg/d div 3–4 ×/d p.c.
Mesalamine (5' aminosalicylate)*	30–50 mg/kg/d div 2–3 ×/d p.c.
Topical mesalazine enema	2–4 g h.s.
Mesalazine suppository	0.5 g h.s.
Corticosteroids	
Prednisone	
(Initial)	1–2 mg/kg/d p.o.
(Maintenance)	Gradual taper (alt. day v discont.)
Intravenous methylprednisolone	1–1.5 mg/kg/d
Rectal hydrocortisone foam	80 mg h.s.
Hydrocortisone enema	50–100 mg 1–2 ×/d
Metronidazole *(C difficile)*	10–15 mg/kg/d div. p.c.
6-Mercaptopurine	1.0–1.5 mg/kg/d
Azathioprine	1.5–2.0 mg/kg/d
Cyclosporine†	Highly selected cases
(Initial)	2.0 mg/kg b.i.d. or cont. infusion
(Maintenance)	4–6 mg/kg po b.i.d.
Methotrexate‡	Limited data available 5–25 mg once weekly

*New 5' ASA preparations should be prescribed in children with a history of sulfa sensitivity or side effects from sulfasalazine.

†Cyclosporine blood levels, blood pressure, and renal function must be carefully monitored.

‡Blood count (including platelet count) must be checked prior to each weekly dose for the first 4 weeks, then every 2 weeks for 1 month and then every month.

(i.e., corticosteroid or mesalamine) or corticosteroid foam.[3, 8, 17, 19, 27, 67, 96, 101, 109] Adolescents often prefer the foam owing to its ease of administration and reduced sensation of rectal distention and urgency. The starting oral dose of SASP is 25 to 40 mg/kg/d and is increased to 50 to 75 mg/kg/d (maximum, 4 g/d) if needed. 5-ASA preparations may be effective in some patients with UC who are unresponsive or sensitive to SASP.[3, 19, 101] In one series, children who initially received olsalazine had a higher rate of subsequent corticosteroid use than a concurrently treated group that received SASP.[17] The side effects of SASP are well known and include headache, gastrointestinal distress (especially nausea), hypersensitivity reactions (e.g., skin eruptions or hemolytic anemia), and exacerbation of bloody diarrhea.[3, 31, 113] Additional rare complications are hepatotoxicity, neutropenia, and thrombocytopenia.[9, 26] Some children show similar reactions with mesalamine and occasional sharp rectal pain with topical preparations.[3] Desensitization to SASP may be successful in some children with selected hypersensitivity reactions.[101] Barden and colleagues compared mesalazine with SASP with regard to tolerance and side effects in children.[3] Of 45 patients who initially received SASP and were subsequently treated with mesalazine, 73% preferred mesalazine because of the ease of administration and reduced nausea and vomiting. However, six children were unable to tolerate mesalazine because of headache or abdominal pain but were successfully treated with SASP. The authors reported that both drugs were equivalent in efficacy in maintaining remission from colitis, whether due to UC or Crohn's colitis.

Limited studies in patients with UC localized to the rectosigmoid have shown beneficial results with butyrate enemas.[87] These preparations are not commercially available in the United States at this time.

Antispasmodic agents, such as loperamide or diphenoxylate with atropine, may help to diminish diarrhea and cramping in children with mild disease. Small doses of these preparations (2 mg) before school and at lunchtime may relieve anxiety due to rectal urgency or incontinence, although some pediatric gastroenterologists avoid prescribing these medications to prevent excessive use and the induction of toxic megacolon.

Moderate to Severe Disease

The presence of frequent diarrheal stools with blood, severe abdominal cramping or tenderness to palpation, fever, anemia, and hypoalbuminemia are indications for corticosteroid therapy. Intravenous methylprednisolone or hydrocortisone at a dose equivalent to 1 to 2 mg/kg/d of prednisone is recommended. Intravenous fluids and medications and some restriction of dietary intake may be necessary to decrease intestinal motility. The effectiveness of certain practices such as continuous infusion of hydrocortisone or corticotropin[61] versus bolus administration in these very sick children is unknown. High-dose pulse methylprednisolone (1 g/d for 3 days) resulted in a lower remission rate and greater likelihood of colectomy than did conventional doses of prednisolone

(64 mg/d) in one study of hospitalized patients with UC.[78] Antibiotics (e.g., an aminoglycoside and metronidazole or second-generation cephalosporin) are often administered in cases of severe UC, although their efficacy has not been established. One recent report suggests that ciprofloxacin reduces the incidence of colectomy in patients who are refractory to corticosteroid therapy.[107] Albumin infusions (1 g/kg/d) and packed red blood cells are provided for patients in whom hypoproteinemic edema or severe anemia with ongoing losses is present. Hematologic and electrolyte monitoring of potassium, calcium, and magnesium levels is essential.

Response to Intensive Medical Therapy

Expectations concerning the time to response of children with severe UC have undergone change since the description by Werlin and colleagues.[112] In that study, 14 children with severe UC and 5 children with severe colitis due to CD received an intensive regimen of intravenous corticosteroids and nutritional support. Clinical signs of improvement were noted within 12 days of medical intervention in most cases. The response in children experiencing their first attack of colitis was much better than in those who had relapsed (83% versus 31% response). The duration of response was short, with only one of the eight who responded initially doing well 24 months later.

Seashore and co-workers[89] studied the effect of parenteral nutrition and intravenous steroids in eight children with severe UC. Four became asymptomatic within 7 to 20 days, and four required surgical intervention. During the follow-up period, two of the four responders remained well and two required additional medications. The authors emphasized that they were unable to identify specific clinical or laboratory features that predicted which patients would respond to medical therapy.

Recently, Gold and colleagues reported more favorable results in 10 children with severe UC who were hospitalized with more than 2 weeks of intensive therapy.[22] During the follow-up period of 27 months, only two patients required surgery, six of ten patients were in remission, and two had active disease.

Maintenance Therapy

Corticosteroids are given on a daily basis until cramping and hematochezia subside. They then are tapered by 2.5 to 5.0 mg every 1 to 2 weeks as tolerated. Tapering of corticosteroids may rarely be followed by the development of severe headaches, signaling pseudotumor cerebri or acute ileus simulating intestinal obstruction.[93] Some pediatric gastroenterologists discontinue corticosteroids entirely, whereas others continue an alternate-day regimen. Prednisone dosages of as many as 40 to 50 mg as a single morning dose every other day may maintain disease remission while allowing normal growth.[82] Powell-Tuck and colleagues observed that alternate-day corticosteroids decrease the frequency of relapse in adult patients who experience frequent exacerbations of UC.[73]

New corticosteroid preparations (e.g., budesonide) that undergo rapid first-pass metabolism in the liver are undergoing clinical trials in patients with IBD.[25, 30, 57, 81] European studies have demonstrated their efficacy as topical preparations (enemas) in patients with distal colitis.[57] The decrease in suppression of the hypothalamic-hypopituitary-adrenal axis in comparison with conventional corticosteroids would be beneficial in reducing the risk of steroid-induced growth failure and bone demineralization in the pediatric population. These drugs are not yet available for use in the United States.

Immunosuppressive Therapy in Children

Azathioprine and 6-Mercaptopurine

Immunosuppressive drugs, such as azathioprine or 6-mercaptopurine (6-MP), suppress disease activity in approximately 70% of steroid-dependent or refractory children, thus allowing reduction or discontinuation of corticosteroids.[59, 110] The long period of time required to produce an effect generally precludes use during acute episodes of severe colitis. Drug-induced complications in pediatric patients have been low and rarely require cessation of drug therapy.[59, 110] Adequate warnings about pancreatitis and the need for regular laboratory monitoring for neutropenia, thrombocytopenia, anemia, or hepatic dysfunction are essential. The author has seen three children (two with UC and one with CD) develop acute pancreatitis within the first 2 weeks of initiating therapy, all of which cases resolved with discontinuation of the drug. The long-term malignant potential does not seem to be greater than that for the general population.[74] The recommended dosage of 6-MP is 1.0 to 1.5 mg/kg/d and 1.5 to 2.0 mg/kg/d for azathioprine. In addition, the author advises parents to notify their child's physician when fever or other signs of infectious illness develop so that appropriate cultures and antibiotic therapy are obtained.

Methotrexate

Methotrexate was recently reported to be beneficial in adult patients with UC or CD,[15, 49, 50] although the effect seems to be more consistent in patients with CD. Its role in pediatric IBD has not been described. A report of 12 children with rheumatoid arthritis who received total dosages of 0.8 to 3.0 g for 84 to 296 weeks noted no hepatotoxicity or evidence of fibrosis.[24]

Cyclosporine

Cyclosporine A has been used in selected adults and a few children with severe refractory UC.[45, 54, 77, 84, 103] Induction of remission may follow either oral[103] or parenteral administration.[45, 54, 77, 84] Improvement is evident within 7 to 10 days in the 60% to 70% of patients who enter remission. Potential side effects include hypertension, tremor, hirsutism, seizures, and potential renal insufficiency. In the author's experience, six of seven children with severe colitis improved sufficiently to be discharged from the hospital.[45] Three achieved transient endoscopic and histologic remission. During follow-up varying from 1 month to 4 years, however, all have suffered relapse or protracted steroid-dependent disease resulting in colectomy. Treem and colleagues reported using oral cyclosporine (mean 8.3 mg/kg/d) in six children with severe UC.[103] All initially improved, but four subsequently elected or required colectomy within 8 months of starting cyclosporine therapy. Thus, the long-term benefit of this expensive and intensive therapy is uncertain. Some investigators have suggested that its real role may be inducing remission in very sick patients until more standard therapies (e.g., 6-MP and azathioprine) are likely to be effective.[77] Ulcerative colitis has developed in patients receiving cyclosporine as a part of their immunosuppression following liver transplantation.[71]

Nutritional Intervention

The importance of nutritional assessment and support in children is highlighted by IBD-related growth retardation. Malabsorption is not a feature of UC and therefore does not account for the nutritional deficits found in these children. Most studies in children have included patients with CD rather than UC. Children with CD tend to reduce dietary intake below that recommended for age to diminish symptoms induced by eating.[39, 41, 100] Reversal of growth failure follows a variety of methods used to enhance caloric intake, whether by enteral or parenteral means.[1, 6, 7, 39, 41, 70, 85, 89, 90, 94] Both elemental and polymeric formulas clearly provide nutritional restitution and stimulate enhanced growth.[1, 6, 7, 41, 70, 85, 90,] Caloric recommendations, if calculated on a per-kg basis, at the onset of therapy are usually higher (70-100 kcal/kg) than for healthy children because patients have usually lost weight and require additional calories for nutritional restitution. Recommendations for protein intake in most studies have been similar to those of healthy children. For normal growth to occur, disease activity and nutritional intake must be adequate for a prolonged period of time, that is, until skeletal maturation is complete.

Infectious Agents as Triggers of Relapse

Despite medical therapy, relapse of UC occurs in the majority of patients. Often, no inciting cause is evident, but sometimes intercurrent infections trigger an exacerbation in disease activity.[18, 32, 37, 48, 88] Gryboski reported a higher-than-expected frequency of *Clostridium difficile* toxin

(16% versus 4%) during exacerbations of IBD in children,[32] but others have not substantiated this finding. Many pediatric gastroenterologists treat children with moderate to severe IBD and toxin-positive stools with vancomycin, 0.5 to 2.0 g/d for 7 to 10 days,[111] or metronidazole, 10 to 15 mg/kg/d (maximum of 1.5 g/d).[4] Clinical response usually occurs within 3 to 6 days, and elimination of toxin within 7 to 10 days.

Viral infections can precipitate disease activity in some children with IBD.[18, 37] Gebhard and colleagues prospectively measured serologic titers for selected enteric viruses (e.g., rotavirus, Norwalk agent, or adenovirus).[18] In the minority of cases in which increasing titers occurred (8 of 77 patients), the relapse was more protracted. In children with ileostomies, rotavirus infection may induce large fluid losses, resulting in hyponatremia.[28]

Respiratory infections also may trigger relapses in children with IBD.[37] A prospective evaluation of 64 children with CD and 18 with UC demonstrated that 42% of infections with influenza A and B, respiratory syncytial virus, *Mycoplasma pneumoniae*, rubella, Epstein-Barr virus, herpes simplex, and adenovirus were associated with an exacerbation of the symptoms of IBD.

Surgical Intervention

Although the emphasis of this article focuses on the medical treatment of IBD in children, an awareness that proper timing of surgery may reduce complications is essential in managing these patients. Telander recently published the primary indications for colectomy in a group of 100 children with UC.[97] The major factors leading to surgery were intractable disease (64%), refractory growth failure (14%), toxic megacolon (6%), hemorrhage (4%), perforation (3%), and cancer prophylaxis (2%).

Michener and colleagues analyzed the risk of developing colon cancer in 333 patients who developed UC during childhood and were followed for a mean of 11.8 years.[62] Nine of the 333 patients developed adenocarcinoma of the colon, with the earliest case diagnosed 11 years after the diagnosis of UC. Ekbom and colleagues noted that in patients with pancolitis, the observed risk of cancer at 35 years after diagnosis was 30% for the group as a whole, but 40% for those diagnosed prior to 15 years of age.[13] In contrast, Langholz and colleagues reported that the cumulative cancer incidence in 1161 UC patients was only 3.1% in those followed to 25 years.[52] This prevalence compares with 3.7% expected for the general Danish population. During the period of observation, 32% of the patients underwent colectomy. The authors concluded that "with an active approach to medical and surgical treatment, as practiced here, patients whose colons are left intact bear no significant increased risk of colorectal malignancy." The explanation for the lower risk for cancer than previously anticipated was proposed to be better control of disease activity through continuous (lifelong) treatment with SASP or

5'aminosalicylic acid. Others have suggested that folate supplementation may contribute to a reduced frequency of adenocarcinoma in patients with longstanding UC.[53] Based on this and other reports, surveillance colonoscopy is recommended beginning 8 years after diagnosis in children with pancolitis.

References

1. Aiges H, Markowitz J, Rosa J, et al: Home nocturnal supplemental nasogastric feedings in growth retarded adolescents with Crohn's disease. Gastroenterology 97:905, 1989
2. Ament ME, Berquist WE, Vargas J, et al: Fiberoptic upper endoscopy in infants and children. Pediatr Clin North Am 35:141, 1988
3. Barden L, Lipson A, Pert P, et al: Mesalazine in childhood inflammatory bowel disease. Aliment Pharmacol Ther 3:597, 1989
4. Bartlett JG: Treatment of clostridium difficile colitis. Gastroenterology 89:1192, 1985
5. Barton JR, Gillon S, Ferguson A: Incidence of inflammatory bowel disease in Scottish children between 1968 and 1983; marginal fall in ulcerative colitis, three-fold rise in Crohn's disease. Gut 30:618, 1989
6. Beattie RM, Schriffrin EJ, Donnet-Hughes A, et al: Polymeric nutrition as the primary therapy in children with small bowel Crohn's disease. Aliment Pharmacol Ther 8:609, 1994
7. Belli DC, Seidman E, Bouthillier L, et al: Chronic intermittent elemental diet improves growth failure in children with Crohn's disease. Gastroenterology 94:603, 1988
8. Biddle WL, Miner PB: Long-term use of mesalamine enemas to induce remission in ulcerative colitis. Gastroenterology 99:113, 1990
8a. Bousvaros A, Werlin S, Tolia V, et al: Effects of ursodeoxycholic acid on biochemical parameters in children with primary sclerosing cholangitis. J Pediatr Gastroenterol Nutr 21:325, 1995
9. Boyer DL, Ulysses B, Li K, et al: Sulfasalazine-induced hepatotoxicity in children with inflammatory bowel disease. J Pediatr Gastroenterol Nutr 8:528, 1989
10. Campbell CA, Walker-Smith JA, Hindocha P, et al: Acute phase proteins in chronic inflammatory bowel disease. J Pediatr Gastroenterol Nutr 1:193, 1982
11. Chong SKF, Blackshaw AJ, Morson BC, et al: Prospective study of colitis in infancy and early childhood. J Pediatr Gastroenterol Nutr 5:352, 1986
12. Duerr RH, Targan SR, Landers CJ, et al: Neutrophil cytoplasmic antibodies: A link between primary sclerosing cholangitis and ulcerative colitis. Gastroenterology 100:1385, 1991
13. Ekbom A, Helmick CG, Zack M, et al: Survival and causes of death in patients with inflammatory bowel disease: a population-based study. Gastroenterology 103:954, 1992
14. Engström I, Lindquist BL: Inflammatory bowel disease in children and adolescents: A somatic and psychiatric investigation. Acta Paediatr Scand 80:640, 1991
15. Feagen BG, Rochon J, Fedorak RN, et al: Methotrexate for the treatment of Crohn's disease. N Engl J Med 332:292, 1995
16. Ferguson A, Ghosh S, Choudari CP: Analysis of disease distribution, activity and complications in the patient with inflammatory bowel disease. L'Internista 2:17, 1994
17. Ferry GD, Kirschner BS, Grand RJ, et al: Olsalazine versus sulfasalazine in mild to moderate childhood ulcerative colitis: Results of the Pediatric Gastroenterology Collaborative Research Group Clinical Trial. Pediatr Gastroenterol Nutr 17:32, 1993
18. Gebhard RL, Greenberg HB, Singh N, et al: Acute viral enteritis and exacerbations of inflammatory bowel disease. Gastroenterology 83:1207, 1982
19. Giaffer MH, O'Brien CJ, Holdsworth CD: Clinical tolerance to three 5-aminosalicylic acid releasing preparations in patients with inflammatory bowel disease intolerant or allergic to sulfasalazine. Aliment Pharmacol Therap 6:51, 1992

20. Gibson GR, Whitacre EB, Ricotti CA: Colitis induced by nonsteroidal anti-inflammatory drugs. Report of four cases and review of the literature. Arch Intern Med 152:625, 1992
21. Gilat T, Hacohen D, Lilos P, et al: Childhood factors in ulcerative colitis and Crohn's disease: An international cooperative study. Scand J Gastroenterol 22:1009, 1987
22. Gold DM, Levine JJ, Pettei MJ: Prolonged medical therapy for severe ulcerative colitis. Gastroenterology 104:A708, 1993
23. Gotlin RW, Dubois RS: Nyctohemeral growth hormone levels in children with growth retardation and inflammatory bowel disease. Gut 14:191, 1973
24. Graham LD, Myones BL, Rivas-Chacon RF, et al: Morbidity associated with long-term methotrexate therapy in juvenile rheumatoid arthritis. J Pediatr 120:468, 1992
25. Greenberg GR, Feagan BG, Martin F, et al: Oral budesonide for active Crohn's disease. N Engl J Med 331:836, 1994
26. Gremse DA, Bancroft J, Moyer MS: Sulfasalazine hypersensitivity with hepatotoxicity, thrombocytopenia and erythroid hypoplasia. J Pediatr Gastroenterol Nutr 9:261, 1989
27. Griffiths A, Koletzko S, Sylvester F, et al: Slow-release 5-aminosalicylic acid therapy in children with small intestinal Crohn's disease. J Pediatr Gastroenterol Nutr 17:186, 1993
28. Grill BB, Andiman WA, Gryboski JD: Rotavirus induced electrolyte losses in a patient with ileostomy. Am J Dis Child 137:1127, 1983
29. Grill B, Hillemeier AC, Gryboski JD: Fecal α1-antitrypsin clearance in patients with inflammatory bowel disease. J Pediatr Gastroenterol Nutr 3:56, 1984
30. Gross V, Roth M, Uberschaer T, et al: Treatment of active Crohn's ileocolitis with enteric coated budesonide. Gastroenterology 106:A694, 1994
31. Gryboski JD, Spiro HM: Prognosis in children with Crohn's disease. Gastroenterology 74:807, 1978
32. Gryboski JD: Clostridium difficile in inflammatory bowel disease relapse. J Pediatr Gastroenterol Nutr 13:39, 1991
33. Gryboski JD: Ulcerative colitis in children 10 years or younger. J Pediatr Gastroenterol Nutr 17:24, 1993
34. Gryboski JD: Crohn's disease in children 10 years old and younger: Comparison with ulcerative colitis. J Pediatr Gastroenterol Nutr 18:174, 1994
35. Holmquist L, Ahren C, Fällström SP: Relationship between results of laboratory tests and inflammatory activity assessed by colonoscopy in children and adolescents with ulcerative colitis and Crohn's disease. J Pediatr Gastroenterol Nutr 9:187, 1989
36. Hyams J: Extraintestinal manifestations of inflammatory bowel disease in children. J Pediatr Gastroenterol Nutr 19:7, 1994
37. Kangro HO, Chong SKF, Hardiman A, et al: A prospective study of viral and mycoplasma infections in chronic inflammatory bowel disease. Gastroenterology 98:549, 1990
38. Kanof MD, Bayless TM: Decreased height velocity in Crohn's disease. Gastroenterology 88:1437, 1985
39. Kelts DG, Grand RJ, Shen G, et al: Nutritional basis of growth failure in children and adolescents with Crohn's disease. Gastroenterology 76:720, 1979
40. Kirschner BS, Voinchet O, Rosenberg IH: Growth retardation in children with inflammatory bowel disease. Gastroenterology 75:504, 1978
41. Kirschner BS, Klich JR, Kalman SS, et al: Reversal of growth retardation in Crohn's disease with therapy emphasizing oral nutritional restitution. Gastroenterology 80:10, 1981
42. Kirschner BS, DeFavaro MV, Jensen W: Lactose malabsorption in children and adolescents with inflammatory bowel disease. Gastroenterology 81:829, 1981
43. Kirschner BS, Sutton MM: Somatomedin-C levels in growth-impaired children and adolescents with chronic inflammatory bowel disease. Gastroenterology 91:830, 1986
44. Kirschner BS: Inflammatory bowel disease in children. Pediatr Clin North Am 35:189, 1988
45. Kirschner BS, Whitington PF, Malfeo-Klein R: Experience with cyclosporin A (CyA) in severe non-specific ulcerative colitis (ulcerative colitis). Pediatr Res 25:A117, 1989

46. Kirschner BS: Consequences for growth and development in chronic inflammatory bowel disease. Acta Paediatr Scand 366:98, 1990
47. Kirschner BS, Uebler N, Sutton MM: Growth after menarche in pediatric patients with chronic inflammatory bowel disease. Gastroenterology 104:A629, 1993
48. Kirschner BS: Does acute infection trigger chronic inflammation in pediatric patients with chronic inflammatory bowel disease? Gastroenterology 104:A725, 1993
49. Korzarek AR, Patterson DJ, Gelfand MD, et al: Methotrexate induces clinical and histologic remission in patients with refractory inflammatory bowel disease. Ann Intern Med 110:353, 1989
50. Kozarek RA: Review article: immunosuppressive therapy for inflammatory bowel disease. Aliment Pharmacol Ther 7:117, 1993
51. Kühn R, Löhler J, Rennick D, et al: Interleukin-10-deficient mice develop chronic enterocolitis. Cell 75:263, 1993
52. Langholz E, Munkholm P, Davidsen M, et al: Colorectal cancer risk and mortality in patients with ulcerative colitis. Gastroenterology 103:1444, 1992
53. Lashner BA, Heidenreich PA, Su GL, et al: Effect of folate supplementation on the incidence of dysplasia and cancer in chronic ulcerative colitis - a case control study. Gastroenterology 97:255, 1989
54. Lichtiger S, Present D, Kornbluth A, et al: Cyclosporine in severe ulcerative colitis refractory to steroid therapy. N Engl J Med 330:1841, 1994
55. Lindsey CB, Schaller JG: Arthritis associated with inflammatory bowel disease in children. J Pediatr 84:16, 1974
56. Lloyd-Still JD, Cahan J: Liver disease associated with childhood inflammatory bowel disease (IBD), abstr. Hepatology 7:1088, 1987
57. Löfberg R, Thomsen O Ostergaard, Langholz E, et al: Budesonide versus prednisolone retention enemas in active distal ulcerative colitis. Aliment Pharmacol Ther 8:623,1994
58. MacDermott RP, Nash GS, Bertovich MJ, et al: Alterations of IgM, IgG, and IgA synthesis and secretion by peripheral blood and intestinal epithelial cells in humans. Gastroenterology 81:844, 1981
59. Markowitz J, Rosa J, Grancher K, et al: Long-term 6-mercaptopurine treatment in adolescents with Crohn's disease. Gastroenterology 99:1347, 1990
60. Markowitz J, Kahn E, Grancher K, et al: Atypical rectosigmoid histology in children with newly diagnosed ulcerative colitis. Am J Gastroenterol 88:2034, 1993
61. Meyers S, Sachar DB, Goldberg JD, et al: Corticotropin versus hydrocortisone in the intravenous treatment of ulcerative colitis: A prospective, randomized, double-blind clinical trial. Gastroenterology 85:351, 1983
62. Michener WM, Farmer RG, Mortimer EA: Long-term prognosis of ulcerative colitis with onset in childhood or adolescence. J Clin Gastroenterol 1:301, 1979
63. Michener WM, Whelan G, Greenstreet RL, et al: Comparison of the clinical features of Crohn's disease and ulcerative colitis with onset in childhood or adolescence. Cleveland Clin Quart 49:13, 1982
64. Mir-Madjlessi SH, Michener WM, Farmer RG: Course and prognosis of idiopathic ulcerative proctosigmoiditis in young patients. J Pediatr Gastroenterol Nutr 5:570, 1986
65. Mombaerts P, Mizoguchi E, Grusby MJ, et al: Spontaneous development of inflammatory bowel disease in T cell receptor mutant mice. Cell 75:275, 1993
66. Motil KJ, Grand RJ, Davis-Kraft L, et al: Growth failure in children with inflammatory bowel disease: A prospective study. Gastroenterology 105:681, 1993
67. Mulder CJJ, Tygat GNJ, Wiltink EHH, et al: Comparison of 5-aminosalicylic acid (3 g) and prednisolone phosphate enemas (30 mg) in the treatment of distal ulcerative colitis: A prospective, randomized, double-blind trial. Scand J Gastroenterol 23:1005:1988
68. Murch SH, Lamkin VA, Savage MO, et al: Serum concentrations of tumour necrosis factor in childhood chronic inflammatory bowel disease. Gut 32:913, 1991
69. National Center for Health Statistics Percentiles. National Center for Health Statistics (NCHS), Hyattsville, Maryland, 1980
70. Navarro J, Vargas J, Cesard JP, et al: Prolonged constant rate elemental enteral nutrition in Crohn's disease. J Pediatr Gastroenterol Nutr 1:541, 1982

71. Passfall J, Distler A, Riecken EO, et al: Development of ulcerative colitis under the immunosuppressive effect of cyclosporine. Clin Invest 70:611, 1992
72. Passo MH, Fitzgerald JF, Brandt KD: Arthritis associated with inflammatory bowel disease in children: Relationship of joint disease to activity and severity of bowel lesion. Dig Dis Sci 31:492, 1986
73. Powell-Tuck J, Brown RL, Chambers TG, et al: A controlled trial of alternate day prednisolone as a maintenance treatment for ulcerative colitis. Digestion 22:263, 1981
74. Present DM, Meltzer SJ, Krumholz MP, et al: 6-Mercaptopurine in the management of inflammatory bowel disease: Short and long-term toxicity. Ann Int Med 111:641, 1989
75. Probert CSJ, Jayanthi V, Hughes AO, et al: Prevalence and family risk of ulcerative colitis and Crohn's disease: An epidemiological study among Europeans and South Asians in Leicestershire. Gut 34:1547, 1993
76. Proujousky R, Fawcett PT, Gibney KM, et al: Examination of anti-neutrophil cyto-plasmic antibodies in childhood inflammatory bowel disease. J Pediatr Gastroenterol Nutr 17:193, 1993
77. Ramakrishna J, Langhans N, Calenda K, et al: Combined use of cyclosporine A (CSA) and azathioprine (AZA) in pediatric inflammatory bowel disease (IBD). Gastroenterology 106:A23, 1994
78. Rosenberg W, Ireland A, Jewell DP: High-dose methylprednisolone in the treatment of active ulcerative colitis. J Clin Gastroenterol 12:40, 1990
79. Rossi T: Endoscopic examination of the colon in infants and children. Pediatr Clin North Am 35:331, 1988
80. Roth M-P, Petersen GM, McElree C, et al: Geographic origins of Jewish patients with inflammatory bowel disease. Gastroenterology 97:900, 1989
81. Rutgeerts P, Löfberg R, Malchow H, et al: A comparison of budesonide with prednisolone for active Crohn's disease. N Engl J Med 331:842, 1994
82. Sadeghi-Nejad A, Senior B: The treatment of ulcerative colitis in children with alternate-day corticosteroids. Pediatrics 43:840, 1968
83. Sadlack B, Merz H, Schorle H, et al: Ulcerative colitis-like disease in mice with a disrupted interleukin-2 gene. Cell 75:253, 1993
84. Sandborn WJ, Goldman DH, Lawson GM, et al: Measurement of colonic tissue cyclosporine concentration in children with severe ulcerative colitis. J Pediatr Gastroenterol Nutr 15:125, 1992
85. Sanderson IR, Udeen S, Davies PSW, et al: Remission induced by an elemental diet in small bowel Crohn's disease. Arch Dis Child 61:123, 1987
86. Sartor RB: Cytokines in intestinal inflammation: Pathophysiological and clinical considerations. Gastroenterology 106:533, 1994
87. Scheppach W, Sommer H, Kirchner T, et al: Effect of butyrate enemas on the colonic mucosa in distal ulcerative colitis. Gastroenterology 103:51,1992
88. Schumacher G, Kollberg B, Sandstedt B, et al: A prospective study of first attacks of inflammatory bowel disease and non-relapsing colitis - Microscopic findings. Scand J Gastroenterol 28:1077, 1993
89. Seashore JH, Hillemeier AC, Gryboski JD: Total parenteral nutrition in the management of inflammatory bowel disease in children: A limited role. Am J Surg 143:504, 1982
90. Seidman EG, Bouthillier L, Weber AM, et al: Elemental diet versus prednisone as primary treatment of Crohn's disease. Gastroenterology 90:A1625, 1986
91. Seibold F, Slametschka D, Gegor M, et al: Neutrophil autoantibodies: A genetic marker in primary sclerosing cholangitis and ulcerative colitis. Gastroenterology 107:532, 1994
92. Steinhausen H-C, Kies H: Comparative studies of ulcerative colitis and Crohn's disease in children and adolescents. J Child Psych 23:33, 1982
93. Stelzer M, Phillips D, Fonkalsrud EW: Acute ileus from steroid withdrawal simulating intestinal obstruction after surgery for ulcerative colitis. Arch Surg 125:914, 1990
94. Strobel CT, Byrne WJ, Ament ME: Home parenteral nutrition in children with Crohn's disease: An effective management alternative. Gastroenterology 77:272, 1979
95. Surawicz CM, Haggitt RC, Husseman M, et al: Mucosal biopsy diagnosis of colitis:

Acute self-limited colitis and idiopathic inflammatory bowel disease. Gastroenterology 107:755, 1994
96. Sutherland LR, Martin F, Greer S, et al: 5-Aminosalicylic acid enema in the treatment of distal ulcerative colitis, proctosigmoiditis and proctitis. Gastroenterology 92:1894, 1987
97. Telander RL: Surgical management of inflammatory bowel disease in children: In Telander R (ed): Problems in General Surgery: Surgical Treatment of Inflammatory Bowel Disease. Philadelphia, JB Lippincott, 1993
98. Tenore A, Berman WF, Parks JS, et al: Basal and stimulated growth hormone concentrations in inflammatory bowel disease. J Clin Endocrinol Metab 44:622, 1977
99. Thomas AG, Holly JM, Taylor F, et al: Insulin like growth factor-I, insulin like growth factor binding protein-I, and insulin in childhood Crohn's disease. Gut 34:944, 1993
100. Thomas AG, Taylor F, Miller V: Dietary intake and nutritional treatment in childhood Crohn's disease. J Pediatr Gastroenterol Nutr 17:75, 1993
101. Tolia V: Sulfasalazine desensitization in children and adolescents with chronic inflammatory bowel disease. Am J Gastroenterol 87:1029, 1992
102. Toyoda H, Wang S-J, Yang H-Y, et al: Distinct associations of the HLA class II genes with inflammatory bowel disease. Gastroenterology 104:741, 1993
103. Treem WR, Davis PM, Hyams JS: Cyclosporine treatment of severe ulcerative colitis in children. J Pediatr 119:994, 1991
104. Tripathi RC, Kirschner BS, Kipp MA, et al: Corticosteroid treatment for inflammatory bowel disease in pediatric patients increases intraocular pressure. Gastroenterology 102:1957, 1992
105. Tripathi RC, Kipp MA, Tripathi BJ, et al: Ocular toxicity of prednisone in pediatric patients with inflammatory bowel disease. Lens and Eye Toxicity Research 9:469, 1992
106. Truelove SC, Witts LS: Cortisone in ulcerative colitis: Final report on a therapeutic trial. Br Med J i:387, 1959
107. Turunen U, Färkkilä M, Vouristo M, et al: A double-blind controlled six-month ciprofloxacin treatment improves prognosis in ulcerative colitis. [Abstract] Gastroenterology 106:A786, 1994
108. Tysk C, Lindberg E, Jänerot G, et al: Ulcerative colitis and Crohn's disease in an unselected population of monozygotic and dizygotic twins. A study of the heritability and the influence of smoking. Gut 29:990, 1988
109. Van Hees PAM, van Lier HJJ, van Elteren PH, et al: Effect of sulfasalazine in patients with active Crohn's disease: A controlled double-blind study. Gut 22:404, 1981
110. Verhave M, Winter HS, Grand RJ: Azathioprine in the treatment of children with inflammatory bowel disease. J Pediatr 117:809, 1990
111. Viscidi RP, Bartlett JG: Antibiotic-associated pseudomembranous colitis in children. Pediatrics 17:381, 1981
112. Werlin SL, Grand RJ: Severe colitis in children and adolescents: Diagnosis, course, and treatment. Gastroenterology 73:828, 1977
113. Werlin SL, Grand RJ: Bloody diarrhea - a new complication of sulfasalazine. J Pediatr 92:450, 1978
114. Winter HS, Landers CJ, Winkelstein A, et al: Anti-neutrophil cytoplasmic antibodies in children with ulcerative colitis. J Pediatr 125:707, 1994
115. Yang H, Rotter JI, Toyota H, et al: Ulcerative colitis: A genetically heterogeneous disorder defined by genetic (HLA class II) and subclinical (antineutrophil cytoplasmic antibodies) markers. J Clin Invest 92:1080, 1993

Address reprint requests to:

Barbara S. Kirschner, MD
Wyler Children's Hospital
5825 South Maryland Avenue, MC-4065
Chicago, IL 60637

0031–3955/96 $0.00 + .20

CROHN'S DISEASE IN CHILDREN

Jeffrey S. Hyams, MD

Only a little more than 60 years ago, the first comprehensive review of the clinical and pathologic manifestations of Crohn's disease involving the small bowel was written.[9] Twenty-five years ago, it was recognized that Crohn's disease unequivocally affects the colon. During the past 20 years, clinicians have come to recognize the protean manifestations of this illness, with its inconsistent response to medical therapy and a strong tendency to recur despite removal of all obvious disease at the time of surgery. This article briefly reviews the current understanding of the epidemiology, pathogenesis, and pathology of Crohn's disease, and then focuses on its clinical manifestations, diagnosis, treatment, and long-term prognosis.

EPIDEMIOLOGY

Data regarding the frequency with which Crohn's disease affects children of different geographic regions are limited. The peak frequency of new cases in the pediatric population seems to occur in the mid- to late teens, with an age-specific incidence of approximately 16 per 100,000 persons.[26, 44] Some investigators have suggested that the incidence of Crohn's disease in the adult populations in the Western hemisphere increased from 1950 through 1980, with a decrease in the past 10 years. Anecdotal evidence suggests similar trends in children. In the mid-1980s, the prevalence of Crohn's disease in British and Scottish children ranged from 9.5 to 11.0 per 100,000 persons fewer than 18 years of age.[14]

Males and females are equally affected, and whites are more com-

From the Department of Pediatrics, University of Connecticut School of Medicine; and the Division of Digestive Diseases, Connecticut Children's Medical Center, Hartford, Connecticut

monly affected than non-whites. Crohn's disease seems to be more common in Jews than non-Jews, and in the Jewish population, the disease is more common in families of middle European origin relative to those of Polish or Russian origin. In the United States, Crohn's disease is more frequent in northern compared with southern areas and urban compared with rural areas.[58]

PATHOGENESIS

The etiology of Crohn's disease, like that of ulcerative colitis, remains unknown. Whether these two disorders are different manifestations of a single disease process, or whether they represent two entirely different diseases with similar clinical manifestations is unknown also.

Since Crohn's disease seems to be far more common in first-degree relatives of affected individuals than in the general population, some investigators have suggested that a genetic predisposition may exist for this disorder. The risk of developing Crohn's disease approaches 50% in the twin sibling of a monozygotic twin compared with 3% for a dizygotic twin.[57] At the time of diagnosis, the likelihood of finding inflammatory bowel disease in a first-degree relative of a proband is 5% to 25%.[5] Siblings of individuals with Crohn's disease are 17 to 35 times more likely to develop the disease than those in the general population.

Crohn's disease occurs with a higher frequency in patients with Turner's syndrome, Hermansky-Pudlak syndrome, and glycogen storage disease type Ib. HLA studies have generally been nonrevealing, but an association with HLA-DR4 has been suggested.[57]

Infectious etiologies have also been entertained, although no convincing and reproducible evidence to date has identified a specific pathogen. Some investigators have suggested that atypical mycobacteria might be important because the pathologic expression of mycobacterial intestinal infection may be similar to that observed in patients with Crohn's disease. An intriguing report from France of the clustering of Crohn's disease in two families was believed to suggest the possibility of an infectious process.[63]

Most recent efforts have focused on proposed abnormalities in the intestinal mucosal immune system and dysregulation of intestinal inflammation.[55] As seen schematically in Figure 1, an antigenic stimulus, either of microbial or dietary origin, stimulates the normally rich immune system of the intestinal mucosa. Mucosal inflammation occurs in a controlled and protective fashion ("physiologic inflammation"), and in a normal host the inflammation is self-limited. In a genetically predisposed host, or in someone with previous mucosal injury, the inflammatory cascade is not self-limited, and the continued production of inflammatory mediators by activated immune cells leads to tissue injury and fibrosis.

This cascade of events suggests that a particular target cell may not be involved in tissue injury in Crohn's disease. Rather, tissue destruction

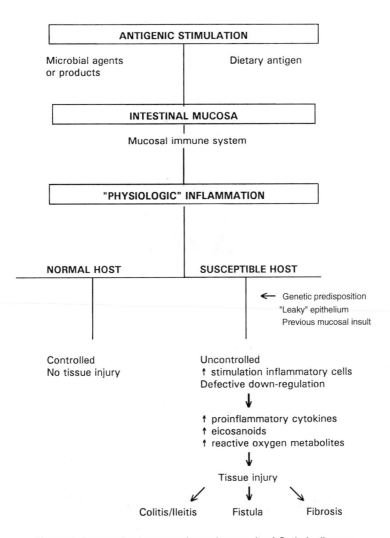

Figure 1. Proposed schema on the pathogenesis of Crohn's disease.

might occur in an "innocent bystander" fashion.[56] Bacterial products, such as endotoxin (lipopolysaccharide), peptidoglycan polysaccharide, and N-formyl-methionyl-leucyl-phenylalanine (FMLP), are potent activators of inflammatory cells.[13] Recent data have shown that diversion of the fecal stream at the time of ileal resection greatly decreases the likelihood of recurrent disease in the "neoterminal" ileum, which suggests that stimulation by the fecal stream is crucial to the pathogenesis of recurrent disease at the anastomotic site.[51]

Inflamed intestinal tissue contains markedly increased concentrations of proinflammatory cytokines such as interleukin (IL)-1, IL-6, and IL-8. These cytokines have multiple local effects, including the recruitment of inflammatory cells through the increased expression of vascular adhesion cell molecules, increased neutrophil eicosanoid production, eosinophil degranulation, induction of nitric oxide synthase in macrophages and neutrophils, and increased collagen production.[12] IL-1 and IL-6 are potent stimuli of hepatic production of acute phase reactants. Reactive oxygen metabolites produced by neutrophils participating in the local inflammatory response are potent cytotoxins and cause cell injury or death.[65] Products of inflammatory cells such as histamine, prostaglandins, and leukotrienes cause chloride secretion by epithelial cells contributing to diarrhea.[43]

Stimulated mononuclear cells that produce the potent proinflammatory cytokine, IL-1, also produce IL-1 receptor antagonist (IL-1ra) that blocks the effect of IL-1 on target cells.[11] Preliminary observations have suggested that the normal excess of IL-1ra to IL-1 in intestinal mucosa is diminished in active intestinal inflammation.[29] Whether this finding is of primary importance to the pathogenesis of Crohn's disease is not known. Additional immunoregulatory cytokines, such as IL-4 and IL-10, also may control the inflammatory response.

PATHOLOGY

The initial pathologic event in Crohn's disease seems to be localized ulceration over a lymphoid follicle (aphthous lesion). As the disease progresses, mucosal ulcers may coalesce to form broader linear ulcer beds. Mucosal inflammation extends into the deeper tissue layers with significant infiltration of lymphocytes, histiocytes, and plasma cells. Marked submucosal inflammation may occur with edema, lymphatic dilatation, and collagen deposition. Crypt abscesses and goblet-cell depletion may occur but are usually less prominent than in ulcerative colitis. Characteristically, there is segmental involvement of the bowel with varying degrees of microscopic involvement. Granuloma need not be present to establish a diagnosis of Crohn's disease, although they may be found in approximately 50% of resection specimens.

Over time, the bowel wall becomes thickened secondary to edema, chronic inflammation, and fibrosis. The degree of wall thickening may be severe enough that the lumenal diameter is sufficiently compromised to cause obstruction. "Skip" areas are common with more or less extensively involved areas. Loops of adjacent bowel may become matted together owing to serosal and mesenteric inflammation. Fistulas arise when transmural bowel inflammation extends through the serosa into adjacent structures such as contiguous bowel, bladder, vagina, or perineum. With bowel, mesentery, and lymph node involvement an inflammatory mass or phlegmon may develop. This may progress into a chronic active abscess cavity.

Three general patterns of gross bowel involvement are common in Crohn's disease in children.[24] Approximately 50% to 60% of affected individuals have involvement of the terminal ileum and variable segments of the colon, most commonly the ascending colon. Approximately 30% to 35% have small bowel involvement only, most of whom have disease in the terminal ileum. Approximately 10% to 15% of children have disease limited to the large bowel. Gastroduodenal disease as documented by mucosal biopsy is present in more than one third of all patients.[37] Although these patterns of gross bowel involvement are used for disease classification, it is important to appreciate that Crohn's disease may involve any portion of the alimentary system, and biopsy of macroscopically uninvolved areas frequently reveals evidence of microscopic inflammation.

PATHOPHYSIOLOGY OF GASTROINTESTINAL SYMPTOMS

Active mucosal inflammation in the small and large bowel initiates a series of events that lead to diarrhea, gastrointestinal bleeding, and abdominal pain. Inflamed mucosa secretes increased quantities of electrolytes and water and concomitantly is impaired in its ability to absorb these substances. Inflammatory mediators, such as prostaglandins and leukotrienes, alter bowel permeability and electrolyte transport. Malabsorbed fatty acids entering the colon impair electrolyte and water absorption. Abnormal terminal ileal function may result in bile acid loss, with an eventual decrease in lumenal bile acid concentration leading to steatorrhea. Bile salts also may impair colonic absorption of electrolytes. Bacterial overgrowth in the small bowel from obstruction or enteroenteric fistula may lead to mucosal damage, bile salt deconjugation, and further worsening of diarrhea.

Diffuse mucosal disease leads to exudation of serum proteins, resulting in protein-losing enteropathy. More extensive mucosal disease leads to mild blood loss, and ulceration penetrating into deeper bowel layers may affect larger blood vessels potentially resulting in massive hemorrhage. Abdominal pain usually ensues from either gut distention associated with obstruction, or inflammation of the serosa resulting from transmural inflammation.

CLINICAL FEATURES

While gastrointestinal symptoms are usually present at diagnosis, extraintestinal manifestations may be observed in 25% to 35% of patients and may represent the initial manifestation for some subjects (Table 1).[27] A prolonged interval (> 6 months) commonly exists between onset of symptoms and diagnosis in children with Crohn's disease.

Table 1. PRESENTING CLINICAL FEATURES OF CHILDREN WITH CROHN'S DISEASE

Feature	Percentage
Abdominal pain	75
Diarrhea	65
Weight loss	65
Growth retardation	25
Nausea/vomiting	25
Rectal bleeding	20
Perirectal disease	15
Extraintestinal manifestations	25

Data compiled from refs. 3, 7, 24, 48, and 50.
From Hyams JS: Crohn's disease. *In* Wyllie R, Hyams JS (eds): Pediatric Gastrointestinal Disease. Pathophysiology, Diagnosis, Management. Philadelphia, WB Saunders, 1993, p 746.

Gastrointestinal Symptoms

Abdominal pain and diarrhea are present in the majority of affected children.[3, 7, 24, 48, 50] The pain is commonly in the right lower quadrant and may be associated with tenderness on palpation together with a fullness or mass. Periumbilical or left-sided pain may also be observed. In the presence of esophageal or gastroduodenal involvement, epigastric discomfort, often of a "dyspeptic" nature, may be noted.[21] Frequently, the abdominal pain associated with Crohn's disease is severe and may wake the child from sleep.

Diarrhea may be variable in severity, ranging from one or two loose stools daily to marked diarrhea (> 6 stools/day), occurring both at night and during the day. Gross blood in the stool is more common with colonic than small bowel involvement, although deep small bowel ulceration may precipitate severe hemorrhage. Anorexia, nausea, and vomiting are common. Perirectal disease (e.g., fistulae, fissures, and tags) are observed in approximately 15% to 30% of patients.[39]

Extraintestinal Symptoms

Systemic manifestations, such as fever, fatigue, and weight loss, are noted in a majority of patients. A listing of the extraintestinal manifestations of inflammatory bowel disease is shown in Table 2. The most common target organs are the skin, joints, liver, eye, and bone.[27]

Erythema nodosum is more common in Crohn's disease than ulcerative colitis and usually reflects active bowel inflammation. In approximately 75% of patients in whom erythema nodosum develops, arthritis also develops. Pyoderma gangrenosum is rare in patients with Crohn's disease.

Two forms of joint involvement may be observed, including a peripheral form called *enteropathic synovitis* or *colitic arthritis*, and an

Table 2. EXTRAINTESTINAL MANIFESTATIONS OF INFLAMMATORY BOWEL DISEASE

Skin	**Joints**	**Cardiac**
Erythema nodosum	Arthralgia	Myocarditis
Pyoderma	Arthritis	Pericarditis
gangrenosum	Ankylosing spondylitis	**Musculoskeletal**
Perianal disease	Sacroiliitis	Granulomatous myositis
Erythema multiforme	Granulomatous	Dermatomyositis
Cutaneous vasculitis	synovitis	Vasculitic myositis
Polyarteritis nodosa	Hypertrophic	Steroid-induced
Metastatic cutaneous	osteoarthropathy	myopathy
Crohn's disease	**Eye**	**Extraintestinal cancer**
Crohn's disease of the	Uveitis	Acute myelocytic
vulva	Episcleritis	leukemia
Pellagra	Scleritis	Lymphoma
Psoriasis	Corneal ulcers	Myelodysplastic
Epidermolysis bullosa	Blepharitis	syndromes
acquisita	Conjunctivitis	**Neurologic**
Pyoderma vegetans	Keratitis	Peripheral neuropathy
Vesiculopustular	Serous retinal	Perineuritis
eruption	detachment	Spinal epidural
Hermansky-Pudlak	Choroidal infiltrates	abscesses
syndrome with	Retrobulbar neuritis	Seizures
albinism	Cataract	Stroke
Alopecia	Orbital myositis	**Growth**
Acrodermatitis	Orbital pseudotumor	Delayed growth
enteropathica	Increased intraocular	Delayed puberty
Scrotal cellulitis	pressure	**Hematologic**
Acne	**Vascular**	Iron deficiency anemia
Mouth	Thrombophlebitis	Folate deficiency
Aphthous stomatitis	Vasculitis	Vitamin B_{12} deficiency
Glossitis	Polyarteritis nodosa	Autoimmune hemolytic
Cheilitis	Takayasu's arteritis	anemia
Pyostomatitis vegetans	Portal vein thrombosis	Anemia of chronic
Granulomatous tonsillitis	Budd-Chiari syndrome	disease
Liver/biliary tract	Pulmonary vasculitis	Heinz body anemia
Fatty infiltration	Giant cell arteritis	Neutropenia
Sclerosing cholangitis/	CNS thromboembolism	Thrombocytosis
pericholangitis	**Pancreas**	Thrombocytopenia
Chronic hepatitis	Pancreatitis	**Renal/urologic**
Cirrhosis	Acute	Nephrolithiasis
Granulomatous hepatitis	Chronic	Obstructive
Cholelithiasis	Pancreatic insufficiency	hydronephrosis
Hepatic abscess	**Pulmonary**	Enterovesical fistula
Budd-Chiari syndrome	Pulmonary vasculitis	Urinary tract infection
Acalculous cholecystitis	Fibrosing alveolitis	Immune complex
Biliary tract carcinoma	Eosinophilic pneumonia	glomerulonephritis
Amyloidosis	Pneumomediastinum	Perinephric abscess
Portal vein thrombosis		Amyloidosis
Bone		Hypertension
Osteopenia		
Osteonecrosis		
Osteoporosis		
Osteomalacia		

From Hyams JS: Extraintestinal manifestations of inflammatory bowel disease. J Pediatr Gastroenterol Nutr 19:8, 1994; with permission.

axial form, including ankylosing spondylitis or sacroiliitis. The knees, ankles, and hips are the more commonly involved peripheral joints. Because 50% of patients with inflammatory bowel disease in whom arthritis develops also develop ocular inflammation, routine ophthalmologic evaluation is warranted. Hypertrophic osteoarthropathy or clubbing is noted in as many as 30% of patients.

Abnormal serum aminotransferases are noted in approximately 15% of children with inflammatory bowel disease during their course.[31] Transient elevations are frequently associated with disease flares; medications such as 6-mercaptopurine or sulfasalazine; parenteral hyperalimentation; and hepatic steatosis from corticosteroids, malnutrition, or massive weight gain. Two more serious chronic conditions that may arise include chronic active hepatitis and sclerosing cholangitis. These complications develop in less than 1% of all children with Crohn's disease but may result in cirrhosis of the liver and liver failure.

Ocular complications frequently are observed in the setting of other extraintestinal manifestations. Patients with colonic involvement are more likely than those with small bowel disease to develop uveitis, scleritis, or episcleritis. The chronic administration of high-dose daily corticosteroids may be complicated by the development of increased intraocular pressure and cataracts.

Diminished bone density has been reported in patients with Crohn's disease at diagnosis[16] and during the disease course.[8] Factors that might be operative include poor diet with protein-calorie deprivation, inadequate calcium intake or malabsorption, vitamin D deficiency, excessive cytokine production by inflamed bowel that interferes with bone metabolism, and corticosteroid inhibition of calcium absorption and direct inhibition of bone formation. Accelerated bone mineral loss may occur with prolonged bed rest and corticosteroid-induced hypercalciuria.

Additional extraintestinal complications of note include right-sided hydronephrosis in the setting of ileocolic inflammation when an inflammatory mass encases the right ureter, hypercoagulability with venous thrombosis, pancreatitis, autoimmune anemia, and vasculitis.[27]

Growth Abnormalities and Nutritional Deficiencies

In 20% of children with Crohn's disease, a decrease in growth velocity may precede overt gastrointestinal symptoms by months or years.[34] Absolute height deficits are observed in as many as 40% of children,[19] with almost 50% of patients having weight-for-age measurements less than 90% of those expected.[42] Factors that have been proposed to contribute to poor growth in these children include chronic malnutrition, corticosteroid administration, and a still poorly defined growth-retarding effect of chronic inflammation (Table 3). Malnutrition occurs because of suboptimal dietary intake, increased gastrointestinal losses, and malabsorption. Although most studies have not shown increased basal caloric requirements in patients with Crohn's disease, factors such

Table 3. CONTRIBUTING FACTORS TO GROWTH ABNORMALITIES IN CHILDREN WITH CROHN'S DISEASE

Factor	Reason
1. Suboptimal intake	Fear of worsening GI symptoms, anorexia, delayed gastric emptying
2. Stool losses	Mucosal damage or resection leading to protein-losing enteropathy, steatorrhea
3. Increased nutritional needs	Fever, chronic deficits
4. Corticosteroid therapy	Inhibition of bone formation, increased calcium losses
5. Disease activity	Possible role of circulating inflammatory cytokines in inhibiting bone metabolism

as fever may increase caloric demands. Anorexia is very common and is not always secondary to fear of precipitating gastrointestinal symptoms. A central appetite-reducing effect of circulating proinflammatory cytokines has been suggested but not proven. Delayed gastric emptying in some children may lead to early satiety.[23]

Growth hormone levels have been found to be normal in children with growth delay secondary to Crohn's disease.[59] Serum insulin-like growth factor-1 (IGF-1) levels are low in most patients with growth abnormalities and likely reflect a poor nutritional state.[35, 60] IGF-binding protein 1 (IGF-BP 1) serum levels are similar in growth-retarded and normally growing children with Crohn's disease.[60]

Daily corticosteroid therapy may inhibit growth at several levels.[28] Corticosteroids may inhibit the biologic activity of IGF-1, inhibit several steps in collagen synthesis, and promote negative calcium balance by decreasing intestinal absorption and increasing urinary loss. Alternate-day corticosteroid therapy, however, does not seem to inhibit growth.[32] Serum levels of the C-terminal propeptide of type I collagen and the N-terminal propeptide of type III collagen are significantly lower in children with slow growth velocity who are on daily corticosteroids, regardless of disease activity.[33] However, it is often difficult to separate the relative contributions of disease activity from corticosteroid usage in the pathogenesis of slow linear growth.[22, 33, 42] It should be emphasized that the eradication of gastrointestinal symptoms by high-dose daily corticosteroid therapy with the concomitant compromise of growth is not considered successful medical management.

DIAGNOSIS

The diagnosis of Crohn's disease is tentatively established by obtaining a detailed history and performing a thorough physical examination (Table 4). Laboratory tests are then used to confirm the diagnosis

Table 4. ESTABLISHING A DIAGNOSIS OF CROHN'S DISEASE

I. History	IV. Contrast radiography
Abdominal pain	Skip areas
Diarrhea	Ileal string sign
Fever	Fistula
Rectal bleeding	Nodularity
Arthritis	Ulceration
Rash	**V. Endoscopy**
(+) Family hx IBD	Patchy inflammation
II. Physical examination	Aphthous lesions
Abdominal tenderness	Cobblestoning
Right lower quadrant mass	Linear ulcers
Clubbing	Rectal sparing
Perirectal disease	
Stomatitis	
Erythema nodosum	
Growth percentiles	
III. Laboratory evaluation	
Anemia	
Elevated ESR	
Hypoalbuminemia	
Thrombocytosis	
(+) Stool guaiac	

Adapted from Hyams JS: Crohn's disease. *In* Wyllie R, Hyams JS (eds): Pediatric Gastrointestinal Disease: Pathophysiology, Diagnosis, Management. Philadelphia, WB Saunders, 1993, p 751.

and establish the severity of complications such as anemia and nutritional deficiencies.

Physical Examination

Abdominal tenderness is found in the majority of children with Crohn's disease. If the terminal ileum and cecum are involved, a fullness in the right lower quadrant or a mass may be present and usually represents a phlegmon. Frank peritoneal signs are unusual. Careful inspection of the perirectal area and a digital rectal examination with stool guaiac are mandatory. The presence of stomatitis, clubbing, arthritis, or erythema nodosum supports a diagnosis of inflammatory bowel disease. Height and weight values should be carefully obtained and compared with previous values to calculate growth velocity.

Laboratory Evaluation

A "screening" complete blood count, erythrocyte sedimentation rate, and biochemical profile often are performed in the evaluation of children with chronic gastrointestinal symptoms to establish supporting data for a diagnosis of inflammatory bowel disease. Anemia (70% of cases), elevated erythrocyte sedimentation rate (80%), hypoalbuminemia (60%), and thrombocytosis (60%) are the most frequent abnormalities noted in patients with Crohn's disease.[61] Normal laboratory results do not exclude a diagnosis of Crohn's disease.

Although anemia is most frequently secondary to iron deficiency, other potential causes include folic acid deficiency, vitamin B_{12} deficiency, malnutrition, and rarely autoimmune hemolysis. The anemia of chronic disease characterized by a decreased serum iron and iron-binding capacity, a decreased percentage saturation of serum iron-binding capacity, normal or increased serum ferritin, and increased bone marrow storage–iron also may be observed. Proinflammatory cytokines, such as IL-1, interferon-gamma, and tumor necrosis factor-α, which are produced in large quantities by inflamed bowel, may circulate and inhibit erythropoiesis by progenitor erythroid cells, inhibit erythropoietin production, and impair iron metabolism.[41]

In malnourished patients, measurement of serum calcium, phosphorus, magnesium, and zinc may be helpful. Serum aminotransferases should be determined. Breath hydrogen testing for carbohydrate malabsorption may be useful in guiding subsequent dietary management. Urinalysis should be performed to exclude pyuria or infection associated with enterovesical fistula.

Radiographic Evaluation

Radiographic studies are used to confirm a diagnosis of Crohn's disease, evaluate the distribution of bowel involvement, and aid in distinguishing Crohn's disease from ulcerative colitis. Barium enema is used less frequently than colonoscopy to evaluate colonic disease.

Because small bowel involvement is observed in more than 80% of cases, upper gastrointestinal series with small bowel follow-through is mandatory. Careful fluoroscopy and abdominal palpation are used to reveal irregular, nodular (cobblestoned), and thickened bowel loops and stenotic areas (string sign), deep ulcers, and fistulas (Fig. 2). Terminal ileal nodularity is common in Crohn's disease and may be difficult to distinguish from nodular lymphoid hyperplasia (NLH), although in NLH the nodules are usually 3 mm or less in diameter.

When a tender mass is present in the right lower quadrant, it is important to differentiate bowel phlegmon from abscess. Ultrasound examination may reveal bowel wall thickening and extraluminal fluid, suggesting abscess. Computed tomography may be more helpful in revealing relationships between adjacent organs and loops of bowel particularly, regarding fistulization to the bladder and vagina. Radioisotope studies are limited by the large dose of radiation involved.

Endoscopic and Histologic Evaluation

Endoscopy and mucosal biopsy have become indispensable tools in the diagnosis and monitoring of inflammatory bowel disease. In many

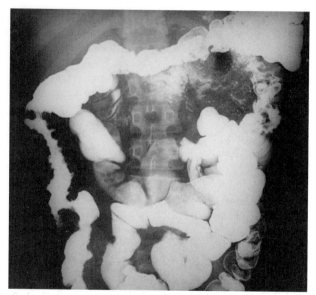

Figure 2. Radiographic findings in Crohn's disease involving the terminal ileum and ascending colon.

cases, direct visualization of the colon frequently allows differentiation of Crohn's disease from ulcerative colitis in children who present with bloody diarrhea in the presence of negative cultures for enteric pathogens. Colonoscopy is more sensitive than radiographic studies for detecting mild mucosal disease and provides the opportunity to obtain tissue for histologic examination.

Although the endoscopic appearances of ulcerative colitis and Crohn's disease occasionally are similar, certain features of Crohn's disease are distinctive. Rectal sparing is rare in patients with ulcerative colitis but common in those with Crohn's disease. Aphthous lesions (small ulcers on an erythematous base) in the midst of normal-appearing mucosa may be observed. Patchiness to inflammation with abnormal areas interspersed with grossly normal-appearing areas is characteristic of Crohn's disease of the colon. Deep fissuring ulcers and heaped-up edematous mucosa (pseudopolyps) may be present. The ileocecal valve may appear granular, friable, and edematous. If intubation of the ileocecal valve can be accomplished during colonoscopy, marked nodularity and inflammation of the terminal ileum (Fig. 3) may be present.

In as many as 30% of cases of Crohn's disease in children, there may be symptoms of upper gastrointestinal tract disease, such as epigastric pain, early satiety, and pyrosis.[21] Esophagogastroduodenoscopy and biopsy are more sensitive than radiologic evaluation for detecting Crohn's disease of the esophagus, stomach, and duodenum.

Histologic examination of tissue obtained by mucosal biopsy during endoscopic procedures is important. Frequently, grossly normal-appearing areas still may reveal evidence of inflammation. Colonic mucosal granulomas are found in approximately one third of cases of Crohn's disease.

DIFFERENTIAL DIAGNOSIS

The protean manifestations of Crohn's disease at presentation lead to a long differential diagnosis (Table 5). Infection, appendicitis, ovarian pathology, neoplasm, mesenteric adenitis, and intussusception may present with right lower quadrant pain, although more commonly in an acute fashion. More chronic pain is often considered to be irritable bowel syndrome, recurrent functional abdominal pain, carbohydrate intolerance, peptic disease, or urinary tract pathology. In young children bloody diarrhea and abdominal cramping also raise the specter of Henoch-Schönlein purpura and hemolytic-uremic syndrome. Extraintestinal manifestations may further compound the diagnostic dilemma.

MANAGEMENT

There is currently no cure for Crohn's disease. Treatment is directed toward controlling symptoms, addressing complications, and trying to

Table 5. DIFFERENTIAL DIAGNOSIS OF PRESENTING SYMPTOMS OF CROHN'S DISEASE

Primary Presenting Symptom	Diagnostic Considerations
Right lower quadrant abdominal pain, with or without mass	Appendicitis, infection (e.g., Campylobacter, Yersinia), lymphoma, intussusception, mesenteric adenitis, Meckel diverticulum, ovarian cyst
Chronic periumbilical or epigastric abdominal pain	Irritable bowel, constipation, lactose intolerance, peptic disease
Rectal bleeding, no diarrhea	Fissure, polyp, Meckel diverticulum, rectal ulcer syndrome
Bloody diarrhea	Infection, hemolytic-uremic syndrome, Henoch-Schönlein purpura, ischemic bowel, radiation colitis
Watery diarrhea	Irritable bowel, lactose intolerance, giardia, cryptosporidium, sorbitol, laxatives
Perirectal disease	Fissure, hemorrhoid (rare), streptococcal infection, condyloma (rare)
Growth delay	Endocrinopathy
Anorexia, weight loss	Anorexia nervosa
Arthritis	Collagen-vascular disease, infection
Liver abnormalities	Chronic hepatitis

From Hyams JS: Crohn's disease. *In* Wyllie R, Hyams JS (eds): Pediatric Gastrointestinal Disease: Pathophysiology, Diagnosis, Management. Philadelphia, WB Saunders, 1993, p 754.

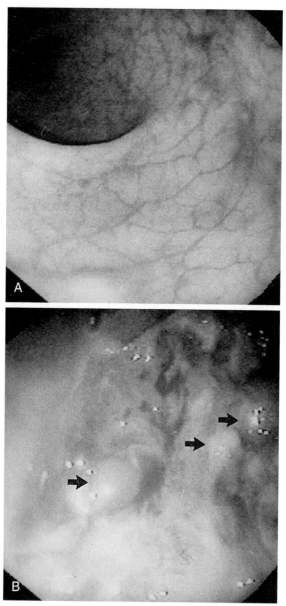

Figure 3. *A*, Normal colon. Note prominent vascular pattern. *B*, Severe Crohn's colitis with pseudopolyps *(arrows)*, exudate, and spontaneous hemorrhage.

Illustration continued on opposite page

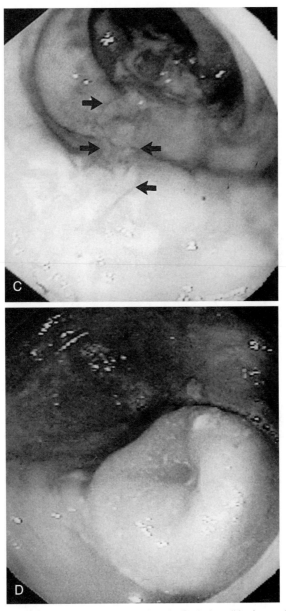

Figure 3 *(Continued). C,* Serpiginous linear ulcer in Crohn's colitis *(arrows). D,* Cecum in Crohn's colitis. Note granularity of mucosa, loss of normal vascular pattern, and markedly swollen ileocecal valve.

prevent recurrent or worsening disease. Treatment should be directed toward the patient's symptoms rather than abnormal laboratory tests, biopsies, or radiographs. Considerable dissociation often exists between endoscopic and radiographic findings and an individual's symptoms. Treatment of Crohn's disease is divided into four categories: (1) pharmacologic, (2) nutritional, (3) surgical, and (4) psychosocial.

Pharmacologic

Several classes of medications are currently being used in the treatment of Crohn's disease, including corticosteroids, 5-aminosalicylate (ASA) preparations, immunomodulators, and antibiotics (Table 6). Novel pharmacologic agents are being investigated and are mentioned later.

Corticosteroids

Corticosteroids have profound effects on the body's immune system and inflammatory response. Important proposed effects that may be useful in patients with Crohn's disease include inhibition of T-cell proliferation, decreased IL-1 production by macrophages, decreased IL-2 production by T cells, decreased leukotriene production by monocytes and macrophages, decreased expression of adhesion molecules by endothelial cells, and decreased vascular permeability leading to reduced migration of neutrophils from the blood to the site of inflammation.[1]

Corticosteroids are able to induce remission in most patients with either small or large bowel disease. Therapy is initiated with daily

Table 6. PHARMACOLOGIC TREATMENT OF CROHN'S DISEASE

Drug	Daily Dose	Indications	Comment
Prednisone	1–2 mg/kg max. 40–60 mg	Small or large bowel disease	Once remission achieved lower by 5 mg q week. Attempt to achieve q.o.d. schedule. Continue to taper and then stop.
5-ASA agents	30–50 mg/kg		—
Sulfasalazine	(max. 3 g)	Colon	May have prophylactic value.
Mesalamine	(max. 3.6 g)	Colon/sm. bowel	
Mesalazine	(max. 4.8 g)	Colon/sm. bowel	
Metronidazole	15–20 mg/kg (max. 1 g)	Perirectal or colonic disease	May require prolonged use; Neurotoxicity important.
6-Mercaptopurine or azathioprine	1–2 mg/kg (max. 100 mg)	Severe disease Corticosteroid toxicity	Effect may be delayed for 3–6 months. Need careful monitoring.

administration of prednisone or methylprednisolone (1–2 mg/kg/d). In "sicker" patients, intravenous corticosteroids are often used because of anecdotal experience suggesting increased effectiveness compared with oral therapy. Following symptomatic improvement, the daily dose is slowly weaned over several weeks to an alternate-day dose (0.2–0.5 mg/kg prednisone). The eventual goal is to stop the use of corticosteroids totally.

High-dose corticosteroids may mask signs of intra-abdominal sepsis or perforation. Significant side effects associated with chronic use include growth suppression, acne, facial puffiness (moon facies), hirsutism, striae, posterior subcapsular cataracts, aseptic necrosis of the femoral head, vertebral collapse, hypertension, and depression. The more serious complications of corticosteroid therapy often can be avoided by the coadministration of other anti-inflammatory or immunomodulatory drugs (discussed later) to minimize the dose of prednisone and the earlier consideration of surgery for refractory symptoms.

Because the side effects of corticosteroids often limit their use, attempts have been made to formulate corticosteroid medications that have high topical anti-inflammatory activity and low systemic activity because of rapid hepatic inactivation. Budesonide, a corticosteroid structurally related to 16α-hydroxyprednisolone, is efficacious against active Crohn's disease of the ileum and colon in adults.[20, 53] Side effects seem to be less than with prednisone. Its utility in children has not been determined.

5-Aminosalicylate Agents

Although sulfasalazine is still being used widely in the treatment of Crohn's disease, newer 5-ASA agents (i.e., mesalamine and mesalazine) that have greater efficacy against small bowel inflammation and better safety profiles are increasingly being used. These compounds have been shown to have several anti-inflammatory effects, including inhibiting eicosanoid production by inflammatory cells, inhibiting oxygen radical production by activated neutrophils, serving as oxygen radical scavengers, and inhibiting the binding of FMLP to human neutrophils.[45]

5-ASA agents are currently being used to induce remission in active disease and to prevent recurrence induced by medical treatment or surgery. Mild to moderate colonic disease usually responds well to all 5-ASA agents. Small bowel disease, especially that of the terminal ileum, is currently being treated with mesalamine and mesalazine, which are partly released into the small bowel in contradistinction to sulfasalazine, which is primarily released in the colon. Several studies have shown that mesalamine and mesalazine may decrease the likelihood of recurrent disease over a 2-year follow-up period by almost 50% compared with placebo following a medical or surgical remission.[15, 49] The dose of 5-ASA agent used seems to be critical. Although exact data in pediatric patients are lacking, a dose of 50 mg/kg/d seems to be appropriate.

Immunomodulatory Agents

Agents that currently are being used to treat Crohn's disease include 6-mercaptopurine, azathioprine, methotrexate, and cyclosporine. Considerable pediatric experience with 6-mercaptopurine and azathioprine exists, although double-blind, placebo-controlled trials of its use in this population are lacking. It seems to have particular efficacy in facilitating corticosteroid reduction in patients dependent on high corticosteroid dosage.[40, 64] Although the mechanism of action of these agents in Crohn's disease is unclear, they significantly affect lymphocyte metabolism and activation. The dose ranges from 1 to 2 mg/kg/d. Bone-marrow suppression and pancreatitis are the two most important side effects.

No published data exist concerning the use of methotrexate or cyclosporine in Crohn's disease in children, although these agents have been used in the pediatric population.[62] Cyclosporine has been shown to have efficacy in severe Crohn's disease in adults, although recurrent symptoms were common on discontinuation of the drug.[6] A recent report suggested a role for cyclosporine in treating severe fistulous disease.[25] The long-term use of the agents in children must still be approached with caution, because long-term toxicity data need to be collected.

Antibiotics

Antibiotic therapy is used in several ways. Intra-abdominal abscess developing as a result of fistulization is treated with broad-spectrum coverage directed against stool flora and commonly include ampicillin, gentamicin, and clindamycin or metronidazole. Similar therapy is offered in many cases, even in the absence of obvious abscess formation in patients presenting with right lower quadrant tenderness with fever because of the presumption of "microfistulization" and localized infection.

Perianal fistulous disease is treated frequently with metronidazole, which also may have more general use for severe colonic disease. This potent antianaerobe antibiotic also seems to affect the ability of neutrophils to migrate to sites of inflammation.[2] Antibiotics may alter bowel flora and diminish antigenic stimulation to the gut's mucosal immune system.

Newer Agents

Therapeutic agents are being assessed that target specific events in the initiation and perpetuation of the intestinal inflammatory cascade. These include drugs that are leukotriene-synthesis inhibitors, adhesion-molecule modulators, soluble receptors for proinflammatory cytokines, antibodies to proinflammatory cytokines, and cytokine-receptor antagonists.

Nutritional

Nutritional intervention can be used as primary or adjunctive therapy. Conflicting data exist on whether the administration of an elemental diet is comparable with corticosteroid therapy in inducing remission in mild to moderate disease.[18, 38, 54] Because elemental diets are unpalatable, especially in children, they often need to be administered by nasogastric tube infusion.

The greatest use of nutritional treatment in children with Crohn's disease is in addressing malnutrition as a cause of growth failure. Multiple studies document successful reversal of growth failure in Tanner I and II patients treated with intensive caloric supplementation.[4, 47]

Surgical

Within 10 to 15 years of diagnosis, approximately 50% to 70% of children with Crohn's disease require surgery.[10] The indications for surgery are shown in Table 7. Unfortunately, resectional surgery is not curative, and the likelihood of relapse seems to increase with length of follow-up postoperatively. After terminal ileal resection, endoscopic evidence of recurrent disease is found in the neoterminal ileum in more

---

Table 7. INDICATIONS FOR SURGERY IN CROHN'S DISEASE

1. Failure of medical therapy
   Intractable symptoms
   Corticosteroid toxicity
   Social invalidism
2. Obstruction—Acute or chronic
   Gastroduodenal
   Small bowel
   Large bowel
3. Hemorrhage
   Small bowel lesion
   Large bowel lesion
   Fulminant colitis, with or without toxic megacolon
4. Perforation
   Free
   Closed, with abscess
5. Fistula
   Intractable perirectal disease
   Enteroenteric
   Enterocutaneous
   Enterovesical
   Enterovaginal
6. Growth retardation
7. Carcinoma
8. Obstructive uropathy

From Hyams JS: Crohn's disease. *In* Wyllie R, Hyams JS (eds): Pediatric Gastrointestinal Disease: Pathophysiology, Diagnosis, Management. Philadelphia, WB Saunders, 1993, p 757.

than 70% of adults at 1 year, and 35% are symptomatic.[52] The recurrence rate after panproctocolectomy and ileostomy depends partly on the presence or absence of ileal disease at the time of surgery. Those with ileocolitis have a 70% relapse rate within 10 years compared with 15% for those with colitis alone.[30]

The child who has undergone multiple surgical operations presents a significant management problem. To prevent the loss of substantial bowel length because of multiple resections, strictureplasty has been developed. In this procedure, a longitudinal incision is made through stenotic bowel, and the opening is then closed transversely. The obstruction is relieved without sacrificing bowel. The presence of severe inflammation, abscess, or phlegmon at the operative site is a contraindication to this procedure.

Psychiatric Therapy

As with any chronic illness, Crohn's disease may have a significant social impact not only on the affected child but also on the family. For adolescents trying to achieve independence from their parents, the situation may be particularly difficult because of potential conflict with parents concerning compliance with medication regimens and avoiding dietary indiscretion. It is imperative to try to allow children and adolescents with Crohn's disease to participate fully in age-appropriate activities. Peer support groups can be very helpful.

PROGNOSIS

For most children with Crohn's disease, the disease course is one of exacerbation and remission. A small minority (5%) of patients have what seems to be one period of symptoms (at diagnosis) followed by a prolonged remission. A smaller minority (< 5%) have recalcitrant disease requiring continual aggressive medical therapy and multiple surgical procedures. Although the causes of most exacerbations are unclear, intercurrent viral illness seems to be a common precipitating factor.

The natural history of Crohn's disease will change as newer, more effective anti-inflammatory medications become available. For those patients with longstanding Crohn's disease of the colon who are not treated with surgical resection, the risk of malignancy may be similar to that found in chronic ulcerative colitis.[17] Colonoscopic surveillance may be appropriate for these subjects. With appropriate management, death from Crohn's disease is extremely rare in the pediatric population.

References

1. Andus T, Targan SR: Glucocorticoids. In Targan SR, Shanahan F (eds): Inflammatory Bowel Disease: From Bench to Bedside. Baltimore, Williams & Wilkins, 1994, pp 487–502

2. Arndt H, Palitzsch KD, Grisham MB, et al: Metronidazole inhibits leukocyte-endothelial cell adhesion in rat mesenteric venules. Gastroenterology 106:1271, 1994
3. Barton JR, Ferguson A: Clinical features, morbidity and mortality of Scottish children with inflammatory bowel disease. Q J Med 75:423, 1990
4. Belli DC, Seidman E, Bouthillier L, et al: Chronic intermittent elemental diet improves growth failure in children with Crohn's disease. Gastroenterology 94:603, 1988
5. Bennett RA, Rubin PH, Present DH: Frequency of inflammatory bowel disease in offspring of couples both presenting with inflammatory bowel disease. Gastroenterology 100:1638, 1991
6. Brynskov J, Freund L, Norby Rasmussen S, et al: Final report on a placebo-controlled, double-blind, randomized multicentre trial of cyclosporine treatment in active chronic Crohn's disease. Scand J Gastroenterol 26:689, 1991
7. Burbige EJ, Huang SS, Bayless TM: Clinical manifestations of Crohn's disease in children and adolescents. Pediatrics 55:866, 1975
8. Clements D, Motley RJ, Harries A, et al: Longitudinal study of cortical bone loss in patients with inflammatory bowel disease. Scand J Gastroenterol 27:1055, 1992
9. Crohn B, Ginzburg L, Oppenheimer G: Regional ileitis: Pathologic and clinical entity. JAMA 99:1323, 1932
10. Davies G, Evans CM, Whand WS, et al: Surgery for Crohn's disease in childhood: Influence of site of disease and operative procedure on outcome. Br J Surg 77:891, 1990
11. Dinarello CA: Interleukin-1 and interleukin-1 antagonism. Blood 77:1627–1652, 1991
12. Dinarello CA, Wolff SM: The role of interleukin-1 in disease. N Engl J Med 328:106–113, 1993
13. Doerfler ME, Danner RL, Shelhammer JH, et al: Bacterial lipopolysaccharides prime neutrophils for enhanced production of leukotriene B_4. J Clin Invest 83:970, 1989
14. Ferguson A, Rifkind EA, Doig CM: Prevalence of chronic inflammatory bowel disease in British children. In McConnell RB, Rozen P, Fiocchi C: Cytokines and animal models: A combined path to inflammatory bowel disease. Gastroenterology 104:1202, 1993
15. Gendre JP, Mary JY, Florent C, et al: Oral mesalamine (Pentasa) as maintenance treatment in Crohn's disease: A multicenter placebo-controlled study. Gastroenterology 104:435, 1993
16. Ghosh S, Cowen S, Hannan WJ, et al: Low bone mineral density in Crohn's disease, but not in ulcerative colitis, at diagnosis. Gastroenterology 107:1031, 1994
17. Gillen CD, Walmsley RS, Prior P, et al: Ulcerative colitis and Crohn's disease: A comparison of the colorectal cancer risk in extensive colitis. Gut 35:1590, 1994
18. Gonzalez-Huix F, de Leon R, Fernandez-Banares F, et al: Polymeric enteral diets as primary treatment of active Crohn's disease: A prospective steroid-controlled trial. Gut 34:778, 1993
19. Grand RJ, Motil KJ: Growth failure in inflammatory bowel disease. In Bayless TM (ed): Current therapy in Gastroenterology and Liver Disease, 2nd ed. Toronto, BC Dekker, 1986, pp 223–229
20. Greenberg GR, Feagan BG, Martin F, et al: Oral budesonide for active Crohn's disease. N Engl J Med 331:836, 1994
21. Griffiths AM, Alemayehu E, Sherman P: Clinical features of gastroduodenal disease in adolescents. J Pediatr Gastroenterol Nutr 8:166, 1989
22. Griffiths AM, Nguyen P, Smith C, et al: Growth and clinical course of children with Crohn's disease. Gut 34:939, 1993
23. Grill BB, Lange R, Markowitiz R, et al: Delayed gastric emptying in children with Crohn's disease. J Clin Gastroenterol 7:216, 1985
24. Gryboski JD, Spiro HM: Prognosis in children with Crohn's disease. Gastroenterology 74:807, 1978
25. Hanauer SB, Smith MB: Rapid closure of Crohn's disease fistulas with continuous intravenous cyclosporine A. Am J Gastroenterol 88:646, 1993
26. Haug K, Schrumpf EH, Halvorsen JF, et al, and the Study Group of Inflammatory Bowel Disease in Western Norway: Epidemiology of Crohn's disease in Western Norway. Scand J Gastroenterol 24:1271, 1989
27. Hyams JS: Extraintestinal manifestations of inflammatory bowel disease in children. J Pediatr Gastroenterol Nutr 19:7, 1994

28. Hyams JS, Carey DE: Corticosteroids and growth. J Pediatr 113:249, 1988
29. Hyams JS, Fitzgerald J, Wyzga N, et al: Relationship of interleukin-1 receptor antagonist to mucosal inflammation in inflammatory bowel disease. J Pediatr Gastroenterol Nutr 21:419, 1995
30. Hyams JS, Grand RJ, Colodny AH, et al: Course and prognosis after colectomy and ileostomy for inflammatory bowel disease in childhood and adolescence. J Pediatr Surg 17:400, 1982
31. Hyams JS, Markowitz J, Treem WR, et al: Characterization of hepatic abnormalities in children with inflammatory bowel disease. Inflammatory Bowel Disease 1:27, 1995
32. Hyams JS, Moore RE, Leichtner AM, et al: Relationship of type I procollagen to corticosteroid therapy in children with inflammatory bowel disease. J Pediatr 112:893, 1988
33. Hyams JS, Treem WR, Carey DE, et al: Comparison of collagen propeptides as growth markers in children with inflammatory bowel disease. Gastroenterology 100:971, 1991
34. Kanof ME, Lake AM, Bayless TM: Decreased height velocity in children and adolescents before the diagnosis of Crohn's disease. Gastroenterology 95:1523, 1988
35. Kirschner BS, Sutton MM: Somatomedin-C levels in growth impaired children and adolescents with chronic inflammatory bowel disease. Gastroenterology 91:830, 1986
36. Langman MJS, Gilat T (eds): The Genetics and Epidemiology of Inflammatory Bowel Disease (Front Gastrointest Res 11), Basel, Karger, 1986, pp 69–72
37. Lenaerts C, Roy CC, Vaillancourt M, et al: High incidence of upper gastrointestinal tract involvement in children with Crohn's disease. Pediatrics 83:777, 1989
38. Lochs H, Steinhardt HJ, Klaus-Wentz B, et al: Comparison of enteral nutrition and drug treatment in active Crohn's disease. Results of the European Cooperative Crohn's disease study IV. Gastroenterology 101:881, 1991
39. Markowitz J, Daum F, Aiges H, et al: Perianal disease in children and adolescents with Crohn's disease. Gastroenterology 86:829, 1984
40. Markowitz J, Rosa J, Grancher K, et al: Long-term 6-mercaptopurine treatment in adolescents with Crohn's disease. Gastroenterology 99:1347, 1990
41. Means RT Jr, Krantz SB: Progress in understanding the pathogenesis of the anemia of chronic disease. Blood 80:1639, 1992
42. Motil KJ, Grand RJ, Davis-Kraft L, et al: Growth failure in children with inflammatory bowel disease: A prospective study. Gastroenterology 105:681, 1993
43. Musch MW, Chang EB: Diarrhea in inflammatory bowel disease. In Targan SR, Shanahan F (eds): Inflammatory Bowel Disease: From Bench to Bedside. Baltimore, Williams & Wilkins, 1994, pp 239–254
44. Olafsdottir EJ, Gjermund F, Haug K: Chronic inflammatory bowel disease in children in western Norway. J Pediatr Gastroenterol Nutr 8:454, 1989
45. Peppercorn M: Antiinflammatory agents. In Targan SR, Shanahan F (eds): Inflammatory Bowel Disease: From Bench to Bedside. Baltimore, Williams & Wilkins, 1994, pp 478–486
46. Phillips SF: Pathophysiology of symptoms and clinical features of inflammatory bowel disease. In Kirsner JB, Shorter RG (eds): Inflammatory Bowel Disease, ed 3. Philadelphia, Lea and Feabiger, 1988, pp 239–256
47. Polk DB, Hattner JT, Kerner JA Jr: Improved growth and disease activity after intermittent administration of a defined formula diet in children with Crohn's disease. J Parenter Enter Nutr 16:499, 1992
48. Posthuma R, Moroz SP: Pediatric Crohn's disease. J Pediatr Surg 20:478, 1985
49. Prantera C, Pallone F, Brunetti G, et al: Oral 5-aminosalicylic acid (Asacol) in the maintenance treatment of Crohn's disease. Gastroenterology 103:363, 1992
50. Raine PAM: BAPS collective review: Chronic inflammatory bowel disease. J Pediatr Surg 19:18, 1984
51. Rutgeerts P, Geboes K, Peeters M, et al: Effect of faecal stream diversion on recurrence of Crohn's disease in the neoterminal ileum. Lancet 337:771, 1991
52. Rutgeerts P, Gebhoes K, Vantrappen G, et al: Predictability of the postoperative course of Crohn's disease. Gastroenterology 99:956, 1990
53. Rutgeerts P, Lofberg R, Malchow H, et al: A comparison of budesonide with prednisolone for active Crohn's disease. N Engl J Med 331:842, 1994

54. Ruuska T, Savilahti E, Maki M, et al: Exclusive whole protein enteral diet versus prednisolone in the treatment of acute Crohn's disease in children. J Pediatr Gastroenterol 19:175, 1994
55. Sartor RB: Cytokines in intestinal inflammation: Pathophysiological and clinical considerations. Gastroenterology 106:533, 1994
56. Shanahan F: Pathogenesis of inflammatory bowel disease: A perspective. Autoimmunity Forum. Gastroenterology 1:3, 1989
57. Sofaer J: Crohn's disease: The genetic contribution. Gut 34:869, 1993
58. Sonnenberg A, McCarty DJ, Jacobsen SJ: Geographic variation of inflammatory bowel disease within the United States. Gastroenterology 100:143, 1991
59. Tenore A, Berman WF, Parks JS, et al: Basal and stimulated serum growth hormone concentrations in inflammatory bowel disease. J Clin Endocrinol Metab 44:622, 1977
60. Thomas AG, Holly JMP, Taylor F, et al: Insulin-like growth factor-I, insulin like growth factor binding protein-1, and insulin in childhood Crohn's disease. Gut 34:944, 1993
61. Thomas DW, Sinatra FR: Screening laboratory tests for Crohn's disease. West J Med 150:163, 1989
62. Treem WR, Hyams JS: Cyclosporine therapy for gastrointestinal disease. J Pediatr Gastroenterol Nutr 18:270, 1994
63. Van Kruiningen HJ, Colombel JF, Cartun RW, et al: An in-depth study of Crohn's disease in two French families. Gastroenterology 104:351, 1993
64. Verhave M, Winter HS, Grand RJ: Azathioprine in the treatment of children with inflammatory bowel disease. J Pediatr 117:809, 1990
65. Yamada T, Grisham MB: Pathogenesis of tissue injury: Role of reactive metabolites of oxygen and nitrogen. *In* Targan SR, Shanahan F (eds): Inflammatory Bowel Disease: From Bench to Bedside. Baltimore, Williams & Wilkins, 1994, pp 133–150

Address reprint requests to
Jeffrey S. Hyams, MD
80 Seymour Street
Hartford, CT 06102

ENCOPRESIS AND SOILING

Vera Loening-Baucke, MD

Constipation, encopresis, and fecal incontinence represent common problems in children. *Encopresis* is fecal soiling in the presence of *functional constipation* (constipation not due to organic and anatomic causes or intake of medication) after the child has reached the age of 4 years.[15, 28] It is the involuntary loss of formed, semiformed, or liquid stool into the child's underwear. *Fecal incontinence* is fecal soiling in the presence of an organic or anatomic lesion, such as anal malformation, anal surgery or trauma, meningomyelocele, and some muscle diseases. *Fecal soiling* is any amount of stool deposited in the underwear, independent of whether an organic or anatomic lesion is present.

The aims of this article are to describe the symptoms of functional constipation in young children, to describe the symptoms of functional constipation and encopresis in older children, to present the differential diagnosis of constipation with or without fecal incontinence, to describe the evaluation and treatment of these children, and to report on treatment outcome.

ANATOMY AND PHYSIOLOGY

Very special control mechanisms are developed in the body to prevent loss of wind, stool, and urine. Unconscious regulation of bowel movements is a normal phenomenon after birth. Conscious regulation of bowel movements is achieved at an average age of 28 months.[7]

This work was supported by The Children's Miracle Network Telethon Fund and grant M01-RR-00059 from the General Clinical Research Center Program, Division of Research Resources, National Institutes of Health.

From the Division of General Pediatrics, Department of Pediatrics, University of Iowa, Iowa City, Iowa

Fecal continence is the body's ability to recognize when the rectal ampulla fills; to discriminate whether the content is formed stool, liquid stool, or gas; and to retain the content until emptying is convenient. The major structures responsible for continence and defecation are the external anal sphincter, puborectalis muscle, internal anal sphincter, and rectum. The factors that are responsible for maintaining fecal continence and that also facilitate defecation are the high pressure zone in the anal canal, the anal and rectal sensory and reflex mechanisms, the visco-elastic properties of the rectum, and stool volume and consistency. Fecal material can be retained by contraction of the external sphincter and puborectalis muscle. Fecal material is expelled by the combination of increased intra-abdominal pressure produced by closure of the glottis, fixation of the diaphragm, and contractions of the abdominal muscles, with relaxation of the internal and external anal sphincters and rectal contractions.

FUNCTIONAL CONSTIPATION WITH OR WITHOUT ENCOPRESIS

Ninety-five percent of children seen in the Encopresis Clinic at the University of Iowa in Iowa City, Iowa, have functional constipation; no underlying cause for the constipation can be identified. Weaver and Steiner[68] found that 85% of 1- to 4-year-old children passed stools once or twice a day, and 96% did so three times daily to once every other day, a pattern that persists to old age. Constipation is usually defined in terms of alterations in the frequency, size, consistency, or the ease in passage of stool. Constipation in children can be defined by a stool frequency of less than three per week, or painful bowel movements often accompanied by severe discomfort, screaming, and stool withholding maneuvers in young children, or stool retention with or without enco-presis, even when the stool frequency is three or more per week.

Stool retention results when stool expulsion has not occurred for several days. When stool retention persists, then formed, soft, or semiliq-uid stools leak to the outside around the accumulated firm stool mass. When stool retention remains untreated for a prolonged period of time, the rectal wall becomes stretched and a megarectum develops. The intervals between bowel movements become increasingly longer, and the rectum becomes so large that the stored stool can be felt as an abdominal mass that sometimes reaches up to the umbilicus (*megarec-tum*). In some cases, stool distends the whole colon, a *megacolon*.

No single mechanism is responsible for chronic functional constipa-tion. Constitutional and inherited factors, such as intrinsic slow motility, and psychological factors contribute to chronic constipation.[9, 16, 61] If defecation is painful, the child avoids the pain-producing activity by withholding stool. The rectum adjusts to the contents, and the urge to defecate gradually passes. As the cycle is repeated, successively greater amounts of stool are built up in the rectum with longer exposure to its drying action, and a vicious cycle is started. A pain-based cause is supported by data that 63% of children with encopresis had a history of painful defecation beginning before 36 months of age.[49]

Infants and Preschool Children

In a study by Issenman and colleagues,[22] 16% of parents of 22-month-old children reported constipation in their toddlers. Most often, constipation is short-lived and of little consequence; however, chronic constipation most often follows an inadequately managed acute problem.[16] Constipation can develop gradually in some children as a result of a progressive decrease in the frequency of bowel movements and a progressive increase in the difficulties in passing an excessively firm stool. In other children, an acute episode of constipation can follow a change in diet or environment, febrile illness, period of dehydration, or bed rest. The passage of these formed stools becomes painful, and the child begins to withhold stool in an attempt to avoid discomfort. The passage of the resultant harder and larger stool comes with even greater pain, often expressed by screaming and severe stool withholding maneuvers. Infants tend to extend the body and contract the anal and gluteal muscles, whereas toddlers often rise on their toes, hold their legs and buttocks stiffly, and often rock back and forth while holding on to a piece of furniture. Refusal to sit on the toilet, particularly during times of pain, is typical. The male to female ratio for chronic constipation in children less than 4 years of age is 1:1.[33]

School-Age Children

In general, the constipated school-age child is brought to medical attention because of encopresis, often of many years' duration, or because of abdominal pain. In the United States, only 25% to 30% of children are reliably toilet-trained by the age of 2 years,[60] and the average age at which initial toilet training is accomplished is 28 months.[7] The relatively wide range in age for achieving bowel control among normal children influences the definition of encopresis to children who are at least 4 years of age. Encopresis is reported to affect 2.8% of 4-year-old children, 2.2% of 5-year-old children, 1.9% of 6-year-old children, 1.5% of 7- to 8-year-old children, and 1.6% of 10- to 11-year-old children.[1, 5, 55, 56] The male to female ratio for encopresis ranges from 2.5:1 to 6:1.[5, 27, 35, 50, 62] Some children have daily bowel movements but evacuate incompletely, as evidenced by periodic passage of very large amounts of stool. Only half of parents have recognized that their children suffer from constipation, and few parents relate soiling to constipation. Parents often assume that encopresis is caused by the reluctance of the child to use the toilet. The frequency of encopresis varies among children and for an individual child and can occur occasionally, once a day, or many times a day. Some children have intermittent soiling. A period free of soiling may occur after a large bowel movement, and soiling resumes only after several days of stool retention. Usually the consistency of stool found in the underwear is loose or clay-like. Sometimes the core of the impaction breaks off and is found as a firm stool in the underwear. Encopresis frequently occurs in the afternoon when the child is in an upright position, especially during exercise or during the walk home from school. Many children with encopresis deny the presence of stool in their underwear and the accompanying foul and penetrant odor, and many children hide their soiled underwear. Parents usually find this situation frustrating, and soiling becomes a major issue of contention between the parent and the child. Encopresis is a complication of long-standing constipation and is involuntary.

Severe attacks of abdominal pain can occur either just before a bowel movement, for several days prior to a large bowel movement, or daily. Many constipated children suffer from vague chronic abdominal pain. Some patients with large stool masses throughout the entire colon may not experience any abdominal pain. Anorexia is present in many children with severe constipation. Daytime urinary incontinence is present in 20% of encopretic children, bed wetting in 33%; recurrent urinary tract infections in 10% of girls are common complaints.[35]

FECAL INCONTINENCE WITH OR WITHOUT CONSTIPATION

Fecal incontinence, soiling in the presence of an organic disease or an anatomic abnormality, can include loss of liquid, solid, or gaseous matter. The list of organic and anatomic causes in children is given in Table 1. Fecal incontinence is rare in children; 1 in 5000 children is born with Hirschsprung's disease and only some have fecal incontinence prior to or after surgery; 1 in 1000 children is born with meningomyelocele and most have fecal incontinence; and 1 in 8000 children is born with anorectal malformation, in whom incontinence depends on the severity of the abnormality.

Hirschsprung's Disease

Hirschsprung's disease (i.e., congenital aganglionic megacolon) is rare but needs to be considered in the differential diagnosis of any child of any age with severe constipation. Boys are affected four times more commonly than girls. Hirschsprung's disease is a congenital abnormality. The mean age at diagnosis decreased from 19.0 months during the 1960s to 2.6 months in the 1980s[23] due to more awareness of the disease, the availability of anorectal manometry, and better staining methods for the biopsy specimen.

The usual presentation of neonatal Hirschsprung's disease is consti-

Table 1. CAUSES OF CONSTIPATION WITH OR WITHOUT FECAL SOILING

Functional constipation in 95%
Neurogenic constipation
  Hirschsprung's disease
  Chronic intestinal pseudo-obstruction
  Disorders of the spinal cord, such as myelomeningocele or tumor
  Cerebral palsy, hypotonia
Constipation secondary to anal lesions
  Anal fissures
  Anterior location of the anus
  Anal stenosis and anal atresia
Constipation secondary to endocrine and metabolic disorders
  Hypothyroidism
  Renal acidosis
  Diabetes insipidus
  Hypercalcemia
Constipation induced by drugs
  Methylphenidate
  Phenytoin
  Imipramine hydrochloride
  Phenothiazide
  Antacids
  Codeine-containing medication

From Loening-Baucke V: Chronic constipation in children. Gastroenterology 105:1557, 1993; with permission.

pation, abdominal distention, vomiting, or diarrhea. The severity of disease ranges from complete obstruction that is relieved only by surgery to mere transient meconium retention, and some cases are even less severe. Gastrointestinal bleeding and diarrhea are danger signs for enterocolitis of Hirschsprung's disease. Hirschsprung's disease in infants and toddlers often presents with constipation and stools of small diameter (i.e., ribbon-like stools). Rectal examination reveals the rectum to be small in diameter and empty of stool. Although many children with Hirschsprung's disease have failure to thrive, not all are sickly, underweight, and anemic. Table 2 shows the differences in presentation of

Table 2. FUNCTIONAL CONSTIPATION VERSUS HIRSCHSPRUNG'S DISEASE IN CHILDREN FEWER THAN 4 YEARS OF AGE

	Functional* Constipation	Hirschsprung's Disease
Boys : girls	1 : 1	1 : 5
Stool size	Large in 74%	Normal to ribbon-like
Failure to thrive	5%	Common
Constipation from birth	24%	50%
Constipation prior to age 1 yr	84%	90%
Stool withholding	97%	Rare
Abdominal fecal mass	42%	95%
Stool in the rectum	Most	Uncommon
Size of rectal ampulla	Normal to large	Small to large

*Results from 174 children with functional constipation fever than 4 years of age.

children fewer than 4 years of age with functional constipation and Hirschsprung's disease. Prediagnosis-enterocolitis is no longer as prevalent and thus not as great a danger as before 1960,[23] probably because Hirschsprung's disease now is diagnosed much earlier in life. Post–pull-through enterocolitis still causes significant morbidity.

The chief complaint of older children, adolescents, and adults with Hirschsprung's disease is severe constipation. It is sometimes difficult to differentiate older patients with Hirschsprung's disease from patients with functional megacolon by history and even physical examination. Patients with either disease present with infrequent bowel movements and abdominal distention. Table 3 lists the differences in presentation between children with functional constipation and those with Hirschsprung's disease who are at least 5 years of age.

The absence of the rectosphincteric reflex during anorectal manometry,[39] a transition zone in the unprepped barium enema study, and the absence of ganglion cells on rectal biopsy differentiate between patients with Hirschsprung's disease and those with functional megacolon. The primary defect in patients with Hirschsprung's disease is the absence of ganglion cells from the submucosal and myenteric plexuses. The extent of bowel involved with aganglionosis varies. In 58% of patients, the rectum with or without the sigmoid was involved; in 26%, a longer segment was involved; and in 12%, the total colon and sometimes even small bowel was involved.[23] The treatment for Hirschsprung's disease is surgical.

Pseudo-Obstruction

Intractable constipation is observed in children with chronic intestinal pseudo-obstruction, a rare but devastating disease.[2, 64] Chronic intestinal pseudo-obstruction can be either localized or disseminated and results in motor dysfunction at various levels of the gastrointesti-

Table 3. FUNCTIONAL CONSTIPATION VERSUS HIRSCHSPRUNG'S DISEASE IN CHILDREN AT LEAST 5 YEARS OF AGE

	Functional Constipation (n = 215)	Hirschsprung's Disease (n = 15)
Boys : girls	1 : 3.3	1 : 2
Stool size	Large in 98%	Small to large
Failure to thrive	3%	Uncommon
Constipation from birth	10%	53%
Constipation prior to 1 year of age	49%	67%
Stool withholding	71%	Rare
Abdominal pain	51%	87%
Abdominal fecal mass	42%	93%
Rectal impaction	96%	27%
Size of rectal ampulla	Large in 80%	Small to large
Fecal soiling	90%	33%

nal tract, involving the esophagus, stomach, duodenum, small bowel, and/or large bowel. Patients with large bowel involvement commonly present with severe constipation with megacolon. The term *chronic intestinal pseudo-obstruction* covers a variety of different disorders. In some cases, a specific myopathy is present[2]; in others, a degeneration of the ganglia or the nerves occurs,[47, 59] and in some cases, no specific pathologic alteration has been detected. The disorder is familial in some cases. Onset often occurs in childhood. In many patients, symptoms are recurrent and mainly include constipation, diarrhea, and gaseous abdominal distention.

A cause of intestinal pseudo-obstruction is neuronal intestinal dysplasia.[13, 24, 44, 52] Clinical neuronal intestinal dysplasia type A mimics Hirschsprung's disease in the neonatal period with symptoms of intestinal spasticity, diarrhea, bloody stools, enterocolitis, and stool retention. The abnormalities on the rectal biopsy are hyperplasia of the submucosal and myenteric plexuses, but not every ganglia is involved a moderate increase in acetylcholinesterase activity, and mucosal inflammation.[13] Clinical improvement occurs with time in localized disease, and sometimes bowel resection is necessary.

Neuronal intestinal dysplasia type B presents first in children 6 months to 6 years of age as chronic constipation and megacolon. Some cases present in the newborn period with a meconium plug. Biopsy shows numerous ganglia in the submucosal and myenteric plexuses, consisting of giant and small ganglion cells and a moderate increase in acetylcholinesterase activity.[13] Although a considerable megacolon develops, the clinical course is often benign.

Most patients with neuronal intestinal dysplasia can be managed medically (see section on management). Patients with most other forms of pseudo-obstruction do not respond well to medical or surgical treatment. Temporary improvement is sometimes observed after surgery.

Myelomeningocele

Myelomeningocele is a congenital neural tube defect that occurs in approximately 1 in 1000 births. As a result of aggressive medical and surgical treatment, 80% to 90% of children survive. Fecal incontinence occurs in 90% of children with myelomeningocele. Many patients suffer from severe constipation with overflow fecal incontinence; others have incontinence due to diarrhea.

Varying degrees of nerve impairment exist in these patients, the most common being loss of anal or rectal sensation. Many such patients are unable to differentiate sensations produced by gas and that produced by liquid or solid feces. The second most common impairment is loss of external anal sphincter function. The sphincter cannot be squeezed voluntarily.[3, 41, 65, 69, 70] The reflex relaxation of the internal anal sphincter and the absence of external sphincter contraction permit a rectal contraction to propel a bolus of feces through the anal canal.

Cerebral Palsy and Hypotonia

Constipation is observed in many children with cerebral palsy, generalized hypotonia, or mental retardation, particularly in those who are neurologically devastated. In tube-fed children, the absence of dietary fiber may be constipating. In other children, poor defecatory efforts are due to poor skeletal muscle tone and poor coordination.

Anorectal Lesions

Fistula, abscess, and hemorrhoids rarely occur in children. The passage of large, formed stools may be painful and promote stool-withholding maneuvers.

Anorectal Malformations

The reported overall incidence of anorectal anomalies ranges from 1 in 3000 to 1 in 15,000 live births. Anorectal malformations are classified into low (i.e., translevator), intermediate, and high (i.e., supralevator) types.

Anterior location of the anus, which is the mildest form of anorectal malformation, has been proposed as a cause of constipation.[19, 26, 54, 63] Anterior location of the anus is more common in girls and is associated with a posterior shelf that interferes with evacuation. Surgical repositioning of the anus into a more posterior location supposedly corrects the presence of the posterior shelf and facilitates the passage of stool.[19, 26, 63] The concept that an anteriorly placed anus and a posterior rectal shelf causes constipation does not stand the test of objective critical analysis.[57] Many girls have an anterior location of the anus without constipation, and few patients benefit from anoplasty.

The presence of a rectal opening located anterior to the center of the anal sphincter is well known and is called *perineal fistula*. In many cases, the orifice is narrow and is not surrounded by sphincter muscles. The sphincter muscles are located in the normal position. Most of these patients suffer from constipation, but some just from fecal incontinence. These patients benefit from surgical positioning of the anal opening into the center of the sphincter muscles.

Anal stenosis is characterized by passage of stools of small diameter. A tight anal canal is felt during the rectal examination. Anal stenosis is often diagnosed in the newborn nursery or in the first few months of life. Treatment consists of anal dilatation and sometimes surgery.

An anal membrane or an imperforate anus is found during the newborn examination and requires surgery. Identification of the sometimes small anal sphincters and puborectalis muscle and their location should be done prior to surgery by MR imaging and during surgery by electric stimulation of these muscles. Most patients require medical treatment of fecal incontinence or constipation after successful surgery. Anal stenosis and secondary megacolon are observed in many children following surgical correction of imperforate anus and require anal dilation and, often, anoplasty.

Anorectal Trauma

Although anorectal trauma may be related to an impalement injury, it may be due to child abuse. Presentations are rectovaginal tears, often extending through the anal sphincter; rectovaginal fistula; or destruction of the anus and rectum. Ultrasound and anorectal manometry to assess the external and internal anal sphincters should be performed prior to surgical repair. Treatment for fecal incontinence resulting from anorectal trauma may require surgical repair for sphincter disruption or fistulas and may require a colostomy for those children with loss of their anal sphincters.

Rectal Prolapse

Rectal prolapse involves all of the coats of the rectal wall. It is rare in children, is most common before 3 years of age, and has its highest incidence in infants fewer than 1 year of age. Rectal prolapse occurs most often in children with constipation and other diseases leading to malnutrition, such as cystic fibrosis and celiac disease. Laxatives are given to those with functional constipation (see section on management). Children with rectal prolapse and cystic fibrosis need to have their pancreatic enzymes adjusted. The prolapse in children with celiac disease disappears with better nutrition through adherence to a gluten-free diet.

Other Causes

Occasionally, the author evaluates a child with myotonic dystrophy or muscular dystrophy for fecal incontinence, constipation, abdominal cramping, or abdominal distention. Some of these children may have a fecal impaction. Most patients have low anal resting pressures and squeeze pressures. Pellet stools are observed in children with hypothyroidism and metabolic disorders associated with water depletion, such as renal acidosis, diabetes insipidus, or hypercalcemia.

Drugs such as anticonvulsants (e.g., phenytoin), psychotherapeutic agents (e.g., methylphenidate, imipramine hydrochloride, and phenothiazide), and cough syrups containing codeine can cause constipation. Cow's-milk–protein ingestion seems to be associated with constipation in some infants. Switching to a cow's-milk–free formula or an enzymatically hydrolyzed formula alleviates constipation in most infants.

INVESTIGATIONS

History and physical examination should be complete (Table 4). In the history, the intervals, size, and consistency of bowel movements that are deposited into the toilet and into the child's underwear should be elicited. The physical examination confirms constipation. An abdominal fecal mass may be palpated. Sometimes the mass extends throughout the entire colon, but more commonly the mass is felt suprapubically and midline, sometimes filling the left or the right lower quadrant. In many cases, inspection of the perineum shows fecal material. In many patients, the rectum is packed with stool, either of hard consistency or, more commonly, the outside of the fecal impaction feels like clay and the core of the impaction is rock hard. Sometimes the retained stool is soft or loose. No rectal impaction is felt in a few children with a recent large bowel movement. Visual study of the anus and perineum, simple neurologic examination, and determining perianal sensation should be included in the examination. Loss of perianal skin sensation can be associated with various neurologic diseases of the spinal cord. A low anal pressure during digital rectal examination suggests either fecal retention with inhibition of anal resting pressure, a disease involving the external or internal anal sphincter, or both.

Laboratory Investigation

Careful history and physical examination allow the physician to make a decision regarding requirements for blood studies (e.g., deficiency or excess of thyroid or adrenal hormones, electrolyte imbalances, and calcium level), urine culture, radiograph studies, anorectal manometric studies, or rectal biopsy. Most infants and children with functional constipation require minimal work-up.

Radiologic studies usually are not indicated in uncomplicated con-

Table 4. ENCOPRESIS AND SOILING

History	Physical Examination
Complete with special attention to:	Complete with special attention to:
Stooling habits	Abdominal examination
Character of stools in toilet	Anal inspection
Character of stools in underwear	Rectal digital examination
Stool withholding maneuvers	Neurologic examination, including perianal
Age of onset of constipation or soiling	sensation testing
Abdominal pain	
Dietary habits	
Urinary symptoms	
Day wetting	
Bed wetting	
Urinary tract infections	

stipation. A plain abdominal film can be very useful in assessing the presence or absence of retained stool, its extent, and whether the lower spine is normal in encopretic children with absence of a fecal mass on abdominal and rectal examination, in children who vehemently refuse rectal examination, or in children who are markedly obese. Fecal incontinence is not likely related to spinal disease without urinary symptoms or neurologic abnormalities of the lower limbs.

Anorectal manometric assessment of children with mild constipation is not necessary. The main role of anorectal manometry is in the evaluation of children with severe constipation in whom the diagnosis of Hirschsprung's disease needs to be excluded and in patients with fecal incontinence in whom anal pressure and rectal sensation should be assessed. In patients with Hirschsprung's disease, the internal anal sphincter does not relax during rectal balloon distention and the rectosphincteric reflex is absent.[32]

Numerous manometric studies have been performed in children with functional constipation and encopresis.[31, 35, 39, 40, 45, 66] The abnormalities found in the author's laboratory in these children include increased threshold to rectal distention and decreased rectal contractility as compared with controls.[31, 35, 39, 40] In follow-up, after 3 years of therapy, most children show continued abnormalities of anorectal function, leaving them at risk for recurrent problems.[39] Another abnormality is the failure of the external anal sphincter and pelvic floor to relax during defecation attempts.[12, 35, 39, 40, 42, 66] This abnormality is found in many constipated children who respond poorly to treatment.[35]

When history (e.g., early onset of severe constipation, absence of fecal soiling, or stools of small diameter) or physical examination (e.g., failure to thrive or empty or small rectal ampulla with impacted stools in the proximal colon) suggests Hirschsprung's disease or when constipation is persistent despite adherence to the treatment program, then anorectal manometry should be performed. If the rectosphincteric reflex is absent or atypical, then barium enema and rectal biopsy need to be performed to evaluate for Hirschsprung's disease and other neuronal disorders.

Barium enema is unnecessary in uncomplicated cases of constipation; however, it is helpful in the assessment of Hirschsprung's disease in which a transition zone between aganglionic bowel and ganglionic bowel may be observed, in other neuronal disorders in which extensive bowel dilatation may be observed, and in the evaluation of the postsurgical patient operated on for anal atresia or Hirschsprung's disease.

Histologic and histochemical information is obtained through rectal biopsy. The presence or absence of ganglion cells can be evaluated from superficial suction rectal biopsy.[44] False-negative results are possible. Absence of ganglion cells with increased staining of nerve trunks with acetylcholinesterase stain is diagnostic for Hirschsprung's disease. Full-thickness biopsies are necessary for the evaluation of other abnormalities of both the myenteric and submucosal plexuses, such as in hypoganglionosis or hyperganglionosis.[4, 13, 44, 57]

MANAGEMENT

Most children with chronic constipation with or without fecal soiling benefit from a precise, well-organized plan. Few patients require surgery, as was reported in the section describing the different diseases. Nonsurgical treatment includes various forms of behavioral therapy and psychological approaches and is designed to clear fecal impaction, prevent future impaction, and promote regular bowel habits. The treatment of constipation with or without fecal soiling is comprehensive and has four phases, including (1) education; (2) disimpaction; (3) prevention of reaccumulation of stools; and (4) reconditioning to normal bowel habits.[9, 10, 11, 15, 16, 28, 30, 34, 48, 49, 58, 61]

Education

The stooling problem is not caused by a disturbance in the psychological behavior of the child and is not the parents' fault. Soiling occurs involuntarily and usually without the knowledge of the child. In most cases, a detailed plan eliminates parents' and children's frustration and improves compliance for the prolonged treatment that is necessary. Some parents do not possess the skills necessary to effectively manage their child's behavior, specifically in relation to following a demanding regimen. These parents need to be identified so that educational efforts can be optimized. In addition, a caring relationship is established. Therapy should be appropriate for the severity of the constipation and the age of the child.

Disimpaction

For disimpaction, a hypertonic phosphate enema can be used, with 30 mL/5 kg body weight in young infants. An adult-sized enema (135 mL) can be used for children weighing more than 20 kg. In most children, one to two enemas result in good bowel clean-out. Hypernatremia, hyperphosphatemia, hypocalcemia, hypokalemia, and dehydration have occurred in few children after hypertonic phosphate enemas.[17] Normal (i.e., isotonic) saline enemas may be used but are often not effective. Cleansing soap-suds enemas should be avoided because they can result in bowel necrosis, perforation, or death.[6] Tap-water enemas should be avoided because they can cause water intoxication, hypervolemia, dilution of serum electrolytes, seizures, or death.[71] Children with megarectum or megacolon who do not respond to phosphate enemas can be disimpacted with a hyperosmolar milk-of-molasses enema (1:1 milk and molasses) with the infusion stopped when the child indicates discomfort (200–600 mL). The milk-of-molasses enema may need to be repeated. Lavage solutions given orally or by nasogastric tube until clear fluid is excreted through the anus can be used for disimpaction. An average of 12 L given over 23 hours at a rate of 14 mL to 40 mL/kg/h is required for disimpaction.[21] Other[25] physicians have used 750 mL to 1000 mL/h of lavage solution for children more than 12 years of age until fecal effluent consisted of clear fluid. It is recommended to give metoclopramide 5 mg to 10 mg orally 15 minutes prior to the lavage solution to reduce nausea and vomiting.[25]

Gilger and colleagues[18] reported an efficient, comfortable, and safe way for disimpaction using pulsed irrigation-enhanced evacuation. Five gallons of warm water were given more than 25 to 30 minutes as automated small pulses (25 mL) lasting a few seconds, alternating with gravity drainage of feces and water into a sealed bag. Although disimpaction was not complete after the procedure, all patients continued to empty their colon afterwards. All patients were effectively disimpacted 12 hours later. For a child who vehemently fears enemas, the fecal mass can be softened and liquefied with large quantities of mineral oil or osmotic agents with the administration continued until the fecal mass is passed. Soiling increases dramatically, and abdominal pain and cramping may increase during oral disimpaction.

Prevention of Reaccumulation of Stools

Even though the role of dietary fiber in the treatment of functional constipation is controversial, the author recommends fiber found naturally in many foods to parents of infants fewer than 1 year of age, such as pureed fruits, vegetables, and infant cereal. The parents of older children are encouraged to give several servings daily from a variety of fiber-rich foods, such as whole-grain breads and cereals, fruits, vegetables, and legumes. Dietary fiber increases water retention and provides substrate for bacterial growth. It is beneficial for children with fecal incontinence who also have loose stool consistency.

Switching from cow's-milk formula to a formula containing whey protein alleviates constipation in most infants. In most constipated patients, daily defecation is maintained by the daily administration of laxatives beginning on the evening of the clinic visit. Laxatives should be used according to age, body weight, and severity of the constipation. Suggested dosages of commonly used laxatives are given in Table 5. The choice of medication for functional constipation does not seem as important as children's and parents' compliance with the treatment regimen. There is no set dosage for any laxative. There is only a starting dosage for each child that must be adjusted to induce one to two bowel movements per day that are loose enough to ensure complete daily emptying of the lower bowel and prevent soiling and abdominal pain. Once an adequate dosage is established, it is continued for approximately 3 months to help the distended bowel to regain some of its function. Usually, regular bowel habits are established by that time. Then, the dosage may be reduced in small decrements while maintaining a daily bowel movement without soiling. Laxatives need to be continued

Table 5. SUGGESTED DOSAGES OF COMMONLY USED LAXATIVES

Laxative	Age	Dose
Malt soup extract	Infant	Breast-fed: 5–10 mL in 2–4 oz of water or fruit juice twice daily Bottle-fed: 7.5–30 mL in day's total formula or 5–10 mL in every second feeding
Karo syrup	Infant	Dose is the same as that of malt soup extract
Milk of magnesia	> 6 months	1–3 mL/kg body weight/d, divide in 1–2 doses
Mineral oil	> 6 months	Dose the same as that of milk of magnesia
Lactulose or sorbitol	> 6 months	Dose the same as that of milk of magnesia
Senna syrup	1–5 years	5 mL with breakfast, maximum 5 mL twice daily
	5–15 years	10 mL with breakfast, maximum 10 mL twice daily

Adapted from Loening-Baucke V: Chronic constipation in children. Gastroenterology 105:1557, 1993; with permission.

for several months and sometimes years at the right dosage to induce daily soft stools.

For young infants, malt-soup extract (Maltsupex) or an osmotic laxative, such as Karo syrup, can be added to the milk. The mechanism of action of milk of magnesia is the relative nonabsorption of magnesium and the resultant increase in luminal osmolality. In severe constipation with rock-hard stools, the starting dosage of milk of magnesia is 2 to 3 mL/kg/d given with the evening meal. In children who have fecal retention of mostly soft-formed stools, usually 1 mL/kg body weight daily is adequate.

Mineral oil is converted into hydroxy fatty acids, which induce fluid and electrolyte accumulation. Dosages are similar to those for milk of magnesia.[11, 16, 27, 67] Mineral oil should never be force-fed or given to patients with dysphagia or vomiting because of the danger of aspiration pneumonia. Anal seepage of the mineral oil is an undesirable side effect, especially in children going to school. Long-term use of mineral oil has been reported to be safe.[8]

Lactulose, a nonabsorbable carbohydrate, is hydrolyzed to acids by the colonic flora, causing increased water content by the osmotic effects of lactulose and its metabolites. It is used commonly in Germany, Britain, and France and used rarely in the United States because of high cost. Sorbitol (70%) is another nonabsorbable carbohydrate that is inexpensive and easily taken by children when mixed in soft drinks.

Senna has an effect on intestinal motility and on fluid and electrolyte transport and stimulates defecation. Senna is used when liquid stools produced by osmotic laxatives are retained; when the child refuses milk of magnesia, mineral oil, and sorbitol; and in children with fecal incontinence secondary to organic or anatomic causes. Other centers use senna more frequently to treat patients with functional constipation.[9, 10]

An appropriate treatment plan is developed using the symptoms and the results of the anorectal manometric evaluation for patients with fecal incontinence. Treatment options are medical therapy (e.g., stool softeners, laxatives, suppositories, phosphate enemas, or large-volume saline enemas), frequent manual removal of feces, a constipating diet or medication, behavior modification, biofeedback training, or a combination of these.

Treatment with osmotic laxatives in patients with myelomeningocele or myotonic dystrophy and fecal impaction is rarely successful. Constipation is relieved, but fecal incontinence increases. Increasing dietary fiber; producing regular daily bowel movements with daily administration of senna; or emptying the rectum regularly with suppositories, enemas, or digitally can improve the incontinence in most of these children.

Reconditioning the Child to Normal Bowel Habits by Regular Toilet Use

Toddler

Toilet training attempts are discouraged in children fewer than 2.5 years of age who are resistant to potty sitting. These children can be put back into diapers or pull-ups. First, normal bowel patterns are accomplished and then toilet training can be started or restarted.

Older Child

Defecation trials are very important and are necessary in any treatment program. The child is encouraged to sit on the toilet for 3 to 5 minutes, three to four times a day following meals. The gastrocolic reflex, which goes into effect shortly after a meal, should be used to his or her advantage. The children and their parents need to be instructed to keep a daily record of bowel movements, fecal soiling, and medication use. This helps to monitor compliance and to make appropriate adjustments in the treatment program by parents or physicians. If necessary, positive reinforcement is given by using star charts, little presents, television viewing, or computer game time as rewards.

Psychological Treatment

Adherence to the treatment program improves constipation, encopresis, or fecal incontinence in all children. The presence of coexisting behavioral problems often is associated with poor treatment outcome.[29] If the coexisting behavior problem is secondary to chronic constipation, encopresis, or fecal incontinence, then it improves with treatment. Children who do not improve should be referred for further evaluation, because continued problems can be caused by noncompliance or control issues by children or parents. Psychological intervention, family counseling, and occasional hospitalization of children for 2 to 4 weeks to get a treatment program started have helped some of these unfortunate children.

Biofeedback Treatment

An abnormality occurring in 25% to 53% of constipated patients is *abnormal defecation dynamics*, an abnormal contraction of the external anal sphincter and pelvic floor muscles during defecation.[35, 42, 66] An abnormality observed in many children with fecal incontinence is weak anal sphincters. The external anal sphincter and pelvic floor consist of striated muscles that are under voluntary control. These muscles are amenable to biofeedback treatment and can be trained to relax during defecation and to squeeze for prevention of incontinence.[12, 37, 38, 41, 42, 65, 67, 69, 70]

Follow-up Visits

Because the management of chronic constipation, encopresis, and fecal incontinence requires considerable patience and effort on the part of the child and parents, it is important to provide necessary support and encouragement through frequent office visits. Parents are encouraged to call. Progress should be assessed by reviewing the stool records and repeating the abdominal and rectal examination to be sure that the problem is adequately managed. If necessary, dosage adjustment is made, and the child and parents are encouraged to continue with the regimen. After regular bowel habits are established, the medication dosage is gradually decreased to a dosage that maintains one bowel movement daily and prevents soiling. After 6 months, a further reduction or discontinuation of the medication is attempted.

OUTCOME

Constipation and Encopresis

Long-term follow-up studies (6.9 ± 2.7 years) in 90 young constipated patients who were initially evaluated and treated before the age of 4 years revealed that 63% had recovered.[33] Twelve-month follow-up studies in patients with constipation and encopresis who were more than 5 years of age treated at the Encopresis Clinic at the University of Iowa showed that approximately 50% of patients have discontinued laxatives and have at least three bowel movements per week without soiling.[35, 36, 40] An additional 20% may be weaned off the laxative within 2 years. The remainder requires laxatives for daily bowel movements or continues with soiling for many years and, in some cases, into adulthood. Fifty-one percent of patients in an Australian study had recovered 1 year after receiving laxatives and behavior modification.[48] Clayden[10] evaluated the duration of laxative treatment in more than 300 patients in Britain and showed that 22% of patients required regular laxative use for fewer than 6 months, 44% for fewer than 12 months, and 56% for more than 12 months. Stopping the laxatives too soon is the most common cause for relapse.[10]

Fecal Incontinence

Constipation and fecal incontinence are common problems postoperatively in patients with Hirschsprung's disease. Mishalany and Woolley[46] followed 62 patients with Hirschsprung's disease who had undergone Swenson, Duhamel, or Soave procedure. Constipation was reported in 21% to 69% of patients at 1- to 30-year follow-up, with 69% of patients reporting constipation after the Soave endorectal pull-through procedure. Fecal incontinence was present in 42% to 67% of patients and was highest after the Swenson procedure. Holschneider and colleagues[20] reported that 32% of 439 patients with Hirschsprung's disease had problems postoperatively with constipation on short-term follow-up, and 9% still suffered from constipation, on average, 8 years later. Some of the problems with constipation, fecal incontinence, or recurrent enterocolitis are explained by the type of surgical procedure. But some of the complications, particularly those that are persistent, may be due to neuronal intestinal dysplasia.[14, 53]

The previously described therapies using scheduled toileting, senna, suppositories, enemas, or manual removal of feces and biofeedback training are successful in many, but not all, of the children with myelomeningocele. Most children with nonfunctioning sphincters continue with some degree of incontinence. For those who continue with severe incontinence, a novel technique was introduced by Malone and colleagues.[43] They reported the formation of a continent appendicocecostomy through which the cecum could be intermittently catheterized and an antegrade enema administered. In this way, the colon could be regularly cleaned, rendering the child nonsoiling. As enema, half of a phosphate enema (64 mL) diluted in an equal volume of saline and then washed through with 100 mL to 200 mL saline, is recommended.[43]

The anatomic development of the anal sphincters and rectum determines the degree of fecal incontinence in patients who have undergone surgery for anal atresia. Incontinence is associated with abnormal function of the rectum or the anal sphincters. Patients with low anal atresia generally have good continence, whereas patients with the high type are often stool-incontinent as children but may experience some improvement during the teenage years.

SUMMARY

The author hopes that readers have gained an understanding about constipation, encopresis, and fecal incontinence and have acquired some useful knowledge that may aid in the diagnosis and then in the establishment of a treatment program for these unfortunate youngsters. The author believes that the primary care practitioner can develop an appropriate treatment program for most of his or her patients with fecal soiling. Only a few patients, young patients with severe constipation starting at birth and older patients who do not respond to treatment, should be referred for further diagnosis and management.

References

1. American Psychiatric Association: Diagnostic and Statistical Manual of Mental Disorders, ed 3. Washington, DC, 1987
2. Anuras S, Mitros FA, Soper RT: Chronic intestinal pseudo-obstruction in young children. Gastroenterology 91:62, 1986
3. Arhan P, Faverdin C, Devroede G, et al: Anorectal motility after surgery for spina bifida. Dis Colon Rectum 27:159, 1984
4. Ariel I, Hershlag A, Lernau OZ, et al: Hypoganglionosis of the myenteric plexus with normal Meissner's plexus: A new variant of colonic ganglion cell disorders. J Pediatr Surg 20:90, 1985
5. Bellman M: Studies on encopresis. Acta Paediatr Scand 170(suppl):1, 1966
6. Brandt LJ: The colon. In Brandt LJ (ed): Gastrointestinal Disorders of the Elderly. New York, Raven Press, 1984, p 261
7. Brazelton TB: A child oriented approach to toilet training. Pediatrics 29:121, 1962
8. Clark J, Russel G, Fitzgerald J: Serum betacarotene, retinol, and alpha tocopherol levels during mineral oil therapy for constipation. J Pediatr Gatroenterol Nutr 141:1210, 1985
9. Clayden GS: Chronic constipation in childhood. Postgraduate Update June:1243, 1989
10. Clayden GS: Management of chronic constipation. Arch Dis Child 67:340, 1992
11. Davidson M, Kugler MM, Bauer CH: Diagnosis and management in children with severe and protracted constipation and obstipation. J Pediatr 62:261, 1963
12. Emery Y, Descos L, Meunier P, et al: Constipation terminale par asynchronisme abdomino-pelvien; analyse des données étiologiques, cliniques, manométriques, et des résultats thérapeutiques aprés rééducation par biofeedback. Gastroenterol Clin Biol 12:6, 1988
13. Fadda B, Maier WA, Meier-Ruge W, et al: Neuronal intestinal dysplasia: A critical 10-year analysis of clinical and bioptic results. Z Kinderchir 38:305, 1983
14. Fadda B, Pistor G, Meier-Ruge W, et al: Symptoms, diagnosis, and therapy of neuronal intestinal dysplasia masked by Hirschsprung's disease. Pediatr Surg Int 2:76, 1987
15. Fitzgerald JF: Difficulties with defecation and elimination in children. Clin Gastroenterol 6:283, 1977
16. Fitzgerald JF: Constipation in children. Pediatr Rev 8:299, 1987
17. Forman J, Baluarte HJ, Gruskin AB: Hypokalemia after hypertonic phosphate enemas. J Pediatr 94:149, 1979
18. Gilger MA, Wagner ML, Barrish JO, et al: New treatment for rectal impaction in children: An efficacy, comfort, and safety trial of the pulsed-irrigation enhanced-evacuation procedure. J Pediatr Gastroenterol Nutr 18:29, 1994
19. Hendren WH: Constipation caused by anterior location of the anus and its surgical correction. J Pediatr Surg 13:505, 1978
20. Holschneider AM, Börner W, Buurman O, et al: Clinical and electromanometrical investigations of postoperative continence in Hirschsprung's disease - an international workshop. Z Kinderchir 29:39, 1980
21. Ingebo KB, Heyman MB: Polyethylene glycol-electolyte solution for intestinal clearance in children with refractory encopresis. Am J Dis Child 142:340, 1988
22. Issenman RM, Hewson S, Pirhonen D, et al: Are chronic digestive complaints the result of abnormal dietary patterns? Am J Dis Child 141:679, 1987

23. Klein MD, Philippart AI: Hirschsprung's disease: Three decades' experience at a single institution. J Pediatr Surg 28:1291, 1993
24. Koletzko S, Ballauff A, Hadziselimovic F, et al: Is the histologic diagnosis of neuronal intestinal dysplasia related to clinical and manometric findings in constipated children? Results of a pilot study. J Pediatr Gastroenterol Nutr 17:59, 1993
25. Koletzko S, Stringer DA, Cleghorn GJ, et al: Lavage treatment of distal intestinal obstruction syndrome in children with cystic fibrosis. Pediatrics 83:727, 1989
26. Leape LL, Ramenofsky ML: Anterior ectopic anus: a common cause of constipation in children. J Pediatr Surg 13:627, 1978
27. Levine MD: Children with encopresis: A descriptive analysis. Pediatrics 56: 412, 1975
28. Levine MD: Encopresis: Its potentiation, evaluation and alleviation. Pediatr Clin North Am 29:315, 1982
29. Levine MD, Bakow H: Children with encopresis: A study of treatment outcome. Pediatrics 58:845, 1976
30. Lewis AV, Hillemeier AC: Pediatric constipation: Diagnosis and treatment. Practical Gastroenterology 13:31, 1989
31. Loening-Baucke V: Abnormal rectoanal function in children recovered from chronic constipation and encopresis. Gastroenterology 87:1299, 1984
32. Loening-Baucke V: Anorectal manometry: Experience with strain gauge pressure transducers for the diagnosis of Hirschsprung's disease. J Pediatr Surg 18:595, 1983
33. Loening-Baucke V: Constipation in early childhood: patient characteristics, treatment and long-term follow-up. Am Fam Physician 49:397, 1994
34. Loening-Baucke V: Elimination disorders. In Greydanus DE, Wolraich ML (eds): Behavioral Pediatrics. New York, Springer-Verlag, 1991, p 280
35. Loening-Baucke V: Factors determining outcome in children with chronic constipation and faecal soiling. Gut 30:999, 1989
36. Loening-Baucke V: Factors responsible for persistence of childhood constipation. J Pediatr Gastroenterol Nutr 6:915, 1987
37. Loening-Baucke V: Modulation of abnormal defecation dynamics by biofeedback treatment in chronically constipated children with encopresis. J Pediatr 116:214, 1990
38. Loening-Baucke V: Persistence of chronic constipation in children after biofeedback treatment. Dig Dis Sci 36:153, 1991
39. Loening-Baucke V: Sensitivity of the sigmoid colon and rectum in children treated for chronic constipation. J Pediatr Gastroentrol Nutr 3:454, 1984
40. Loening-Baucke V, Cruikshank B: Abnormal defecation dynamics in chronically constipated children with encopresis. J Pediatr 108:562, 1986
41. Loening-Baucke V, Desch L, Wolraich M: Biofeedback training in patients with meningomyelocele and fecal incontinence. Dev Med Child Neurol 30:781, 1988
42. Louis D, Valancogne G, Loras O, et al: Techniques et indications du biofeed-back dans les constipations chez l'enfant. Psychologie Médicale 17:1625, 1985
43. Malone PS, Ransley PG, Kiely EM: Preliminary report: the antegrade continence enema. Lancet 336:1217, 1990
44. Meier-Ruge W: Epidemiology of congenital innervation defects of the distal colon. Virchows Arch A Pathol Anat 420:171, 1992
45. Meunier P, Marechal JM, Jaubert de Beaujeu M: Rectoanal pressures and rectal sensitivity studies in chronic childhood constipation. Gastroenterology 77:330, 1979
46. Mishalany HG, Woolley MM: Postoperative functional and manometric evaluation of patients with Hirschsprung's disease. J Pediatr Surg 22:443, 1987
47. Nolan T, Debelle G, Oberklaid F, et al: Randomised trial of laxatives in treatment of childhood encopresis. Lancet 338:523, 1991
48. Navarro J, Sonsino E, Boige N, et al: Visceral neuropathies responsible for chronic intestinal pseudo-obstruction syndrome in pediatric practice: Analysis of 26 cases. J Pediatr Gastroenterol Nutr 11:179, 1990
49. Partin JC, Hamill SK, Fischel JE, et al: Painful defecation and fecal soiling in children. Pediatrics 89:1007, 1992
50. Pawl GA: Encopresis. In Kestenbaum CJ, Williams DT (eds): Handbook of clinical assessment of children and adolescents. New York, University Press, 1988, p 711
51. Pena A: Surgical considerations: Lower gastrointestinal motility disorders. In Hyman

PE, DiLorenzo C (eds): Pediatric gastrointestinal motility disorders. Academy Professional Information Services, Inc., New York, NY, 1994, p 403

52. Pistor G, Hofmann-von Kap-herr S, Grussner R, et al: Neuronal intestinal dysplasia. Modern diagnosis and therapy–report of 23 patients. Pediatric Surgery International 2:352, 1987

53. Puri P, Lake BD, Nixon HH, et al: Neuronal colonic dysplasia: An unusual association of Hirschsprung's disease. J Pediatr Surg 12:681, 1977

54. Reisner SH, Sivan Y, Nitzan M, et al: Determination of anterior displacement of the anus in newborn infants and children. Pediatrics 73:216, 1984

55. Rutter M: Helping troubled children. Harmons-Worth, England, Penguin Education, 1975

56. Schaefer CE: Childhood encopresis: Its causes and therapy. New York, Van Nostrand Reinhold, 1979

57. Schärli AF, Meier-Ruge W: Localized and disseminated forms of neuronal intestinal dysplasia mimicking Hirschsprung's disease. J Pediatr Surg 16:164, 1981

58. Schmitt B: Encopresis. Prim Care 11:497, 1984

59. Schuffler MD, Jonah A: Chronic idiopathic intestinal pseudo-obstruction caused by degenerative disorder of the myenteric plexus: The use of Smith's method to define the neuropathology. Gastroenterology 82:476, 1982

60. Stehbens JA, Silber DL: Parental expectations vs. outcome in toilet training. Pediatrics 54:493, 1974

61. Swanwick T: Encopresis in children: A cyclical model of constipation and faecal retention. Br J Gen Pract 41:514, 1991

62. Taitz LS, Water JKH, Urwin OM, et al: Factors associated with outcome in management of defecation disorders. Arch Dis Child 61:472, 1986

63. Tuggle DW, Perkins TA, Tunnel WP, et al: Operative treatment of anterior ectopic anus: The efficacy and influence of age on results. J Pediatr Surg 25:996, 1990

64. Vargas J, Sachs P, Ament ME: Chronic intestinal pseudo-obstruction syndrome in pediatrics–results of a national survey by members of the North American Society of Pediatric Gastroenterology and Nutrition. J Pediatr Gastroenterol Nutr 7:323, 1988

65. Wald A: Use of biofeedback in treatment of fecal incontinence in patients with meningomyelocele. Pediatrics 68:45, 1981

66. Wald A, Chandra R, Chiponis D, et al: Anorectal function and continence mechanisms in childhood encopresis. J Pediatr Gastroenterol Nutr 5:346, 1986

67. Wald A, Chandra R, Gabel S, et al: Evaluation of biofeedback in childhood encopresis. J Pediatr Gastroenterol Nutr 6:554, 1987

68. Weaver LT, Steiner H: The bowel habit of young children. Arch Dis Child 59:649, 1984

69. Whitehead WE, Parker LH, Basmajian L, et al: Treatment of fecal incontinence in children with spina bifida: comparison of biofeedback and behavior modification. Arch Phys Med Rehab 67:218, 1986

70. Whitehead WE, Parker LH, Masek BJ, et al: Biofeedback treatment of fecal incontinence in patients with myelomeningocele. Dev Med Child Neurol 23:313, 1981

71. Ziskind A, Gellis SS: Water intoxication following tap water enemas. Am J Dis Child 96:699, 1958

Address reprint requests to

Vera Loening-Baucke, MD
Department of Pediatrics
University of Iowa Hospitals and Clinics
200 Hawkins Drive - JCP 2555
Iowa City, IA 52242-1083

INDEX

Note: Page numbers of article titles are in **boldface** type.

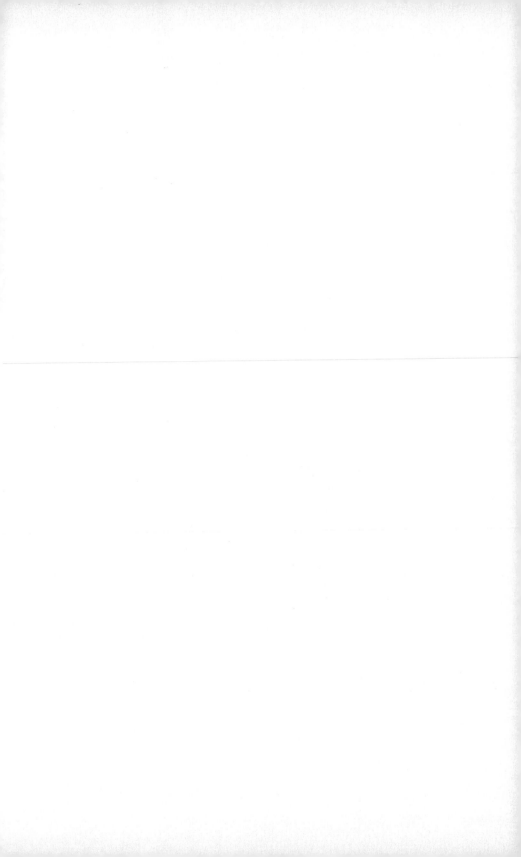

Changing Your Address?

Make sure your subscription changes too! When you notify us of your new address, you can help make our job easier by including an exact copy of your Clinics label number with your old address (see illustration below.) This number identifies you to our computer system and will speed the processing of your address change. Please be sure this label number accompanies your old address and your corrected address—you can send an old Clinics label with your number on it or just copy it exactly and send it to the address listed below.

We appreciate your help in our attempt to give you continuous coverage. Thank you.

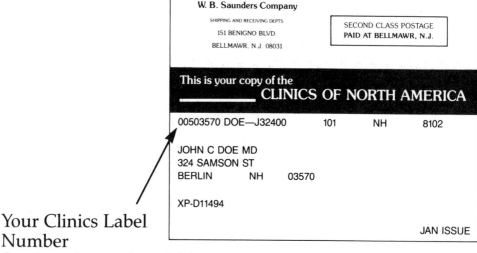

Your Clinics Label Number
Copy it exactly or send your label along with your address to:
W.B. Saunders Company, Customer Service
Orlando, FL 32887-4800
Call Toll Free 1-800-654-2452

Please allow four to six weeks for delivery of new subscriptions and for processing address changes.